ETHICS & ISSUES

In Contemporary Nursing

Fourth Edition

MARGARET A. BURKHARDT
PhD, FNP, AHN-BC

ALVITA K. NATHANIEL
PhD, FNP-BC, FAANP

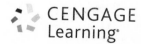
CENGAGE
Learning®

Australia • Brazil • Japan • Korea • Mexico • Singapore • Spain • United Kingdom • United States

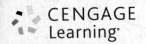
CENGAGE
Learning®

Ethics & Issues: In Contemporary Nursing, Fourth Edition
Margaret A. Burkhardt, Alvita K. Nathaniel

Vice President, Careers & Computing: Dave Garza

Publisher: Stephen Helba

Executive Editor: Maureen Rosener

Director, Development-Career and Computing: Marah Bellegarde

Product Development Manager: Juliet Steiner

Senior Product Manager: Patricia A. Gaworecki

Editorial Assistant: Jennifer Wheaton

Brand Manager: Wendy Mapstone

Market Development Manager: Nancy Bradshaw

Senior Production Director: Wendy Troeger

Production Manager: Andrew Crouth

Senior Content Project Manager: Andrea Majot

Senior Art Director: Jack Pendleton

Media Editor: William Overocker

For product information and technology assistance, contact us at
Cengage Learning Customer & Sales Support, 1-800-354-9706
For permission to use material from this text or product,
submit all requests online at **www.cengage.com/permissions.**
Further permissions questions can be emailed to
permissionrequest@cengage.com

Library of Congress Control Number: 2013936711

Book ISBN-13: 978-1-1331-2916-5

Cengage Learning
200 First Stamford Place, 4th Floor
Stamford, CT 06902
USA

Cengage Learning is a leading provider of customized learning solutions with office locations around the globe, including Singapore, the United Kingdom, Australia, Mexico, Brazil, and Japan. Locate your local office at:
international.cengage.com/region

Cengage Learning products are represented in Canada by Nelson Education, Ltd.

To learn more about Cengage Learning, visit **www.cengage.com.**

Purchase any of our products at your local college store or at our preferred online store **www.cengagebrain.com.**

Printed in the United States of America
1 2 3 4 5 6 7 17 16 15 14 13

Dedication

To Joe and Tim

Contents

PREFACE XVI

ACKNOWLEDGMENTS XX

CONTRIBUTORS XXI

PART I

GUIDES FOR PRINCIPLED BEHAVIOR 1

CHAPTER 1

SOCIAL, PHILOSOPHICAL, AND OTHER HISTORICAL
FORCES INFLUENCING THE DEVELOPMENT
OF NURSING 2

Objectives 2
Introduction 3
The Influence of Social Need 5
Spiritual, Religious, Gender, and Philosophical Influences 8
  Spiritual/Religious Influences 8
  Ancient Times 9
  The Early Christian Era 13
  The Middle Ages 14
  The Renaissance and the Reformation 20
  The Modern Era 22
Summary 24
Chapter Highlights 25
Discussion Questions and Activities 26
References 26

Chapter 2

Ethical Theory   29

Objectives   29
Introduction   30
   Ethics and Nursing   31
Philosophy   32
Morals and Ethics   35
   Philosophical Basis for Ethical Theory   35
Theories of Ethics   38
   Utilitarianism   40
   Deontology   44
   Virtue Ethics   48
   Moral Particularism   51
Summary   53
Chapter Highlights   54
Discussion Questions and Activities   55
References   55

Chapter 3

Ethical Principles   58

Objectives   58
Introduction   59
   Respect for Persons   59
Respect for Autonomy   59
   Recognizing Violations of Patient Autonomy   62
   Informed Consent   64
   Paternalism   65
   Advocacy   67
   Noncompliance   68
Beneficence   69
Nonmaleficence   71
Veracity   73
   Confidentiality   76
   Limits of Confidentiality   79
Justice   81
Fidelity   84
Summary   85

Chapter Highlights 85
Discussion Questions and Activities 86
References 88

PART II

DEVELOPING PRINCIPLED BEHAVIOR 91

CHAPTER 4

VALUES CLARIFICATION 92

Objectives 92
Introduction 93
What Are Values? 93
   Moral Values 93
Acquiring Values 94
Self-Awareness 95
   Enhancing Self-Awareness 96
Values in Professional Situations 98
   Impact of Institutional Values 99
   Clarifying Values with Patients 102
Summary 104
Chapter Highlights 105
Discussion Questions and Activities 105
References 106

CHAPTER 5

VALUES DEVELOPMENT 108

Objectives 108
Introduction 109
Transcultural Considerations in Values Development 109
Beliefs and Values 111
Theoretical Perspectives of Values Development 113
   Piaget's Stages of Cognitive Development 113
   Kohlberg's Theory of Moral Development 114
   Gilligan's Study of the Psychological Development of Women 115
   Fowler's Stages of Faith Development 116
Some Nursing Considerations 120
Summary 122
Chapter Highlights 123

Discussion Questions and Activities   123
References   124

CHAPTER 6

ETHICS AND PROFESSIONAL NURSING   126

Objectives   126
Introduction   127
Professional Status   128
    Nurses as Professionals   130
    Codes of Nursing Ethics   131
Themes of Nursing Ethics   134
    Caring   134
    Expertise   135
    Autonomy   136
Accountability   139
    Mechanisms of Accountability   139
    Authority   143
    Unity   144
Summary   145
Chapter Highlights   145
Discussion Questions and Activities   146
References   147

CHAPTER 7

ETHICAL DECISION MAKING   150

Objectives   150
Introduction   151
Problem Analysis   151
    Moral Uncertainty   152
    Moral/Ethical Dilemmas   152
    Practical Dilemmas   154
    Intervening Factors   154
Ethical Decision Making   158
    Making Decisions   158
Ethical Decision-Making Model   163
    Articulate the Problem   164
    Gather Data and Identify Conflicting Moral Claims   165
    Explore Strategies   166
    Implement the Strategy   166
    Evaluate Outcomes of Action   166

Moral Distress, Moral Outrage, and Moral Reckoning   170
    Moral Distress   170
    Moral Outrage   173
    Moral Reckoning   174
    Ways to Anticipate, Minimize, and Control Moral Reckoning   178
Summary   180
Chapter Highlights   181
Discussion Questions and Activities   181
References   182

PART III

PRINCIPLED BEHAVIOR IN THE PROFESSIONAL DOMAIN   187

CHAPTER 8

LEGAL ISSUES   188

Objectives   188
Introduction   189
Relationship Between Ethics and the Law   189
General Legal Concepts   192
    Sources of Law   193
    Types of Law   194
Contemporary Legal Trends   213
    Legal Trends Involving Managed Care Organizations   214
    Malpractice Claims Against Nurses   215
    Criminalization of Nurses' Professional Negligence   216
    Confidentiality of Electronic Communications   217
Risk Management   219
    Maintaining Communication with Patients   220
    Maintaining Conscientious Practice   221
    Maintaining Autonomy and Empowerment   222
    Liability Insurance   222
Nurses as Expert Witnesses   223
Summary   224
Chapter Highlights   225
Discussion Questions and Activities   226
References   227

CHAPTER 9

PROFESSIONAL RELATIONSHIP ISSUES   230

Objectives   230
Introduction   231
Problem Solving in the Professional Realm   231
   Maintain Attentiveness to Personal Values   232
   Clarify Obligation   232
   Determine the Nature of the Problem   234
   Choose from Alternative Solutions Thoughtfully   237
Nurses' Relationships with Institutions   237
Nurses' Relationships with Other Nurses   240
Nurses' Relationships with Physicians   243
Nurses' Relationships with Subordinates   246
Discrimination and Harassment   248
   Racial Discrimination   248
   Discrimination Against Persons with Disabilities   250
Sexual Harassment and Discrimination   251
Summary   253
Chapter Highlights   253
Discussion Questions and Activities   254
References   255

CHAPTER 10

PRACTICE ISSUES RELATED TO TECHNOLOGY   258

Objectives   258
Introduction   259
Benefits and Challenges of Technology   259
   Quality of Life   260
   Principles of Beneficence and Nonmaleficence   261
Current Technology: Issues and Dilemmas   261
   Treating Patients: When to Intervene and to What End   262
   Issues of Life, Death, and Dying   262
   Medical Futility   266
   Do Not Resuscitate Orders   270
   Artificial Sources of Nutrition and Hydration   273
   Legal Issues Related to Technology   274

Palliative Care   277
Palliative Care Conference   277
Examples of Potential Dilemmas with Other Technology   279
Controversial Technologies   281
Nursing Practice in the Midst of Technology   284
Technology, Privacy, and Confidentiality   284
Attitudes and Values   286
The Importance of Communication: Who Decides?   287
Caring: The Human Focus   288
Summary   289
Chapter Highlights   289
Discussion Questions and Activities   290
References   292

CHAPTER 11

PRACTICE ISSUES RELATED TO PATIENT SELF-DETERMINATION   295

Objectives   295
Introduction   296
Autonomy and Paternalism   296
How Far Does Autonomy Go?   298
Informed Consent   299
Ethical and Legal Elements of Informed Consent   300
Nursing Role and Responsibilities: Informed Consent   301
Advance Directives   304
Decision-Making Capacity   306
Nursing Role and Responsibilities: Advance Directives   310
Choices Concerning Life and Health   312
Choices Regarding Recommended Treatment   313
Controversial Choices   316
Confidentiality   322
Summary   323
Chapter Highlights   323
Discussion Questions and Activities   325
References   326

CHAPTER 12

SCHOLARSHIP ISSUES   329

Objectives   329
Introduction   330

Academic Honesty   330
Research Issues and Ethics   332
    Ethical Issues in Research   333
    Special Considerations: Vulnerable Populations   339
    More Than Protection of Human Rights   341
    Ethical Treatment of Data   343
Summary   344
Chapter Highlights   345
Discussion Questions and Activities   345
References   347

PART IV

GLOBAL ISSUES THAT INTERFACE WITH NURSING PRACTICE   349

CHAPTER 13

GLOBAL CONSCIOUSNESS IN THE TWENTY-FIRST CENTURY   350

Objectives   350
Introduction   351
Earth Ethics and Health   351
    The Earth Charter and Nursing   354
Disaster—Nursing Response and Ethical Considerations   356
Displaced Persons and Victims of Armed Conflict   358
War and Violence   360
Health Care Access and Financing   363
A Brief History of Health Care Delivery: The
    Euro-American Experience   364
    Early Eras of Health Care Delivery   365
    Changes from the Middle Ages to the Industrial Revolution   366
    Changes Influencing Development of Modern Health
    Care in the United States   367
Global Needs and Finite Resources   375
Alternative Traditions of Health Care   379
Challenges for Rural and Urban Aggregates   381
Summary   382
Chapter Highlights   382
Discussion Questions and Activities   383
References   385

CHAPTER 14

HEALTH POLICY ISSUES   388

Objectives   388
Introduction   389
Political Issues   389
Health Policy   393
    The Health Policy Process   395
    Ethics in Policy Making   398
    Research Data in Policy Making   399
Nursing, Policy, and Politics   399
    Policy Goals for Nursing   401
Lobbying   402
    Methods of Lobbying   402
    Political Campaigns   404
Summary   405
Chapter Highlights   406
Discussion Questions and Activities   406
References   407

CHAPTER 15

ECONOMIC ISSUES   409

Objectives   409
Introduction   410
Overview of Today's Health Care Economics   410
Distributive Justice   412
    Entitlement   413
    Fair Distribution   416
    Distribution of Resources   416
    Theories of Justice   417
Recent Trends and Health Economic Issues   419
    Health Care Reform   420
    Managed Care   422
Summary   424
Chapter Highlights   424
Discussion Questions and Activities   425
References   426

CHAPTER 16

SOCIAL ISSUES 428

Objectives 428

Introduction 429

Social Issues 429

    Poverty 429

    Homelessness 431

    Intimate Partner Violence 433

    Human Trafficking 435

    Increasing Elderly Population 436

    Racism 437

Ethical Principles Applied to Social Issues 439

    Justice 439

    Nonmaleficence 439

    Beneficence 440

    Autonomy 440

Personal Impediments to Intervening with Vulnerable Groups 441

    Victim Blaming 441

    Language of Violence 441

Social Issues and Scholarship 442

Summary 443

Chapter Highlights 443

Discussion Questions And Activities 444

References 446

CHAPTER 17

GENDER ISSUES 449

Objectives 449

Introduction 450

Historical Perspectives and Overview of Gender-Based Issues 450

Gender Discrimination in Nursing 452

    Women in Nursing 452

    Men in Nursing 452

    Gender Issues in Women's Health 453

    Gender and Caring 454

Sexual Harassment in Nursing 456

Modern Sexism   457

Sexual Orientation   458

   Caring for Lesbian, Gay, Bisexual, and Transgender Patients   459

Communication Issues Related to Gender   459

   Nurse-Physician Communication   460

   Communicating with Patients   461

Gender and Race   461

Summary   463

Chapter Highlights   463

Discussion Questions and Activities   464

References   465

CHAPTER 18

TRANSCULTURAL AND SPIRITUAL ISSUES   468

Objectives   468

Introduction   469

Transcultural Issues   469

   Understanding Culture   469

   Cultural Values and Beliefs   471

   Culture and the Health Care System   475

   Complementary Therapies   477

   Legal Considerations Related to Transcultural Issues   479

Issues Related to Spirituality and Religion   480

   Approaching Spirituality   480

   Spirituality and Religion   482

   Nurturing Spirit   486

Summary   488

Chapter Highlights   488

Discussion Questions and Activities   489

References   490

PART V

THE POWER TO MAKE A DIFFERENCE   493

CHAPTER 19

EMPOWERMENT FOR NURSES   494

Objectives   494

Introduction   495

Influences on Nursing's Perceptions of Principled Practice   495
    Influence of Mind-Set   495
    Metaphors of Nursing   496
    How Nursing Is Perceived by Others   498
Understanding Power and Empowerment   499
Personal Empowerment   501
Professional Empowerment   504
    Unity in Diversity   506
Re-Visioning Nursing   508
Summary   510
Chapter Highlights   510
Discussion Questions and Activities   511
References   512

CHAPTER 20

FACILITATING PATIENT EMPOWERMENT   515

Objectives   515
Introduction   516
Patients and Empowerment   516
Nurses and Patient Empowerment   516
    Attitudes of Nurses That Facilitate Empowerment   517
    Nursing Knowledge and Skills Necessary for Facilitating Empowerment   517
Enhancing Patient Capacity for Decision Making   518
    Barriers to Empowerment   519
Fostering Patient Empowerment   520
Summary   521
Chapter Highlights   522
Discussion Questions and Activities   522
References   523

APPENDIX A

ONLINE RESOURCES   524

GLOSSARY   525

INDEX   532

Preface

*We who lived in the concentration camps can remember the men who
walked through the huts comforting others, giving away their last piece
of bread. They may have been few in number, but they offer sufficient
proof that everything can be taken from a man but one thing: the last
of his freedoms—to choose one's attitude in any given set of circumstances,
to choose one's own way.*

—V. E. Frankl,
Man's Search for Meaning

As contemporary nurses, we face complex and challenging personal, interpersonal, professional, institutional, and social issues. Appropriate responses to these issues are seldom clear. Ethical dilemmas, in particular, involve choices with no clearly correct solutions. We believe that declaring that there is one correct approach to solving ethical problems risks imposing personal values on others. We must be sensitive to that possibility and recognize that our responses to dilemmas depend on such variables as contextual factors, patient and family values, relationships, moral development, religious beliefs, spiritual perspective, cultural orientation, and legal constraints.

It is our intention in this book to (1) acknowledge that each person is a moral agent, (2) raise awareness of the myriad factors that need to be considered when dealing with ethical decisions, (3) present a decision-making model to help individuals learn to process information and move toward action, and (4) affirm nursing as an ethically responsible profession. We present ethical issues from the perspective of nursing, recognizing that relationships and the authority to make decisions are affected by contextual factors such as professional status; gender; the development of the profession; personal ethical stance; social, economic, institutional, and political climate; and personal and professional empowerment.

Dealing with ethical issues requires skill in the processes of values clarification, ethical decision making, self-awareness, empowerment, transcultural sensitivity, and challenging injustice. The text poses questions about contemporary issues and provides processes for the development of sensitivity and skill in resolving ethical problems. Highlighting nurses in a variety of settings and roles, the exercises and activities are intended to facilitate self-reflection and awareness of personal approaches to issues and decision making. Our goal is that you will become engaged in active learning throughout the text through the use of *Case Presentations* based on real-life situations, *Ask Yourself* and *Think About It* exercises derived from thought-provoking material and case presentations, and *Discussion Questions and Activities.*

Although acknowledging the rich and divergent history of nursing in other cultures, we have chosen to write primarily from the Western perspective. The background that we give explains the many factors that lead to social systems that either encourage or prohibit certain people from critically examining issues and making authoritative decisions. The book begins with a chapter that explores the impact of historical factors, particularly religion and gender, on the profession of nursing in Western culture. We hope that this will help you to understand more fully the context of nursing and question arbitrary and artificial barriers to ethical decision making.

With a strong groundwork of ethical theories and principles in Part I, subsequent chapters deal with various issues as they pertain to ethics and ethical decision making. As you explore political, professional, legal, social, and gender issues, we encourage you to look at the related ethical questions and to continually move back and forth from the concrete to the abstract, from the general to the specific, from the global to the personal, and from issue to principle—recognizing the interrelatedness of many factors.

While continuing to discuss ethical issues from the perspective of nursing, in this fourth edition we have included several new additions. We added more in-depth discussions of the philosophical background of nursing and the development of codes of nursing ethics and added content on ethics committee referrals, human trafficking, the Affordable Care Act, and spirituality assessment. We also included new discussions of current controversial issues such as general HIV screening and care of lesbian, gay, bisexual, and transgender patients.

Principled behavior in personal and professional situations is the organizing theme of this text. Beginning with a brief descriptive history of nursing as it relates to ethics, Part I, *Guides for Principled Behavior,* presents ethical theories, models, and principles that serve as guides for principled behavior. Part II, *Developing Principled Behavior,* discusses personal issues, including values clarification, moral development, and ethical decision making. Part III, *Principled Behavior in the Professional Domain,* presents professional and legal overviews and chapters related to specific issues important to contemporary nursing. This section includes discussions about autonomy, authority, accountability, codes of practice, scholarship issues, practice issues related to health care providers, systems within which nurses work, technology, and patient self-determination. Part IV, *Global Issues That Interface with Nursing Practice*, addresses twenty-first-century issues that require global consciousness as a background for understanding issues that nurses encounter in the contemporary health care system. Considerations related to global health, political, economic, social, gender, transcultural, and spirituality issues are discussed in light of nursing role, potential dilemmas, and professional practice. Part V, *The Power to Make a Difference*, focuses on developing skills to empower both nurses and patients to make principled choices and act with courage.

Throughout this book, we have chosen to refer to the recipient of nursing care as *patient* rather than *client*. Since nurses function as members of interdisciplinary health care teams and the term *patient* is commonly used by other health providers, using a common language fosters better communication, understanding, and collegiality. In addition, the American Nurses Association (2010) *Nursing's Social Policy Statement* notes that although the term *client* is preferred by some nurses, it implies that the recipient of care is able to choose one nurse from among many, a choice that typically does not occur. We recognize that the terms *client*, *person*, or *individual* may be the better choice in some circumstances and encourage the reader to make that distinction if needed.

Although we have written from the Western perspective, we recognize that our culture is a melding of traditions and people from many other cultures. We have attempted to be sensitive in reflecting transcultural situations and issues. In that vein, you will notice that when referring to the dates of historical events, we have used the designation B.C.E. (Before the Common Era) rather than the more familiar B.C.

This book is meant to be very personal. We encourage you to become engaged, examining and questioning your options and values as they relate to real-life situations. As learning is demonstrated by changed behavior, we hope that you will become a more sensitive, capable, courageous, and responsible decision maker and citizen. We believe with Phyllis Kritek (1994) that "the measure of [one's] character and worth is not whether [one has] avoided making poor choices, but how willing [one is] to learn from these errors in an effort to not repeat them, and how [one elects] to attend to their consequences.... Finding meaning, discovering that which is of worth, becomes a searching process where everyone's help is welcome" (pp. 21, 33). This book is offered as a guide to help in the process of learning to make sound choices and act in principled ways in both personal and professional realms. As you use this book, we echo the same sentiment voiced by Florence Nightingale in the preface to her *Notes on Nursing:* "I do not pretend to teach her how, I ask her to teach herself, and for this purpose I venture to give her some hints" (1859, preface).

References

American Nurses Association. (2010). *Nursing's social policy statement: The essence of the profession* (New edition). Silver Springs, MD: Author.

Kritek, P. B. (1994). *Negotiating at an uneven table: A practical approach to working with difference and diversity.* San Francisco: Jossey-Bass.

Nightingale, F. (1859). *Notes on nursing: What it is, and what it is not.* London: Harrison & Sons.

Additional Resources

The **Instructor's Companion Website** is a complete teaching tool to aid instructors in preparing lesson plans, lectures, and assessments. This resource is complimentary to all adopters of *Ethics and Issues in Contemporary Nursing*, Fourth Edition. The Instructor's Companion Website contains these instructional materials:

- Instructor's manual that includes teaching tips and strategies.

- A computerized testbank with over 450 questions. You can use these questions to create your own tests in seconds. And, you have the capability of adding your own questions and modifying existing ones.

- PowerPoint: More than 345 slides designed to help you with your class presentations.

- ISBN: 978-1-1331-2917-2

CourseMate, accessed at **www.Cengage.com/coursemate**, helps the student make the most of study time by offering access in one location to everything needed to succeed. *Ethics and Issues in Contemporary Nursing* CourseMate includes an interactive ebook with highlighting and note-taking ability and an interactive glossary. As an instructor, you can benefit from the engagement tracker to monitor student progress.

To access CourseMate content:

Go to www.cengagebrain.com
For instant access code, ISBN: 978-1-133-12921-9
For print access code, ISBN: 978-1-133-12922-6

Acknowledgments

The journey of writing a book requires solitude and the companionship and support of many people. We express gratitude to the many friends and colleagues who have encouraged us along the way. Special thanks are due to our mentors who have encouraged scholarship and principled behavior. We are grateful to Mary Jo Butler, Sandra L. Cotton, Robin Shirley, and Mary Gail Nagai-Jacobson for their contributions. Thanks go to all those who gave the time and care to review the manuscript at various stages in the writing process, providing us with helpful comments and guidance.

Finally, we are eternally grateful to our families, Joe Golden and Tim, and Josh Nathaniel, and Maggie Belton, for their loving patience, humor, caretaking, and encouragement throughout this challenging and growthful journey.

Contributors

Mary Jo Butler, EdD, RN
Former Associate Professor
and Director
West Virginia University
School of Nursing, Charleston
Division
Charleston, WV

Sandra L. Cotton, DNP, FNP-BC
Director, Faculty Practice Plan
West Virginia University
School of Nursing
Morgantown, WV

Mary Gail Nagai-Jacobson, MSN, RN
Director, Healing Matters
San Marcos, TX

Part

I

Guides for Principled Behavior

Part I lays a foundation for nurses to critically examine issues and systematically participate in ethical decision making. Chapter 1 gives nurses insight into the profession of nursing in Western cultures as part of an overall social system—focusing specifically on the influence of philosophy, the practice of religion, and the status of women in society. Recognizing that knowledge of ethical theories and principles can help the nurse to develop a cohesive and logical system for making individual decisions, Chapters 2 and 3 describe philosophical stances, various classic ethical theories, and ethical principles.

Chapter

1

SOCIAL, PHILOSOPHICAL, AND OTHER HISTORICAL FORCES INFLUENCING THE DEVELOPMENT OF NURSING

You know that the beginning is the most important part of any work, especially in the case of a young and tender thing; for that is the time at which the character is being formed and the desired impression is more readily taken.

(**Plato**, *Republic*)

OBJECTIVES

After completing this chapter, the reader should be able to:

1. Discuss the relationship between social need and the origin of the profession of nursing.

2. Discuss the relationship between moral reasoning and the origin of nursing.

3. Describe the mutually beneficial relationship between the broader society and its professions.

4. Explain the effect of a culture's prevailing belief system on the practice of nursing.

5. Identify how historic spiritual beliefs and religious practices influenced evolutionary changes in nursing.

6. Discuss how the historical background of the status of women in various cultures is related to the practice of nursing.

7. Examine the effect of philosophy on beliefs and practices within society.

8. Make plausible inferences relating the evolution of the practice of nursing to the current state of the profession.

INTRODUCTION

This chapter summarizes the historical beliefs and traditions that are important to a critical examination of the place of nursing in Western society. Ideas, traditions, and beliefs are connected through time. Each period of history is influenced by what came before. Chapter 1 presents the historical relevance of philosophy, religion, and social structures that undergird nursing customs. We ask you to begin to critically examine the role of nursing in ethical decision making. Through this critical examination, it is our hope that you will move beyond tradition toward thoughtful and objective reasoning and thus be better prepared to participate in moral discourse.

This book focuses on the tradition and philosophy of the West because codes of ethics in Western countries flow from these sources. This is not to say that Eastern traditions, religions, and philosophies are of less value. We acknowledge that the East has contributed rich knowledge and wisdom. Brahmanism, Buddhism, Jainism, Confucianism, and Taoism were evolving distinctly Eastern philosophies even before many Western philosophers became popular. These Eastern traditions are important and we encourage you to learn more about them. In an increasingly multicultural environment, it is important that we fully appreciate the beliefs and traditions of others.

It is innate in our nature as humans to accept the beliefs and practices of those around us. We are inclined to assume the values, traditions, and cultural practices of our families and other social groups. We tend to believe what those around us believe and to act in a way that is congruent with our beliefs. Social groups value actions compatible with their beliefs. Since people naturally desire the approval of their social group, traditions become self-perpetuating. The American philosopher Charles Sanders Peirce (1839–1914) discussed methods that people use to solidify or fix their beliefs. We can view much of nursing's history in light of what Peirce called the authority method of fixing belief.

Peirce identified four methods of fixing belief: tenacity, authority, a priori, and reasoning (Houser & Kloesel, 1992). He proposed that truth is the goal of all human inquiry and suggested that inquiry and logic provide the manner in which a person can discover truth. However, Peirce proposed that a person only discovers truth when he or she really questions something. Many people fail to question their beliefs. This allows beliefs to be fixed by the authority method wherein a powerful person or institution forces "correct beliefs" on the people by repeating doctrines perpetually and teaching them to the young. This method has been one of the chief means of upholding theological and political dogmas. We can broadly apply this means of fixing belief to many historical influences on the nursing profession. By examining the history of nursing, you will see how the different methods of fixing belief affected the discipline over time. This deeper understanding will aid you in autonomous moral reasoning as you assume the professional role.

Nursing has been called the "morally central health care profession" (Jameton, 1984, p. xvi). There have always been people who cared for the sick and attempted to cure illness. The development of the nursing profession is difficult to trace since medicine, nursing, and other health care professions all evolved from the same roots. Nevertheless, we understand that moral reasoning is the historical basis for the creation, evolution, and practice of nursing. The spirit and substance of nursing spring from social and individual moral codes. In this chapter, we will look at four historical influences on nursing as a moral discipline—social need, spirituality/religion, philosophy, and the role of women.

Morals and ethics affect nursing on different levels. As nurses, our motivation to care for others is generated by moral reasoning. Collectively, moral beliefs of groups of people produce rules of action, or ethics. These culturally accepted rules are an integral part of both the experience and the profession of nursing. Expressions of ideals, discussions of moral issues, statements of moral principles, and codes of ethics are found throughout the history of nursing. Nursing is morally worthy work since comfort and care for those who suffer is a basic benefit of human culture (Jameton, 1984). As our modern health care technology extends the boundaries of what is possible, all of society is challenged to examine emerging ethical issues. We are faced with ethical tension in a health care system that requires moral decision making, yet sometimes restricts us from legitimate decision-making roles. We examine the history of nursing to help understand our position within the contemporary health care system.

One of our purposes in writing this text is to present nursing ethics in a manner that will encourage empowered decision making. In an examination of nursing empowerment, Fulton (1997) proposes that nurses' perspectives are distorted and constrained by historical forces that impart negative messages. According to Stevens, these distortions and constraints "impede free, equal and uncoerced participation in society" (1989, p. 58). Struggling to cope with impossible situations, nurses continue to believe negative messages about themselves and behave in ways that are neither constructive nor empowered (Hedin, 1986; Roberts, 1983). In other words, we can only understand our present situation in relation to our social and professional history (Harden, 1996). These ideas are related to critical social theory as proposed by Habermas (1971) and Freire (2000). The basic principle of critical social theory is that we can only understand each aspect of a social phenomenon in relation to the history and structure in which it is found. The significance of ideas can be grasped only when we objectively view them in the context of historical and social practices and entanglements of power and interest (McCarthy, 1990). Habermas (1971) proposes that as individuals we can assess the evidence and fully participate only when we are aware of, and free ourselves from the hidden oppressions that affect our lives. Insights gained from the study of nursing history enable us to see these conditions for what they are and to find ways of interpreting them and releasing ourselves from them in order to move forward. To this end, we present some selected historical and social forces that have shaped the contours of our profession.

It is difficult to establish a clear picture of the development of the profession of nursing through history. Medicine and nursing both emerged from a long history of healers. It is not possible for us to know the exact origin of either profession, since the earliest stages of each are so closely interwoven (Donahue, 1996). Even so, we know that the history of nursing is one in which people—usually women—have attempted to relieve suffering. Selanders writes, "Nursing's history is one of people, both ancient and modern. It has not evolved solely because of one individual or one event or with directed purpose. Rather, nursing's current status represents a collective picture of societal evolution in a health care framework" (1998a, p. 227). From the beginning, the motivation of nurses to care for others came from practical, moral, or spiritual influences. Our history is also the story of a profession inescapably linked to the status of women. The history of healers, and subsequently that of nurses, has gone through many phases and has been an important part of social movements. Ours is a narrative of a professional group whose status has always been affected by the prevalent standards of society (Donahue, 1996).

THE INFLUENCE OF SOCIAL NEED

Helping professions find their origin, purpose, and meaning within the context of culturally accepted moral norms, individual values, and perceived social need. By serving others and responding to their needs, we express moral belief. The term **moral thought** relates to the thoughtful examination of right and wrong, good and bad. Moral reasoning includes any level of this type of thinking. It may be complex and well developed, or it may be rudimentary. Why do we care about moral issues? Some moral philosophers propose that empathy is a motive for moral reasoning and action. For example, if we visualize the suffering of another person, we begin to imagine ourselves suffering. Some describe the desire to help others as a natural outcome of social consciousness and motivation similar to the Golden Rule, "Do unto others as you would have them do unto you." A universally popular precept, the Golden Rule is found in some form in most major moral traditions, including Christianity, Judaism, Islam, Confucianism, Hinduism, Buddhism, and Taoism (Honderich, 2005; Spooner, 1914). Some say that we follow the Golden Rule both to help someone in need and, to some degree, in the hope that someone will show us consideration if we are unfortunate enough to find ourselves in similar circumstances. On the other hand, if we base our moral reasoning on pure religious belief, we may be motivated by a desire to obey a commandment, fulfill what we believe to be a duty to God, or gain spiritual rewards. Whether our original motivation of ethical action is based on a desire to help others or a religious duty, the outcome of the action is the same: meeting the health needs of others. As the morally central health care profession, nursing has historically responded to human suffering.

ASK YOURSELF

What Is the Motivation for Helping?

Imagine a utopian world in which all people are happy and healthy, and have satisfying relationships. There is neither illness nor death. Each person's needs are entirely met without the help of other people. Within this model society, because everyone is satisfied, healthy, and happy, there is no social disorder and no need for any helping profession: no police, doctors, nurses, lawyers, or social workers. People do not need to think about moral issues. Now, imagine the social disorder that would follow the introduction of serious disease. Individuals who become ill would be unable to care for themselves and to meet their own basic needs.

- How do you imagine society would deal with this problem?
- Are the ill entirely responsible for themselves?
- Do unaffected people continue to live the utopian existence, ignoring the suffering of others, or is the whole of society responsible for helping those in need?
- Does society allow the diseased members to suffer, or do healthy members help those afflicted, thus altering their own "perfect" lives—and in turn the prevailing social order?

It is likely that at least some members of the hypothetical community described in the accompanying *Ask Yourself* exercise will recognize the importance of helping those in need. These people will begin to exercise moral thinking as they examine their beliefs. Ethics will emerge in the form of rules of action that are specifically related to solving the moral problem. Those committed to helping the ill will devise methods to utilize individuals' abilities to the best advantage and to fairly distribute the burden of providing services and resources. As this example implies, nursing is a profession that exists to meet certain needs of individuals and groups, and thus is a product of the moral reasoning of people in society.

As we will see in later chapters, the needs of a society at a given time combined with its technological capabilities and knowledge base determine the existence and parameters of a profession. Societies establish dynamic professional boundaries that move and change as needs change. Nursing is a part of society. To continue to exist, our professional interest must continue to be (and must be perceived as) serving the interests of the "larger whole of which it is a part" (American Nurses Association [ANA], 1980, p. 3). The landmark document *Nursing: A Social Policy Statement* (ANA, 1980) was the profession's first description of its social responsibility. We can use both this document and a subsequent revision, *Nursing's Social Policy Statement* (ANA, 1996), as a framework for understanding the profession's relationship with society and our obligation to those who receive nursing care. These documents express the mutually beneficial relationship between the broader society and its professions as follows:

> A profession acquires recognition, relevance, and even meaning in terms of its relationship to that society, its culture and institutions, and its other members. Professions acquire recognition and relevance primarily in terms of needs, conditions, and traditions of particular societies and their members. It is societies (and often vested interests within them) that determine, in accord with their different technological and economic levels of development and their socioeconomic, political and cultural conditions, and values, what professional skills and knowledge they most need and desire. By various financial means, institutions will then emerge to train interested individuals to supply those needs. Logically, then, the professions open to individuals in any particular society are the property not of the individual but of society. (ANA, 1980, p. 3)

Think About It

What Makes People Service Oriented?

- *Why do you think people are motivated to help those who are in need?*

- *The actions of those who choose to help others in specific situations might be described as based on self-interest, altruism, or a combination of other motives. How would you describe the motivation to care for others within the healing professions today?*

The nursing profession was created by society for the purpose of meeting specific health needs. In response, the profession has made an implicit promise to ensure, by various means, that members are competent to provide the service, and further, that these are the *only* members of society that can qualify to provide the service. The relationship of social need and our motivation to care for others is complementary. It is fortunate that human nature is such that some of us, for whatever reason, are interested in serving others.

SPIRITUAL, RELIGIOUS, GENDER, AND PHILOSOPHICAL INFLUENCES

Spiritual/Religious Influences

The spiritual and religious foundations of past and present cultures determine many aspects of health care. Spiritual belief and religious practice contributed significantly to the moral foundation of nursing and other healing professions; they have also influenced both the gender and, to some degree, much of the activity of healers. Spirituality and religious doctrine influenced beliefs about the value of individuals, life, death, and health. Historically, many of the dominant religious institutions made judgments about the origin and essence of healing and defined who would hold positions as legitimate healers. The path that nursing has taken since ancient times has not been smooth. There have been advances and setbacks, libraries have been destroyed, widely diverse groups have held the title of nurse, and those who were the nurses in some early cultures left few records. Nevertheless, nursing in some form has existed in every culture, and has been influenced by spiritual beliefs, religious practices, and related cultural values.

Gender Influences

The role of women in society is one of the most critical factors that influence nursing practice. In every culture women have been healers. Because nursing has generally been a profession of women (from the beginning,

95 percent to 98 percent of nurses have been women), women's status in society is central to determining the extent of freedom and respect granted to nurses. Contours of the profession have been shaped, in large part, by social forces that determine gender roles in society. Gender stereotyping has always been a problem for nurses. As a result of the perception that women are more humane and more caring by nature, they have been viewed as naturally endowed with nursing talents. Even Florence Nightingale wrote, "Every woman . . . has, at one time or another of her life, charge of the personal health of somebody, whether child or invalid—in other words, every woman is a nurse" (Nightingale, 1859, preface). This kind of stereotyping has been both a blessing and a curse to nursing.

Society either allows or fails to allow women to assume roles of authority, roles that allow independent decision making or limited participation in the decision-making process. There were periods in history in which women were the honored sole practitioners of the healing arts, and there were periods in which women were forced into submissive and subservient healing roles.

Philosophical Influences

From ancient times until today, philosophers have asked important questions and proposed theories that helped to shape cultures. Philosophers ask questions about the nature of truth and reality. They propose theories about morality and the characteristics of the good life. They propose theories of action, interaction, cause and effect that impact the scientific method. Since the first philosophers emerged, they have influenced every element of society.

Ancient Times

Religious Influences and the Role of Women in Ancient Times. The **cosmology** of a culture indirectly determines specific beliefs about the origin of disease and healing (Achterberg, 1990). Cosmology is the overarching belief system of a culture. It describes how people of the culture view the structure, origin, and processes of the universe. Cosmology includes beliefs about the gods. The nature of the gods worshiped in any culture directly affects prevailing healing beliefs. Regarding ancient cultures, Achterberg says,

> When gods lived in the Earth, the whole planet was worshiped as the manifestation of the divine. The rivers, the rocks, and especially humans were the inhabitants of a sacred place. All—what we call living and nonliving alike—was alive and related. All humans breathed the breath of the spirit and drank the waters of the spirit. (p. 188)

Thus, in ancient cultures, the healer was involved with the sacred elements of the Earth and the spirit in healing practices.

Early cultures viewed the vocation of healer in terms associated with the sacred. In ancient times the position of healer was practiced by those thought to have special spiritual gifts. Through the study of relics, we learn that healing arts in the ancient cultures of Sumer, Denmark, Greece, and other societies were performed in sacred ceremonies by priests, priestesses, or shamans. These ancient healers represented the embodiment of the cultures' gods on Earth (Achterberg, 1990). In ancient Persia there are indications that there were three types of healers: those who healed with the knife, those who healed with herbs, and those who healed with sacred words. Practitioners who used sacred words were considered to have the greatest prestige (Dolan, 1973). Archeological evidence suggests that in all early cultures the position of the healer was associated with the sacred.

Whenever the reigning deity in ancient times had a feminine, bisexual, or androgynous nature, women were leaders in the healing arts. Many diverse and widely placed cultures left evidence that there was a very early time when women served in the esteemed roles of healer and priestess. As the world became a harsher place and the gods assumed a masculine nature, the role of women as independent, primary healers was taken away (Achterberg, 1990).

Asclepius, or Asklepios, was the ancient Greek mythical god of medicine and healing. Asclepius was regarded as a deity, but some believe that he may have been a real person, known for his humane remedies. It is said that Asclepius learned the art of surgery; the use of drugs, incantations, and love potions; and the secrets to raising the dead. According to mythology, Asclepius had a number of children, including Hygieia, the goddess of health (from whose name comes the word "hygiene"); Panaceia, the goddess of healing (from whose name comes the word "panacea," which means universal remedy); Iaso, the goddess of medicine; and others. Asclepius's followers established temples of healing, sometimes referred to as "asclepieions," where the sick spent the night while the proper remedies were "revealed" to the priests of the temple. Those who were cured made a sacrifice to Asclepius, usually a rooster (Hart, 2000).

Romans worshipped Asclepius from about 800 BCE to 400 CE, but his influence continued throughout the centuries. Some believe that Hippocrates may have studied at an asclepieion. The Hippocratic Oath begins with the words, "I swear by Apollo, the healer, Asclepius, Hygieia, and Panacea, and I take to witness all the gods, all the goddesses, to keep according to my ability and my judgment, the following Oath and agreement. . . ." (Temkin & Temkin, 1987, p. 6). Plato, the ancient philosopher most revered by Florence Nightingale, paid homage to Asclepius in *Phaedo* when he reported that Socrates's last words were "Crito, we owe a cock to Asclepius; make this offering to him and do not forget" (Plato, trans 1997, p. 99). Even today, the official symbol of medicine recognized by the American Medical Association and the American Osteopathic Association is the Staff of Asclepius, a depiction of one snake ascending a roughly hewn staff. Perhaps the relationship between Asclepius and his daughters Hygieia, Panaceia, and Iaso contributed to the paternalistic, male-dominated system perpetuated through much of history.

Having a great influence on Western thought, early Hebrew teaching codified health practices as an integral part of the religion. The Mosaic health code applied to every aspect of individual, family, and community life. It included principles related to rest, sleep, cleanliness, hygiene, and childbearing (Dolan, Fitzpatrick, & Herrmann, 1983). The code required inspection of food, detection and reporting of disease, methods of disposal of excreta, feminine hygiene, and isolation of those with communicable illness. It specified particular methods of hand washing and care of food. The Hebrew high priest served in the capacity of priest-physician, and the people were admonished to honor him. Thus, for the early Hebrews, that which was "right" to do in regard to health was mandated by religious doctrine.

The ancient physician Hippocrates (ca. 460 BCE–ca. 377 BCE) is universally recognized as the father of Western medicine. His teachings revolutionized healing arts in ancient Greece and established medicine as a profession, distinct from other disciplines (Garrison, 1966). Differing from the prevailing superstitions that illness and healing derived from religious or magical sources, Hippocrates believed that care of the sick should include observation of symptoms, rational conclusions, and predictable prognoses (Grammaticos & Diamantis, 2008; Yapijakis, 2009). He approached healing passively, relying on the healing power of nature. Hippocrates was influenced by Pythagoras's theory that proposed that nature was made of four elements: water, earth, wind, and fire. Thus, he proposed that the body consisted of the four humors black bile, yellow bile, phlegm, and blood. It was the physician's purpose, he thought, to reinstate a healthy balance of humors by promoting the healing work of benevolent nature (Yapijakis, 2009). In his writings, Hippocrates proposed strict professionalism. He recommended that physicians be well groomed, honest, calm, understanding, and serious (Garrison, 1966). Most sources attribute the Hippocratic Oath, which continues to be discussed in relation to medical ethics, to Hippocrates himself.

Philosophy in Ancient Times. Between the sixth and fourth centuries BCE, in every corner of the globe, an extraordinary development was occurring. Some brilliant, creative thinkers were dissatisfied with popular beliefs and explanations. These early *philosophers* began to question the religious beliefs, mythologies, and folklore that had been established for centuries. Seeking wisdom, philosophers employed abstract thinking and ambitious questions. They questioned popular notions about nature and its relationship to the whims of gods and goddesses. They asked questions about the origins and the nature of all things. They pondered the nature of reality and truth. They explored ideas about the right way for humans to live (Soloman & Higgins, 1996). The ideas generated by these early philosophers have influenced all facets of society throughout the centuries.

Socrates, Plato, and Aristotle proposed new and exciting ideas about truth, reality, relationships, ethics, and the good life. Socrates (470–399 BCE) was arguably the greatest philosopher of ancient times. The first recorded full body of philosophical work was Plato's dialogues between Socrates and various other people. Socrates believed that knowledge leads to the "good life." Socrates proposed that one must seek knowledge and develop the inner self in order to experience a good life. He believed that a person should do what is right, even when opposed by others. Socrates and Plato believed that there was one specific type of good life that was not dependent upon humans' desires, wishes, or opinions. They believed people could acquire it only through study and contemplation (Soloman & Higgins, 1996).

One of Socrates's major contributions was the *Socratic method* of teaching. Demonstrated throughout Plato's dialogues, the Socratic method consists of a *dialectic* in which two people present opposing opinions. In contrast to an argument or debate, however, revelations occur as the two people talk and ask each other questions, and their ideas move closer to *truth*. In this way, students learn to think through a problem in a systematic and objective manner. Teachers today commonly use the Socratic method. Class discussions and the *Think About It* and *Ask Yourself* elements of this textbook can be used for students to learn via the Socratic method.

Aristotle, a student of Plato, proposed ideas that were different from those of his teachers. He believed that virtuous behavior consisted of attaining the "golden mean." For example, he believed that the virtue of courage is the mean between cowardice and foolhardiness. Aristotle proposed that the aim of the good life is *eudaimonia* (translated as happiness or flourishing). He proposed that eudaimonia can only occur through a life of virtue and excellence, one in which the person fulfills the aim of life. Aristotle wrote that that the aim of a flautist is to play the flute, of the carpenter is to build, and so forth. Although this is a simplification of Aristotle's teachings, these examples seem to indicate that happiness or flourishing only occurs when the person focuses on excellence toward a goal. He wrote, "in life it is those who act rightly who will attain what is noble and good" (Aristotle, trans. 2000, p. 14).

The Early Christian Era

Religious Influences and the Role of Women in the Early Christian Era. Arguably the most profound religious influence on healing beliefs and practices in Western civilization occurred with the advent of the Christian era. The effect of Christian belief and organized Christian religion on the history of healing is multifaceted. It is interesting to closely examine textbooks on nursing history and recognize divergent opinions among authors. The pendulum swings from some authors' biases that present only the positive aspects of the Christian influence on the history of nursing, to those that condemn Christianity as a destructive, misogynistic force that hindered nursing progress.

In a text on nursing history originally published in 1916, Dolan writes, "Man and the universe were made to exist in the profound execution of the plan of Creation" (1973, p. 3). Dolan uses the New Testament of the Bible to describe Jesus's message about caring for others in the following way: (1) caring for others represents caring for Jesus; (2) there is spiritual reward to be gained by caring for others; (3) even in a world of selfishness and hatred one should love God and one's neighbor; (4) every person, even the "poorest and most miserable," is an important member of the Kingdom of God; and (5) every person has worth and dignity. As this example shows, nursing texts, in Western culture, often reflect the prevailing influence of early Christian teaching on healing practices and the nursing profession.

Early Christian nurses were frequently women of high social status and often became independent practitioners. Many set aside special places in their homes for hospitality and care of the sick. These places were called *Christrooms* (Dolan, 1973; Dolan et al., 1983). Early Christians exhibited caring and respect for the intrinsic value of each human.

As centuries passed, the path of healing practices assumed a winding course. Jeanne Achterberg describes the first 500 years after the birth of Christ as the "calm before the storm." She says, "These were fluid times, when religion was a satisfying and exotic blend of ingredients taken from pre-Christian, pagan, and folk traditions" (1990, p. 39). As time passed, war, disease, and the influence of religious dogma effectively altered the course of the healing traditions.

When religious belief moved toward a single male god, women's healing role changed from that of sacred healer to subservient caregiver. By the time Jesus lived, the place of women in the healing arts was minimal. Jesus challenged the patriarchal tradition by associating freely with women. He selected the most "compassionate, maternal images from the Jewish tradition, creating a Christian god as androgynous . . . as any male god in history. In some of the early sects, God was even seen as a dyadic being (mother-father), rather than the trinity (father-son-holy spirit)" (Achterberg, 1990, p. 38). As a result, women enjoyed renewed acceptance as healers. Their intellect and contribution to the religious movement were respected by the early Christians. This resurgence of power and respectability, however, only lasted for a few centuries after the birth of Christ.

Philosophy in the Early Christian Era. Many—if not most—of the Western philosophers of the early Christian years were Christians struggling with the challenges and practical concerns of the new religion. The most influential philosopher of the early years of Christianity was St. Paul. Educated in the Greek tradition, Paul agreed with earlier, non-Christian moral philosophers that there is a natural law of conscience inherent in each person (Solomon & Higgins, 1996). St. Augustine was another important philosopher during the early Christian era. He devoted himself to integrating Christian doctrine with Plato's philosophy. He believed that true reality was spiritual and that all Being comes from God. He contributed to Western philosophy an emphasis on one's personal, inner life. St. Augustine proposed that the goal of human existence is the contemplation of God in awe and reverence (Soloman & Higgins, 1996). In addition, he devoted much attention to examination of the passions of the soul, including love and faith, as well as the urges, impulses, and vices such as lust, pride, and curiosity that occur in every person.

The Middle Ages

Philosophy in the Middle Ages. Much of the Middle Ages coincided with the Dark Ages, a period of social disruption and cultural deterioration. The Church maintained a stronghold on society, so what little philosophy did emerge was almost entirely theological. St. Augustine's writings were highly regarded. During this period, Thomas Aquinas synthesized Greek rationalism and Christian doctrine. His work during this time became a cornerstone of Catholic philosophy (Russell, 1967). Later in the Middle Ages, energy was invested in retranslating Plato and Aristotle.

Religious Influences in the Middle Ages. As the early Middle Ages began, many people believed that the world was falling into ruin. During this time, disease, large-scale food shortages, and war interacted to produce a predictable sequence: war drove farmers from their fields and destroyed their crops; destruction of the crops led to famine; and the starved and weakened people were easy victims of the onslaught of disease (Cartwright, 1972). The established social structure was deteriorating, and disorganized communities turned to feudalism, monasticism, and, in certain regions, Islam as solutions to the chaos they were experiencing. During this time, monasticism and other religious groups offered the only opportunities for men and women to pursue careers in nursing. Much of hospital nursing was carried out by repentant women and widows called sisters, and by male nurses called brothers. Deaconesses, matrons, and secular nursing orders were among the organized groups that had religious foundations and offered nursing services.

These early nurses believed they were following the command of God to imitate Jesus, who had spent his life ministering to those in need. For many, this service was viewed as a means of securing salvation. Dolan quotes a Sisters of Charity founder, Saint Louise de Marillac, who wrote in a letter dated 1633, "We do not want those who have no desire to work at their spiritual perfection in the service of God. They should have no motive in coming except the one of serving God and their neighbor" (1973, p. 100). Women who entered nursing orders donated their property and wealth to the Roman Catholic Church and devoted their lives to service. Believing that "charity" was synonymous with "love," many early Christians sold their possessions and gave everything to the Church or the poor. Although in many cases "nursing" care was given by slaves or servants, religious orders offered the only route through which respectable women and men could serve as nurses.

The overall belief system of a culture influences the extent to which members accept various healing methods and health care practices. An example of this can be seen in historical accounts of the healing arts in the Middle Ages. The term **empirical** relates to knowledge gained through the processes of observation and experience. Many people, especially those involved with the Church, had deeply anti-empirical beliefs. Consequently, people were more likely to seek healing through religious interventions such as touching religious relics, visiting sacred places, chanting, and other methods approved by the Church. Because of the religious fervor at the time, empirical treatment (particularly if provided by anyone not explicitly sanctioned by the Church), even if it was successful, was thought to be produced by the devil, since the position of the Church was that only God and the devil had the power to either cause illness or promote healing.

An increasingly influential Christian doctrine led to a constant war waged against the flesh. People during the Middle Ages believed that they should "mortify the flesh" in the name of honoring the spirit. There was little attention to physical needs. People were dirty and covered with rashes and "foul eruptions." These problems were made worse by rough, dirty, woolen clothing and the constant presence of ticks and fleas. Thus, as a direct result of religious teaching, health care practices during the Middle Ages actually caused the spread of disease, intensified health problems, and limited effective empirical healing practices (Achterberg, 1990).

The Crusades, which began in 1096 and lasted nearly 200 years, brought many changes in the health of the population. These holy wars led to deplorable sanitary conditions, fatigue, poor nutrition, diarrhea, and the spread of communicable diseases. Health problems led to a demand for more hospitals and greater numbers of health care providers. Military nursing orders were formed in response to the compelling need. These orders drew large numbers of men into the field of nursing (Dolan, 1973).

Another direct result of the Crusades was the collection of relics by the Church. Believed to offer the potential of healing miracles, the spoils of war included body parts of Crusade martyrs. The Church obtained significant wealth and power through the sale of these relics. Achterberg (1990) compares this time to the time of an earlier Roman mythology in which large numbers of deities or sainted mortals, their relics, and pilgrimages to their sacred sites were believed to hold the key to health.

For most of the Middle Ages, the Roman Catholic Church held tremendous influence over the people and governments of all European countries. Powerful leaders within the Church determined the appropriateness of various healing practices. Official credentialing of physicians, nurses, and midwives was left in the hands of the Church. After civic legislation became common, the Church continued to enforce the law and monitor practitioners (Achterberg, 1990). As we will see in the following section, this power was also used to enforce religious doctrine that influenced the status of women in society.

Accounts of the actual treatment of patients in early times vary. In some hospitals operated by religious orders, patients were treated as welcome guests. People sometimes pretended to be ill to be admitted. In contrast, some groups of patients were treated inhumanely, even by members of nursing orders. If these nurses believed their duty was to God and to the spiritual rather than physical needs of the patients, they may have been less attentive to physical, emotional, and comfort needs.

The treatment of the mentally ill was based for centuries on the idea that they were possessed by devils or that they were being punished for their sins (Dolan, 1973). They were often put in chains, starved, and kept under filthy conditions. There was even a time when it was thought that torture was useful in driving out madness. Because the public perception of mental illness was based on religious beliefs related to demon possession and punishment for sin, the mentally ill were treated inhumanely.

Women in the Middle Ages. During the Middle Ages, the status of women also declined. In many ways this was directly related to Church doctrine. St. Thomas Aquinas, ironically known within the Church as the "angelic doctor" (Donahue, 1996), wrote that one should "only make use of a necessary object, woman, who is needed to preserve the species or to provide food and drink. . . . Woman was created to be man's [helper], but her unique role is in conception. . . since for all other purposes men would be better assisted by other men" (Aquinas as cited by Achterberg, 1990, p. 68). Centuries earlier another Church leader, St. Jerome, who was frequently recognized for his support of matrons in their calling as nurses, remarked that "woman is the gate of the devil, the path of wickedness, the sting of the serpent, in a word a perilous object" (Heer, 1961, p. 322). These religious leaders were setting the stage for the persecution of women that would last for hundreds of years and leave a persistent legacy of misogyny.

Religious and Church-sanctioned secular nursing orders afforded the only legitimate avenue for women wishing to be nurses during the Middle Ages. The Church popularized the ideals of virginity, poverty, and a life of service. By the end of the thirteenth century, an estimated 200,000 women served as nurses within these orders (Achterberg, 1990). Caring for pilgrims in improvised infirmaries and clinics, women's nursing orders were particularly welcome during the Crusades. As was often the case, these orders were subordinate to the men's communities (Donahue, 1996). Nevertheless, some speculate that within the structure of the Church, these women exercised a degree of independence and autonomy. There is no doubt that they made a great contribution to the health care of the time.

Also during the Middle Ages, the Church and the newly formed medical profession were actively engaged in the elimination of lay female healers. Women were excluded from universities. Except for those devoting their lives to serving in religious nursing orders, women were not allowed by the Church to practice the healing arts. During a revival of learning in the thirteenth century, the Church imposed strict controls on the new profession of medicine and officially prohibited women from its practice (Achterberg, 1990). Nevertheless, some women continued to secretly practice the healing arts, both within and outside the home. They used knowledge handed down for generations, empirical knowledge, and intuition.

It was a popular religious view that women were essentially evil by nature. The pain of childbirth was believed to be punishment for Eve's transgression, and served the purpose of reminding women of their original sinful nature. Those who dared provide pain relief to others during childbirth were severely punished (Achterberg, 1990). Later, the Original Sin of Eve would be used to justify torturing and murdering thousands of women during the witch hunts.

The medical profession was officially sanctioned by the Church, and male physicians began to be trained in the university setting. Even so, there was very little scientific knowledge. The physician relied solely on superstition (Ehrenreich & English, 1973). University-trained physicians used bloodletting, astrology, alchemy, and incantations. Their patients were almost exclusively wealthy. Physicians' treatments were usually ineffective, often dangerous, and inaccessible to the majority of the poor.

Women Healers and Social Turmoil. Peasant women were often the only healers for people who suffered bitterly from poverty and disease (Ehrenreich & English, 1973). Folk healers had extensive knowledge about cures that had been handed down for generations via oral tradition. They constantly improved their practice through empirical methods of observation, trial, and evaluation. While physicians continued to rely on superstition, these women developed an extensive understanding of bones and muscles, herbs, drugs, and midwifery (Barstow, 1994; Ehrenreich & English, 1973). Some authorities believed that peasant folk healers were actually practicing some form of magic or witchcraft (Barstow, 1994). Others speculated that these women were honoring the old pagan religions and worshipping the old gods who (according to Church authorities) had assumed the persona of the devil (Achterberg, 1990). It is likely that these women were simply caring for others in a manner that was consistent with prevailing folk belief. After all, almost everyone in medieval Europe believed in the reality of magic (Barstow, 1994). This atmosphere set the stage for Church-sanctioned crimes against women in the form of the witch hunts.

In their sweep across Europe, the witch hunts lasted from the fourteenth century to the seventeenth century. The atmosphere that led to the witch hunts was a critical mixture of war, disease, and poverty combined with religious fervor, superstition, and political unrest. The witch trials were accomplished through an organized partnership among the Church, state, and emerging medical profession. Women, particularly women healers, represented a political, religious, and sexual threat to both Church and state. An atmosphere of superstition and the widespread belief in magic set the stage that would allow terrible crimes to be perpetrated against women (Achterberg, 1990; Barstow, 1994; Ehrenreich & English, 1973).

Armed with papal authorization to purge Germany of witches, Dominican inquisitors Kramer and Sprenger wrote *Malleus Maleficarum* (Barstow, 1994). This witch hunters' manual expressed virulent anti-feminine and anti-sexual opinions. They claimed that women are "liars, more superstitious than men, more impressionable, wicked minded, and in need of constant male supervision" (Barstow, 1994, p. 172). They wrote, "If a woman dare to cure without having studied she is a witch and must die" (Kramer & Sprenger as cited by Ehrenreich & English, 1973, p. 19), and "No one does more harm to the Catholic Church than midwives" (p. 13). They also wrote, "When a woman thinks alone, she thinks evil. . . . Women are intellectually like children" (Kramer & Sprenger as cited by Barstow, 1994, p. 172). Kramer and Sprenger defined witchcraft as treason against God, and described it as female rebellion. According to Barstow, "the document reeks with fear and hatred of women, concluding with thanks to God 'who has so far preserved the male sex from so great a crime' " (1994, p. 62). *Malleus Maleficarum* was printed in four languages and at least 29 editions between the years of 1486 CE and 1669 CE.

ASK YOURSELF

Healing or Witchcraft?

Imagine yourself the parent of a small child in the sixteenth century. You believe the church doctrine about the origin of the knowledge of healing. Your family and neighbors are aware of the growing problem of witchcraft in the region. Your child becomes ill and you recall a remedy that your mother used successfully with the same ailment.

- Will you openly attempt to alleviate your child's suffering and risk being accused of witchcraft?
- How would you feel about having to make this decision?

What were the crimes of which the women were accused? Any woman who treated an illness, even if she applied a soothing salve to the diseased skin of her child, was likely to be accused of witchcraft. If the treatment failed, she was thought to have cursed the patient. If the treatment succeeded, she was believed to be in consort with the devil. Although women were permitted to practice midwifery (no one else wanted to do it), these women were in danger of being accused of witchcraft if anything went wrong with either mother or baby.

No one knows how many women were killed during the witch trials. When records were kept, they were abysmal. Often names were not used, and occasionally the verdict and sentence were not recorded. The most authoritative estimate of the number of executions is 200,000. Some estimates are as high as 10 million. Women comprised 85 percent to 95 percent of those killed (Barstow, 1994). During the twelfth century in Russia, when looking for witches, authorities simply rounded up all the women in an area. Some small European towns were left with essentially no women at all (Achterberg, 1990; Barstow, 1994; Ehrenreich & English, 1973).

It is difficult to comprehend the effect of the witch hunts on European society. Women silently watched the public humiliation, torture, disfigurement, and death of other women. Barstow believes that this public acknowledgment of the evil nature of the female sex left all women humiliated and frightened. Because both the accused and those viewing the proceedings were powerless to prevent the torture and executions, the witch craze served to undermine women's belief in the ability and power of women. Indeed, this was likely the inference made by all of society. Achterberg writes, "women were never again given full citizenship in any country, nor was their role in the healing professions reinstated" (1990, p. 98). Even after the end of this terrible time, women were prohibited from the independent healing professions by law in every country in Europe. This created a climate by which, under the protection and patronage of the ruling classes, males became the authoritative medical professionals (Ehrenreich & English, 1973). Although accounts of the witch hunts are absent in most popular nursing history texts, these events probably influenced the future of the profession more than any other single factor. As Ehrenreich and English write, "It was to become a theme of our history" (1973, p. 6).

The Renaissance and the Reformation

The fourteenth through the early sixteenth centuries were known for two great movements: the Renaissance and the Reformation. The Reformation was a religious movement precipitated by the widespread abuses that had become a part of Church life and doctrinal disagreement among religious leaders. This period left little of the old Church intact (Collison, 2006). The Renaissance, sometimes called the Enlightenment, produced an intellectual rebirth that ushered in the scientific era.

The sixteenth-century Reformation was one of the greatest religious revolutions of all times. At the start of the sixteenth century, western Europe had only one religion—Roman Catholicism. During the Middle Ages, the church had amassed remarkable wealth and perpetrated many kinds of abuses. Martin Luther sparked a movement in the sixteenth century that resulted in the establishment of Protestantism and the loss of the Roman Catholic Church's stronghold on Western culture. Gradually releasing the people from oppressive control of the Roman Catholic Church, the Reformation allowed new types of thinking and opened the door for the Renaissance. Philosophy and science no longer needed to justify themselves to religion.

The Reformation produced unrest. Widespread abuses and differences in belief among church leaders led to a struggle between Catholic and Protestant groups across Europe. One outcome was that the laws and customs in Protestant countries discouraged the humane care of the poor and vulnerable (Donahue, 1996). Religious nursing orders were driven out of hospitals, and many of these orders were ultimately closed. During this era hospitals became places of horror. There was no qualified group to take the place of the religious nursing orders. Unqualified and undesirable women were assigned nursing duties. Conditions were at their very worst between 1550 and 1850—the "Dark Period of Nursing"—when convalescent patients, prostitutes, prisoners, and drunkards provided hospital nursing care (Donahue, 1996).

The Renaissance fostered the scientific revolution and a new era in the healing arts. Beginning its gradual escape from the control of the Church, the scientific community made advances in mathematics and the sciences. Philosophical humanism emerged during the Renaissance. Humanism established humans, rather than God, as a focus of interest. This new perspective enabled a scientific outlook that viewed the universe as governed by general laws. Copernicus theorized that the Earth was not the center of the universe. The philosopher and scientist Galileo used direct observation to gain new knowledge about astronomy. Advances in science during the Renaissance inspired the philosophers of the time. They came to believe that genuine knowledge was accessible to individuals through careful observation of empiric phenomena and subjective reasoning (Solomon & Higgins, 1996).

Some have argued that the Renaissance benefited men, but not women. Although released from the grip of fear produced by the witch hunts, women of the Renaissance continued to live in subordination to men. Their day-to-day lives changed little. Most women were denied educations and, for the most part, none were allowed to become legitimate members of any profession.

Think About It

Who Has the Right to Make Ethical Decisions?

Ethical decision making is not the sole domain of the physician. Nurses may be better prepared and have more opportunities to discuss moral problems with patients and families.

- *Can you describe an instance in which the physician assumed the authority to make an ethical decision, denying nurses (and perhaps the patient and family) participation in the decision-making process?*

- *If you feel you have an important contribution to make in a particular circumstance, and your opinion is not considered, how do you react?*

- *How do you think nurses can overcome the strong heritage of subjugation?*

The Modern Era

The **Modern Era** immediately followed the Renaissance and is generally thought to include the late sixteenth through the late eighteenth centuries. This era ushered in tremendous advances in science, politics, and philosophy. Many modern philosophers' ideas directly influence the profession of nursing as we know it today. Among these philosophers were Emmanuel Kant, who proposed an ethical system based on duty and moral imperatives, and John Stuart Mill, who described a new way of thinking about ethics and justice. Kant and Mill are discussed in depth in Chapters 2 and 3. Another philosopher, René Descartes, proposed new theories that changed the course of science for all times.

Descartes is credited with proposing a theory that quickly altered philosophic beliefs about the separation of mind and body. He proposed that the universe is a physical thing and that everything in the universe is like a machine, which can be analyzed and understood. Descartes further theorized that the mind and body are separate entities, and that people are set against a world of objects that they must seek to master (McCarthy, 1990). Based on Descartes's work, **Cartesian philosophy** began to replace religious beliefs related to the physical and spiritual realms of humankind.

As a result of Cartesian philosophy, a separation was perceived between the acts of caring and curing in the healing arts. Descartes's philosophy elevated the sciences and made scientific inquiry possible, yet it failed to improve the status of nursing. Achterberg identifies this time as an important turning point. She says in regard to Cartesian philosophy, "When spirit no longer is seen to abide in matter, the reverence for what is physical departs. Hence medicine no longer regarded itself as working in the sacred spaces where fellow humans find themselves in pain and peril, and where transcendence is most highly desired" (1990, p. 103). Nursing as we know it today began to emerge in the modern era. Cartesian philosophy effectively created a clear distinction between nurses and physicians and formalized their hierarchical relationship. Nurses' place in the health care system was limited to the "caring" realm. Caring was given lower status than curing within the hierarchy of the healing arts. Some would argue that this legacy still remains with nursing today.

The founder of modern nursing, Florence Nightingale (1820–1910), reflected the influence of the Renaissance and Reformation. Even though she was devoutly religious, Nightingale worked to free nursing from the bonds of the Church, which she called "an over busy mother" (Roberts & Group, 1995). As a person, Nightingale remains an enigma. She viewed nursing as a profession separate from the Church, yet she began her career as the result of a mystic experience (Simkin, 2006). According to Nightingale, God spoke to her four times, calling her into his service when she was 16 years old (Selanders, 1998b). Her experience in the Crimean War was the direct result of her second revelation, which she termed a call from God (Dossey, 2000; Showalter, 1981). Although she was opposed to using Church affiliation as a criterion for admission to nursing programs, her religious beliefs were evident in her dealings with students, whom she admonished to work diligently because "if there is no cross, there is no crown" (Achterberg, 1990; Selanders, 1998b). In addition, Nightingale's description of nursing as caring for the mind and the body implies a rejection of Descartes's philosophy on the separation of these two human spheres.

Florence Nightingale became a model for all nurses. She was a nurse, statistician, sanitarian, social reformer, and scholar. Nightingale was a scholar who studied Plato and helped translate some of his writings into English. She saw corollaries between nursing and Plato's conception of public service. Plato believed that the aim of education is to mold talented people into leading citizens, who will in turn care for the good of the community. Nightingale viewed this orientation to service as the basis for nursing's goal to improve the welfare of people.

Nightingale was politically astute, intelligent, and single-minded. Contrary to the accepted Victorian social order, Nightingale addressed moral issues with courage and conviction. Having strong opinions on women's rights, she was quick to challenge the established male hierarchy. Nightingale argued for the removal of restrictions that prevented women from having careers (Simkin, 2006). Her writings instructed nurses to "do the thing that is good, whether it is 'suitable for a woman' or not" (Nightingale, 1859, p. 76). Although some argue that Nightingale was not a feminist, her writings indicate that she felt women should have a more important place in the social structure. She wrote, "Passion, intellect, moral activity—these three have never been satisfied in woman. In this cold and oppressive conventional atmosphere, they cannot be satisfied" (Nightingale, 1852/1979, p. 29). It is certain that she did not ascribe to the popular Cartesian notion that women do not have minds and souls, and are put on the Earth solely for man's purpose and pleasure (Roberts & Group, 1995).

Lavinia Lloyd Dock (1858–1956) is another of nursing's great modern leaders. Considered a radical feminist, Dock actively engaged in social protest, picketing, and parading for women's rights (Roberts & Group, 1995). She was concerned with the problems plaguing nursing, warning that male dominance in the health field was the major problem confronting the nursing profession. Lavinia Dock's contemporaries ignored her concerns, and twenty-first century nurses have found themselves fighting the same battles.

The mid-1900s brought great advances for nurses. Nurses entered professional, social, and political spheres. Although recurrent themes of paternalism and subjugation continued to affect the nursing profession, twentieth-century women became more politically active. The women's movement encouraged political, social, and economic action to correct the wrongs suffered by women. Roberts and Group (1995) wrote that "Nurses' consciousness of their subordinated and oppressed group status became heightened, propelling some nurses to advocate radical role-breaking, risk-taking behaviors" (p. 187). The profession gained acceptance as a legitimate health care force. In 1958 the first liaison committee was established between the American Nurses Association (ANA) and the American Medical Association (AMA). A historic joint conference was held between the two groups in 1964. Participating in federal policy making, the nursing profession was represented as Medicare was signed into law in 1965 and later enjoyed federal legislation in 1997 that authorized Medicare reimbursement for nurse practitioners and clinical specialists (Zolot & Nelson-Hogan, 2000).

No longer forced into roles of subjugation during the last half of the twentieth century, many nurses began to provide independent health care services and assume institutional and political leadership positions. Perceiving a health care crisis of growing proportions, and recognizing the need for comprehensive, accessible, and affordable health care, society challenged established institutions to foster greater use of nurses in expanded roles. Encouraged by a society in which health care had become a scarce resource, nurse practitioners, nurse midwives, and other advanced nurses began to assert themselves as independent professionals.

Thus entering the twenty-first century, nursing in Western culture is shaped by religious/spiritual and cultural influences of the past. Although many nurses have overcome social and institutional barriers to practicing as full members of the healing professions, others continue to struggle within patriarchal, institutional hierarchies. Recognizing the legitimate need for both the caring and curing aspects of healing, nurses are charged with working together to improve their status and to ensure that the problems of the past are not repeated. Today's health care system is one that is experiencing rapid change. Managed care and other health care reform programs offer nurses both opportunities and challenges. The position of the professional nurse within these systems is far from assured. Recalling lessons from the past, nurses remain acutely aware of threats to newly won professional recognition.

SUMMARY

Nursing is a profession that was created by society for the purpose of meeting specific perceived health needs. The profession belongs to society and therefore is bound by the duty to competently meet the needs for which it was created. Individual nurses, therefore, have a duty to fulfill the promise the profession has made to society.

In all cultures, the nursing profession has been profoundly influenced by various aspects of spirituality and religious practice. The natures of both the healer and the healing act have been influenced by the prevailing cosmology. Until the past two centuries, healing was strongly associated with the sacred. Religious institutions have influenced the parameters and membership of the profession—by either including or excluding particular groups.

From ancient times until today, philosophers have asked important questions and proposed theories that helped to shape cultures. Even when people do not recognize it, culture is influenced by philosophers' ideas. These ideas permeate society, relationships, and professions. Since the first philosophers emerged, no element of society has been free from the influence of philosophy.

In every culture women have been healers. Because nursing is primarily a profession of women, the status of women in society has been an important factor in determining the role of nurses in the health care system. Women's status in society directly determines the freedom they are given to become educated, to think and act independently, and to participate fully in the healing arts. There were periods in history in which women were allowed freedom and responsibility, and there were dark periods in which women lived in subjugation. Nursing today is at a crossroads, free of many of the restrictions of the past, yet not fully franchised as a profession with power and authority.

CHAPTER HIGHLIGHTS

- Throughout history, spiritual beliefs, religious practice, cultural norms, and political factors have influenced evolutionary changes in nursing. These factors continue to influence the practice of nursing today.

- Prevailing philosophical ideas influence every aspect of culture.

- Social need is the criterion for the existence of all professions.

- Moral thinking occurs when individuals or groups desire to meet the needs of others.

- The practice of nursing is focused on meeting the health care needs of others; therefore, the practice of nursing originates in moral thinking.

- Professions exist to meet the needs of society.

- Society grants professionals the exclusive right to practice within defined parameters.

- Professionals have a reciprocal duty to society to practice competently.

- Because nursing is primarily a profession of women, the social status of women affects the status of the profession.
- The status of the nursing profession determines members' ability to practice with freedom and responsibility.

DISCUSSION QUESTIONS AND ACTIVITIES

1. Talk with nurses, physicians, and ministers. Ask their opinions about why some people choose to help others in need. In class, analyze and compare the responses.

2. Discuss the historical developments that caused the separation of the professions of medicine and nursing. How were the distinctions drawn as to the boundaries of the professions? How would you change the boundaries today?

3. Search the Internet for information on Florence Nightingale. Pictures and a short history can be found at http://www.spartacus.schoolnet.co.uk/REnightingale.htm.

4. What is the relationship between the role of women in history and the status of nurses?

5. What is the relationship between the role of women today and the status of nurses?

6. Search out a few retired nurses. Ask them to describe the relationship between nurses and physicians in the mid-1900s. How was this related to the roles of women in society during the same time period?

7. Discuss the relationship between the role of nurses in the health care system today and their role in ethical decision making in the clinical setting.

8. Discuss the challenges that the profession of nursing faces related to attaining or maintaining an authoritative role in the health care system of the future.

REFERENCES

Achterberg, J. (1990). *Woman as healer*. Boston: Shambhala.

American Nurses Association. (1980). *Nursing: A social policy statement*. Kansas City, MO: Author.

American Nurses Association. (1996). *Nursing's social policy statement*. Washington, DC: Author.

Aristotle. (trans. 2000). *Nicomachean ethics* (R. Crisp, Trans. & Ed.). Cambridge, UK: Cambridge University Press.

Barstow, A. L. (1994). *Witchcraze: A new history of the European witch hunts.* San Francisco: HarperCollins.

Cartwright, F. F. (1972). *Disease and history.* New York: Dorset Press.

Collison, P. (2006). *The Reformation: A history.* New York: Modern Library.

Dolan, J. A. (1973). *Nursing in society: A historical perspective* (13th ed.). Philadelphia: Saunders.

Dolan, J. A., Fitzpatrick, M. L., & Herrmann, E. K. (1983). *Nursing in society: A historical perspective* (15th ed.). Philadelphia: Saunders.

Donahue, M. P. (1996). *Nursing: The finest art.* St. Louis, MO: Mosby.

Dossey, B. M. (2000). *Florence Nightingale: Mystic, visionary, healer.* Springhouse, PA: Springhouse.

Ehrenreich, B., & English, D. (1973). *Witches, midwives, and nurses: A history of women healers.* New York: The Feminist Press.

Freire, P. (2000). *Pedagogy of the oppressed* (30th anniversary ed.). New York: Continuum.

Fulton, Y. (1997). Nurses' views on empowerment: A critical social theory perspective. *Journal of Advanced Nursing, 26,* 529–536.

Garrison, F. H. (1966). *History of medicine.* Philadelphia: Saunders.

Grammaticos, P. C., & Diamantis, A. (2008). Useful known and unknown views of the father of modern medicine: Hippocrates and his teacher Democritus. *Hellenic Journal of Nuclear Medicine, 11*(1), 204.

Habermas, J. (1971). *Communication and the evolution of society.* Boston: Beacon Press.

Harden, J. (1996). Enlightenment, empowerment and emancipation: The case for critical pedagogy in nurse education. *Nurse Education Today, 16*(1), 32–37.

Hart, G. D. (2000). *Asclepius: The god of medicine.* London: Royal Society of Medicine Press.

Hedin, B. A. (1986). A case study of oppressed group behavior in nurses. *Image: Journal of Nursing Scholarship, 18*(2), 53–57.

Heer, F. (1961). *The medieval world.* New York: New American Library.

Honderich, T. (Ed.). (2005). *The Oxford companion to philosophy* (2nd ed.). Oxford, England: Oxford University Press.

Houser, N., & Kloesel, C. (Eds.). (1992). *The essential Peirce: Selected philosophical writings* (Vol. 1). Bloomington: Indiana University Press.

Jameton, A. (1984). *Nursing practice: The ethical issues.* Englewood Cliffs, NJ: Prentice-Hall.

McCarthy, T. (1990). The critique of impure reason. *Political Theory, 18*(3), 437–469.

Nightingale, F. (1859). *Notes on nursing: What it is, and what it is not.* London: Harrison & Sons.

Nightingale, F. (1979). *Cassandra.* Old Westbury, NY: Feminist Press. (Original work published 1852)

Plato (trans. 1997). Phaedo. In J. M. Cooper (Ed.) *Plato: Complete works.* (G. M. A. Grube, Trans.). Indianapolis, IN: Hackett Publishing.

Roberts, J. I., & Group, T. M. (1995). *Feminism and nursing: An historical perspective on power, status, and political activism in the nursing profession.* Westport, CT: Praeger.

Roberts, S. J. (1983). Oppressed group behavior: Implications for nursing. *Advances in Nursing Science, 5*(4), 21–30.

Russell, B. (1967). *The history of Western philosophy.* New York: Simon & Schuster.

Selanders, L. C. (1998a). Florence Nightingale: The evolution and social impact of feminist values in nursing. *Journal of Holistic Nursing, 16*(2), 227–243.

Selanders, L. C. (1998b). The power of environmental adaptation: Florence Nightingale's original theory for nursing practice. *Journal of Holistic Nursing, 16*(2), 247–263.

Showalter, E. (1981). Florence Nightingale's feminist complaint: Women, religion, and suggestions for thought. *Journal of Women in Culture and Society, 6*, 395–412.

Simkin, J. (2006). *Florence Nightingale.* Retrieved February 14, 2006, from http://www.spartacus.schoolnet.co.uk/REnightingale.htm

Soloman, R. C., & Higgins, K. M. (1996). A short history of philosophy. New York: Oxford University Press.

Spooner, W. A. (1914). *The Golden Rule.* New York: Scribner's Sons.

Stevens, P. E. (1989). A critical social reconceptualization environment in nursing: Implications for methodology. *Advances in Nursing Science, 11*(4), 56–68.

Temkin, O., & Temkin, C. L. (Eds.). (1987). *Ancient medicine: Selected papers of Ludwig Edelstein.* Baltimore: Johns Hopkins University Press.

Yapijakis, C. (2009). Hippocrates of Kos: The father of clinical medicine, and Asclepiades of Bithynia, the father of molecular medicine. *In Vivo, 23*(4), 505–514.

Zolot, J. S., & Nelson-Hogan, D. (2000). News. *American Journal of Nursing, 100*(10), 32–37.

Chapter

2

ETHICAL THEORY

Within Siddhartha there slowly grew and ripened the knowledge of what wisdom really was and the goal of his long seeking. It was nothing but a preparation of the soul, a capacity, a secret art of thinking, feeling and breathing thoughts of unity at every moment of life. This thought matured in him slowly, and it was reflected in Vasudeva's old childlike face: harmony, knowledge of the eternal perfection of the world, and unity.

(Hesse, 1971, p. 131)

OBJECTIVES

After completing this chapter, the reader should be able to:

1. Discuss the purpose of philosophy.

2. Define the terms *moral philosophy* and *ethics*.

3. Discuss the importance of a systematic study of ethics to nursing.

4. Discuss the importance of ethical theory.

5. Describe utilitarianism.

6. Describe deontological ethics, defining the terms *categorical imperative* and *practical imperative*.

7. Define the terms *virtue* and *virtue ethics*.

8. Discuss moral particularism.

INTRODUCTION

At its core, nursing deals with issues and situations that have elements of ethical or moral uncertainty. A spiraling dependence on technology and the resulting longer lifespans and higher health care costs, coupled with increasing professional autonomy, creates an atmosphere in which nurses are faced with problems of ever-increasing complexity. We need to be able to recognize situations with ethical and moral implications, and make coherent and logical ethical decisions based upon recognized ethical principles and theory. This text will prepare you to examine issues and come to logical, consistent, and thoughtful ethical decisions. The study of ethics will make you more rational, responsible, self-reliant, and effective.

As nurses we need to be able to recognize ethical components of practice and engage in a structured ethical decision-making process. We must have the willingness and courage to participate in work that is emotionally painful. Ethical problems deal with issues of great significance to those involved and, by their very nature, have no easy or obvious solutions. We must have a solid knowledge base that prepares us to identify circumstances that involve ethical components. Knowledge of and insight into personal values, cultural norms, moral development, and ethical theory are necessary for the practicing nurse. We must be sensitive, patient, and insightful. Recognition of subtle clues that may indicate when a situation is laden with ethical components demands that we are attentive to all facets of the predicament. This requires time, focused attention, and sensitivity. We need to be knowledgeable and adept in making logical, fair, and consistent decisions. Ethical decision-making models offer a variety of methods for coming to rational conclusions. Willingness, courage, knowledge, and moral sensitivity must all be present for us to participate effectively in ethical decision making.

Case Presentation

Nursing Students Face an Ethical Dilemma

Tonya and Lydia are two senior nursing students assigned to work in the intensive care unit with a critically ill patient. The patient, Mr. Dunn, is an 87-year-old retired ironworker. He lives alone in an old two-story frame house. Mr. Dunn is diabetic. He is nearly blind and has moderately advanced prostate cancer and Alzheimer's disease. Mr. Dunn was admitted to the intensive care unit after he was

(continued)

discovered unconscious in his home by a neighbor. At that time he was ketoacidotic and had a very severe necrotic wound on his left leg. The surgeon plans to amputate Mr. Dunn's left leg but has been unable to get consent from either Mr. Dunn or his next of kin, a niece who lives out of town.

Tonya is proud of her efficiency as a nursing student. She makes rapid decisions. Tonya insists that Mr. Dunn must have the amputation. She boldly suggests to the physician that he have a surrogate appointed for Mr. Dunn so that the surgery can proceed. The course is clear to her. Lydia, on the other hand, is not certain of the correct course of action. She talks to Mr. Dunn and his niece about his condition. She wonders if the amputation is the best solution to his problem. She thinks about what his quality of life will be after the surgery. She worries about his ability to care for himself and about his state of mind should he be forced to live in a nursing home. She thinks about what she would want for her own father if he were in the same situation. Lydia falls asleep at night pondering these thoughts. She does not know how to go about solving the problem. Tonya is impatient with Lydia. She sees no benefit to the time and energy spent worrying about this problem when the solution is apparent to her. She dislikes wasting her time talking to Lydia about these concerns.

Think About It

Facing Ethical Dilemmas

- *What alerts you to the presence of an ethical dilemma?*
- *How do you feel when confronted with difficult ethical decisions?*
- *To what degree do you think nurses should become involved in making decisions such as the one described in the situation presented previously?*
- *With which qualities of each nurse do you identify?*

In this example, we see nurses at both extremes. Tonya makes quick decisions. In all likelihood she fails to recognize the ethical nature of the problem, the bearing the outcome may have on the people involved, or the conflicting possible solutions. She has great pride in her ability to make decisions, and has confidence in the correctness of those decisions. Lydia, being more insightful and sensitive, recognizes intuitively that the problem presents no clear solution. She is troubled by the situation, but has no tools with which to deal with the predicament. Each of these nurses will benefit from a study of nursing ethics.

Ethics and Nursing

Nursing is a profession that deals with the most personal and private aspects of people's lives. From the beginning of time, nurses—whether called healers, caretakers, nurturers, or nurses—have cared for those in need in a very personal and intimate way. Nurses are attentive to patients' needs over long periods of time. They may have made home visits and may know patients' families. They may care for patients at their bedside for hours and days on end. It is through the intimacy and trust inherent in the nurse-patient relationship that nurses become critical participants in the process of ethical decision making.

As participants in a dynamic profession, we are faced with ethical choices that affect the profession itself. For example, as the needs and demands of society change, boundaries of the domain of nursing contract and expand. This forces us to make decisions about such issues as the delegation of traditional nursing functions to non-nurse caregivers and the expanding boundaries of nursing. Because nursing is self-regulated, we are called on to review and discipline peers. This holds many ethical implications as we attempt to balance this responsibility with our desire to advance the profession, protect the public, and maintain professional cohesiveness.

Nurses may also take part in decision making on a broader scale. More than ever before, we are participating as members of policy-making bodies. Community, state, and national task forces, committees, and boards of advisors are among those health care decision-making groups in which nurses have become integral and respected members. It is imperative that nurses participating in decision making at this level be aware of the ethical implications of the decisions, particularly those dealing with the distribution of goods and services. These decisions are at the very heart of our society's beliefs about the value of the individual and, as such, compel those involved to cautiously deliberate every decision.

This chapter includes a discussion of some prevailing ethical theories. You may ask how you will use these theories in your practice. You will not choose one theory to use exclusively in your career. Instead, you will have a clear awareness of the many nuances and rules that govern moral and ethical decisions. You will better understand decision-making models at the many levels of the health care system, and you will be ready to make clear and consistent ethical choices of your own. You will understand the language of ethics and be empowered as you engage in intra- and interprofessional dialogues.

PHILOSOPHY

Philosophy is the intense and critical examination of beliefs and assumptions. It is both natural and necessary to humanity. Philosophy gives coherence to the whole realm of thought and experience. It offers principles for deciding what actions and qualities are most worthwhile. Philosophy may also show inconsistency in meaning and context (Kneller, 1971). As you were reading Chapter 1, you probably noticed that throughout history there

Think About It

Socratic Questioning

Socrates used questioning to help his students. His questions challenged the accuracy and completeness of their thoughts. Professors today may use the Socratic method to demonstrate new perspectives and to help students organize their thoughts. Professors may use any one of the following types of questions: conceptual clarification questions, questions that probe assumptions, questions that probe reasons and evidence, questions about viewpoints and perspectives, and questions about implications and consequences. Consider the following scenario.

James is a registered nurse who works evenings in the emergency department while completing his bachelor's degree. During a class discussion about professional responsibility, he says, "I would like to see the legislature pass a law to make it illegal to prescribe narcotics to drug addicts." The professor wants to make sure James fully understands the nature of the problem and the implications of such a law. To shed light on factors that might not have been considered, the professor might pose the following questions to James and then open discussion to the entire class:

- *"Are you saying that no controlled substance should ever be prescribed to a person who has an addiction?"*

- *"What evidence do you use to classify a person as a drug addict?"*

- *"Can you imagine a situation in which your judgment about whether a person is a drug addict could be wrong?"*

- *"Do you agree that it is possible for a person who has a drug addiction to also have severe pain?"*

- *"Which classes of people deserve pain relief?"*

- *"Can you think of a situation in which it might be okay to prescribe controlled substances to a drug addict?"*

- *"What would be the long-term social consequences if people who are drug addicts could never receive controlled substances through legitimate sources?"*

- *"Who would benefit from such a law? Who would be harmed?"*

have been many philosophical schools of thought. Because of the nature of philosophy, it is impossible to verify philosophic beliefs or theories; nevertheless, the study of philosophy helps to give order and coherence to beliefs and assumptions. It gives shape to what would otherwise be a random chaos of thoughts, beliefs, assumptions, values, and superstitions.

Philosophers examine questions that deal with the most important aspects of life. Typical questions include the following: What is the meaning of life? Is there a God? What is reality? What is truth? What is the essence of knowledge? How can something be known? How can one describe the relationships among persons, or between humans and the Divine? What is happiness? What is the ideal or virtuous human character? How can one understand human beliefs, values, and morals? Questions such as these have been asked by the most widely studied philosophers. Buddha asked, "How can one find the path that leads to the end of suffering?" Confucius asked, "What is the remedy for social disorder?" Socrates asked, "How should one live?" Through the centuries, philosophy has concerned itself with topics that define the essence of human life. Martin Buber said, "With soaring power [man] reaches out beyond what is given him, flies beyond the horizon and the familiar stars, and grasps a totality" (1965, p. 61). Ayn Rand, author and social philosopher, eloquently expressed her thoughts when she wrote the following:

> A philosophic system is an integrated view of existence. As a human being, you have no choice about the fact that you need a philosophy. Your only choice is whether you define your philosophy by a conscious, rational, disciplined process of thought and scrupulously logical deliberation—or let your subconscious accumulate a junk heap of unwarranted conclusions, false generalizations, . . . undefined wishes, doubts and fears, thrown together by chance, but integrated by your subconscious into a kind of mongrel philosophy and fused into a single weight: self-doubt, like a ball and chain in the place where your mind's wings should have grown. (1982, p. 5)

Philosophy is essentially divided into two branches: the philosophy of knowledge and the philosophy of practice. The philosophy of knowledge focuses on critical examination of assumptions about matters of fact and argument. Included in this branch are epistemology (the study of knowledge), metaphysics or ontology (the study of ultimate reality), philosophy of science, philosophy of the mind, and philosophical logic. Philosophy of practice, on the other hand, focuses on the critical examination of assumptions about norms or values and includes ethics, social and political philosophy, and the philosophy of the law (Raphael, 1994). While epistemology, ontology, and logic provide an important foundation for nursing research, in this text we focus on the philosophy of practice, particularly moral philosophy, because it provides the groundwork for discussion of many of the troubling moral issues facing nurses.

Moral theory provides a framework for cohesive and consistent ethical reasoning and decision making. There are many ethical theories—some more sound than others—and some consisting of combinations of other theories. The best moral theories are part of larger integrated philosophies. Most of them clearly reflect earlier ideas proposed by historical figures such as Plato or Aristotle. This chapter is devoted to an examination of the two moral theories that have had the greatest influence on contemporary bioethics and nursing: utilitarianism and deontology. We also include a description of virtue or character ethics. Theories related specifically to resource allocation, such as libertarianism, are described in Chapter 15. Nurses who are interested in a more detailed examination of specific theories should read works by the original theorists as well as analyses by contemporary writers.

MORALS AND ETHICS

Moral philosophy is the philosophical discussion of what is considered good or bad, right or wrong, in terms of moral issues. Moral issues are those that are essential, basic, or important. They deal with important social values or norms, such as respect for life, freedom, and love; issues that provoke the conscience or such feelings as guilt, shame, self-esteem, courage, or hope; issues to which we respond with words such as *ought, should, right, wrong, good,* and *bad;* and issues that are uncommonly complicated, frustrating, non-resolvable, or difficult in some indefinable way (Jameton, 1984). Morality refers to traditions or beliefs about right and wrong conduct. Morality is a social and cultural institution with a history and code of learnable rules. Morality exists before we are taught its rules—we learn about it in our culture as we grow up (Beauchamp, 2001).

Ethics is concerned with the study of social morality and philosophical reflection about society's norms and practices. Ethics furnishes us with the practical application of moral philosophy, asking the question, "What should I do in this situation?" Professional codes of ethics are tools that offer a formal process for applying moral philosophy. The study of ethics gives us a groundwork for making logical and consistent decisions. These decisions may be based upon morality or formal moral theory. Ethics offers structured guidelines, but it does not tell us what we ought to do in specific situations. We must become familiar with our professional codes of ethics so we are prepared to make well-informed ethical decisions in each case.

Philosophical Basis for Ethical Theory

Similar to the way in which each person's experiences and values contribute to the development of personal ethics, professions strive to develop discipline-specific rules of behavior for members (who are committed to a common ideal). **Professional codes of ethics**, which generally appear when occupations organize themselves into professions, govern professional behavior. Professions have a vested interest in the conduct of their members for a number of reasons, including protecting the people the profession serves, ensuring the competence of members, and safeguarding the integrity and trustworthiness of the discipline. Most ethics codes specify that members conduct themselves honestly, fairly, competently, and benignly, and they provide guidance for ethical conduct in morally ambiguous situations (Bullock & Sangeeta, 2003; Pipes, Holstein, & Aguirre, 2005). As illustrated throughout the following chapters, nursing codes of ethics provide guidance to nurses in their relationships with patients, colleagues, the profession, and society (Pipes et al., 2005; van der Arend, 2003). Specific codes of ethics for nurses, such as those developed by the American Nurses Association (ANA, Appendix A), the Canadian Nurses Association (CNA, Appendix B), and the International Council of Nurses (ICN, Appendix C), serve as guides for nurses in practice. Nursing codes of ethics derive from coherent philosophic foundations and established ethical theories.

ASK YOURSELF

What Are Your Beliefs?

- Do you believe that there are some actions that are absolutely wrong in all circumstances? Give examples.
- Do you believe that you have an innate knowledge of right and wrong?
- How did you learn right and wrong? What was the influence of your parents? Society? Other forces?
- What are your thoughts about how beliefs concerning right and wrong originate?
- To what degree do you believe that rules about right and wrong originate from a universal source? From within oneself?

Unlike mathematics or other empirical sciences, there are no apparent absolute rules governing ethics. Mathematicians can say for certain that two plus two always equals four, regardless of the time factors, circumstances, feelings, or beliefs of those involved in the calculations. Ethical rules are less clear and difficult or impossible to prove. For example, while some people believe that killing for any reason is always wrong, others argue that euthanasia can be beneficial either for the individual or the society, that abortion to save the life of the mother is permissible, or that killing during war is justified. There are reasonable arguments based upon opposing viewpoints that support any of these beliefs. How can rational people reach such different conclusions? The answer to this question may lie in the particular perspectives of the persons involved.

Ethical theories are derived from either of two basic schools of thought: naturalism or rationalism. An examination of these perspectives will help clarify the various theories.

Naturalism

Naturalism is a view of moral judgment that regards ethics as dependent upon human nature and psychology. Naturalism attributes differences in moral codes to social conditions and proposes that nearly all people have similar underlying psychological tendencies (Raphael, 1994). These similarities suggest that there is universality (or near-universality) in moral judgment. This viewpoint allows each group or person to make judgments based upon feelings about particular actions in particular situations. It further suggests that most people's judgments in similar circumstances will be very alike. Naturalism does not explain aberrant, selfish, or cruel choices that are made by apparently rational people. *[handwritten: unusual, atypical, different, abnormal]*

Naturalism holds that, collectively, all people have a tendency to make similar ethical decisions. Though there are many value differences among cultures, the variations are not as great as they may seem. Most people desire to be happy, to experience pleasure, and to avoid pain. There seems to be a natural tendency to sympathize with the wishes and feelings of others and, as a consequence, to approve of helping people in need. Raphael outlines similarities among cultures:

> All societies think that it is wrong to hurt members of their own group at least (or to kill them unless there are morally compelling reasons); that it is right to keep faith; that the needy should be helped; that people who deliberately flout the accepted rules should be punished. (1994, p. 16)

Sympathy is a motivating factor in moral decision making. Sympathy is the sharing, in imagination, of others' feelings. This entails imagining ourselves in the shoes of the other and consequently sharing their feelings.

Think About It

What Would You Do?

If theories about naturalism are true, most people would have similar reactions in certain situations. Think about what you would do in the following situations and ask yourself if most people would act in the same way as you:

- *A toddler wanders into a busy intersection with no parent in sight.*

- *A woman trips and falls into a fountain and lies face down without moving.*

- *A coworker inadvertently chooses an adult strength of Heparin (10,000 u/mL) to administer to a premature infant rather than Heparin (1.0 u/mL).*

Sympathy involves such feelings as pleasure, the tendency to warm toward one who has pleased another, pain, and the tendency to feel hostile toward one who has caused pain to another (Raphael, 1994). Sympathy, according to some, is a natural tendency and is the basis for moral reasoning.

Rationalism

The opposing school of thought is **rationalism**. Rationalists argue that feelings or perceptions, though they may seem similar in many people, may not actually be similar in all people. Rationalists believe, as did Socrates, that there are absolute truths that are not dependent upon human nature. They argue that ethical values have an independent origin in the universe or from God, and that they can be known to humans through the process of reasoning. Rationalists believe there are truths about the world that are necessary and universal, and that these truths are superior to the information that we receive from our senses (Raphael, 1994).

To rationalists, moral rules are necessarily true. Rationalists see the knowledge gained through the senses as only contingently true (Raphael, 1994). For example, the grass is perceived as green, but the actual color may be different—or may be seen as different by some. One who feels bad when hearing of the misfortune of another may not feel the same way about all other people. On the other hand, moral or ethical rules are always true because they originate from a higher source. For example, rationalists argue that it is always good to help those in need, regardless of the circumstances.

The differences in the two schools of thought revolve around the question of the origin of ethics. Is ethics a matter of feeling, or of reason? Are individuals free to make ethical choices based upon a predictable human nature, or is the foundation of ethics based upon universal truth? The comparison between naturalism and rationalism is seen clearly in the study of ethical theories. We challenge you to consider these two viewpoints when reading ethical theory.

THEORIES OF ETHICS

Moral philosophy is the branch of philosophy that examines beliefs and assumptions about certain human values. Ethics is the practical application of moral philosophy; that is, given the moral context of good or bad, right or wrong, "What should I do in this situation?" The philosopher reveals an integrated global vision in which elements, like pieces of a puzzle, have a logical fit. By developing theories of ethics, the philosopher hopes to explain values and behavior related to cultural and moral norms. Each theory is based upon the particular viewpoint of the individual philosopher, and maintains, within itself, philosophical consistency. The discussion related to naturalism and rationalism explains one basic difference among moral philosophers. We choose the ethical theories of utilitarianism and deontology for inclusion in this chapter because they are complete and integrated and are the major theories central to medical ethics, nursing ethics, and bioethics.

The following case implies the differences among various ethical theories. Remember, there are no clear answers in ethical dilemmas. The reader's basic viewpoint is reflected in responses to the questions. If your answers are inconsistent, you may need to identify and strengthen a cohesive ethical basis for practice.

Case Presentation

Conflicting Duties

Ms. Washington is director of a local hospice service. Unrelated to her work with hospice, she serves on a state-wide advisory board that makes recommendations about the allocation of Medicaid services. In response to a dramatic decrease in federal appropriations, the board must cut funding to specific programs. Ms. Washington and other board members are asked to choose between eliminating funding for adolescent well-child screening programs that serve tens of thousands of youths, or eliminating a single costly program that provides catastrophic assistance to only a few individuals. Because of her experience with hospice care, Ms. Washington recognizes the importance of programs to help with catastrophic illness; however, she is hesitant to advise eliminating a program that is proven to help large numbers of children.

Think About It

Resolving Conflicting Duties

- *To what degree does Ms. Washington have a primary duty to see that catastrophic programs benefiting her hospice patients continue to be funded?*

- *As an advisory board member, what is Ms. Washington's responsibility to the large number of adolescents who would be denied health care if the well-child program for adolescents were no longer funded?*

- *What ethical basis should Ms. Washington use for making her decision?*

- *How would you decide what to do in this situation?*

Utilitarianism

As you will see throughout this book, **utilitarianism** is a pivotal form of moral philosophy for health care delivery. Sometimes called **consequentialism**, utilitarianism is a type of teleological theory. *Telos* comes from the ancient Greek language and literally means *end:* Utilitarianism is the moral theory that holds that an action can be considered good or bad in relation to its end result. Utilitarianism is an important ethical philosophy that has its basis in naturalism. According to the utilitarian school of thought, the right action is that which has the greatest **utility** or usefulness. No action is, in itself, either good or bad. Utilitarians hold that the only factors that make actions good or bad are the outcomes, or end results, that are derived from them.

Jeremy Bentham (1748–1832), a leading political philosopher, is considered to be the father of modern utilitarianism. His theories laid the foundations of modern government and social science. According to Bentham's theory, actions are right when they increase happiness and diminish misery, and wrong when they have the opposite effect. Following is Bentham's definition of the "principle of utility":

> By utility is meant that property in any object, whereby it tends to produce benefit, advantage, pleasure, good, or happiness . . . or . . . to prevent the happening of mischief, pain, evil, or unhappiness to the party whose interest is considered: if that party be the community in general, then the happiness of the community: if a particular individual, then the happiness of that individual. (Bentham, 1948, p. 2)

Bentham attempted to create a science derived from the principle of utility. He proposed that we should measure the product of an act in terms of the value of a proposed pleasure. Six criteria used to measure the pleasure included intensity, duration, certainty, propinquity (nearness in place or time), fecundity (the chance of it being followed by sensations of the same kind), and purity (the chance of it not being followed by sensations of the opposite kind). Bentham proposed that each criterion be given a value, and that the sum of the values related to the pleasure be weighed against a similar sum of values related to the pain that might result from any given act. The person should act in accordance with a mathematical formula, resolving ethical decisions based upon the sum total of the value of a given act. Because Bentham's formula to measure utility is complex and cumbersome, it is not used today. Nevertheless, when choosing a course of action a person will tacitly consider some of Bentham's criteria such as the likely intensity, duration, and certainty of the anticipated outcome.

Though many critics describe Bentham as having a hedonistic tendency (his theory is often referred to as hedonistic utilitarianism), it is clear from his writings that his interest extended far beyond physical pleasure. He wrote that *pleasure* is synonymous with many other terms, such as *good, profit, advantage, benefit,* and so forth. In fact, his interest in the common good of the community refutes those who charge that his theory is hedonistic. He describes a type of justice in which action should have a tendency to augment the happiness of the community as a whole, rather than diminish it.

John Stuart Mill (1806–1873) was a leading nineteenth-century British moral philosopher. Like Bentham, Mill was a utilitarian. He described utilitarianism in terms of judging acts according to their end result. He wrote, "All action is for the sake of some end; and rules of action, it seems natural to suppose, must take their whole character and color from the end to which they are subservient" (Mill, 1910, p. 2). The phrase *the end justifies the means* relates to Mill's theory. According to Mill, the only right actions are those that produce the greatest happiness. His "greatest happiness principle" holds that the right action in conduct is not the agent's own happiness, but the happiness of all concerned. He further believed that sacrifice is good only when it increases the total sum of happiness. For Mill, the object of virtue is the multiplication of happiness. He cautioned, however, that we must carefully attempt to avoid violating the rights of some people in the process of maximizing the happiness of others.

Mill defined his concepts in ways that make the meaning of this theory clearer. He described happiness as a state of pleasure that is not restricted to physical pleasure alone. Consistent with Aristotle's ancient philosophy, Mill made a strong argument in favor of prioritizing pleasure, with intellectual pleasure having greater priority than physical pleasure. Further, Mill condemned those who chose sensual indulgences to the injury of health. He described the greatest sources of physical and mental suffering as "indigence, disease, and the unkindness, worthlessness, or premature loss, of objects of affection" (Mill, 1910, p. 14).

Although Mill disagreed with the notion that rules of ethics are edicts from God, he related utilitarianism to Judeo-Christian doctrine. He believed utilitarianism to be in the spirit of the Golden Rule, "do unto others as you would have them do unto you" (Mill, 1910). Thus, the Golden Rule depicts the ideal perfection of the utilitarian morality. Mill further wrote that the happiness of humankind is certainly within the interest of a benevolent God, and that people are given the opportunity to make ethical choices according to these precepts.

Although the works of Bentham and Mill are the most frequently quoted, there are many other utilitarian theories. There are two basic types of utilitarianism. **Act-utilitarianism** suggests that people choose actions that will, in any given circumstance, increase the overall good. **Rule-utilitarianism**, on the other hand, suggests that people choose rules that, when followed consistently, will maximize the overall good.

Case Presentation

Making Decisions Based Upon the Situation

Many years ago, as a junior nursing student, Mary was assigned to observe the labor and delivery department of a small rural hospital. As frequently occurs in small towns, the nurses and physicians were acquainted with many of the women—they knew their backgrounds, home situations, and so forth. During her second day on the unit, Mary attended the delivery of a set of premature twins. After delivering the tiny babies, the physician walked to a nearby room and placed them on a metal utility table. He turned and said to those in attendance, "Nobody is to touch them. This woman has nine children at home. She doesn't need any more babies."

Because these babies were very premature, it is unlikely they would have survived in the best of situations; nevertheless, the nurses struggled with the moral implications. This example raises many ethical questions, and illustrates a case of paternalism and utilitarianism taken to the extreme.

Think About It

Does the End Justify the Means?

- *Utilitarianism holds that an action is judged as good or bad in relation to the consequences or outcomes that are derived from it. If the physician were thinking in terms of utilitarianism, what could have been the arguments to support his actions?*
- *Assume that the twins were rescued. Name as many possible outcomes as you can imagine.*
- *Name four arguments in support of, and four arguments in opposition to, the physician's decision.*
- *Considering her position as a student in the hospital, what were Mary's options?*
- *What thoughts would have gone through your mind if you were in this situation?*

Act-utilitarianism

Act-utilitarianism allows for different, sometimes opposing, actions in different situations. For example, while act-utilitarians probably believe that it is best to tell the truth (or keep promises, or avoid killing, and so on), they recognize that there are times when the overall consequences will be better for everyone concerned if this guideline is not followed, even if the rights of some individuals are violated (Beauchamp & Childress, 2012; Smart, 1997). Act-utilitarians recognize that tenets should be used as rough guidelines rather than strict rules.

Rule-utilitarianism

Rule-utilitarianism, on the other hand, suggests that people should act according to rules that tend to maximize happiness and diminish unhappiness. Rule-utilitarianism requires that people in all circumstances tell the truth, keep promises, avoid killing, and so on, because the overall good is maximized by consistently following such rules. The rules are consistent and easy to learn. For example, there may be times when you wonder if deceiving a patient is acceptable. If an elderly patient who was injured in an automobile accident is critically injured and unstable, should you temporarily deceive him about his wife's death? A rule utilitarian would argue that you should not deceive the patient. Even though you are afraid that this patient's health might be threatened if you tell the truth, a widespread use of deception will eventually cause more harm than good. Thus, though rule-utilitarians recognize that in some instances good might result from a particular act that violates the rules, in the end the overall good is maximized by following strict rules in all situations.

Utilitarianism is widely used in the health care system. It is the basis for many policy-level decisions about the distribution of health care services and can be integral to medical emergency triage decisions. Policy makers attempt to wisely appropriate public funds. The debates about funding are often in the news and include topics on a variety of public programs, such as Medicare, Medicaid, managed care, family planning, pediatric services, mental health, and others. As these programs focus on delivering cost-effective health care to large numbers of people, they serve very specific narrow populations (denying resources to others) and provide or deny very specific services—all based upon utilitarian principles. In emergency situations such as war or natural disasters, utilitarianism may become the default method of making these types of decisions. Consider this e-mail message from a Dallas physician who served on a disaster assistance team set up at the New Orleans airport in the days immediately following Hurricane Katrina. He writes, "We did everything from delivering babies to simply providing morphine and a blanket to septic and critical patients, and allowing them to die" (Vankawala, 2005, p. 13). He continues,

> Our busiest day, we off-loaded just under 15,000 patients by air and ground. At that time, we had about 30 medical providers and 100 ancillary staff. All we could do was provide the barest amount of comfort care. We watched many, many people die. We practiced medical triage at its most basic—"black-tagging" the sickest people and culling them from the masses so that they could die in a separate area. (Vankawala, 2005, p. 8)

Nursing organizations and schools of nursing across the United States also provided emergency care and triage during the hurricane aftermath.

For example, graduate nursing students and faculty at the University of Texas at Austin helped set up temporary first aid stations and identified evacuees to be triaged for medical help, placing more than 3,000 evacuees in cots before the end of the first day (Patillo, 2005). These stories dramatically illustrate the practical use of utilitarianism during catastrophic emergencies. But utilitarianism can also serve as the basis for distribution of services in day-to-day situations. For example, whenever there is a shortfall of critical care beds, someone will likely use utilitarian principles to assign bed space.

Though utilitarianism is a widely accepted ethical theory, there are a few problems inherent in its use. Utilitarianism does not give sufficient thought to respect of persons. In fact, it is possible that harm can be done to minority groups or individuals in the name of the overall good. It gives little recognition to the principle of autonomy, particularly when we consider utilitarian decision making relative to distributive justice, the ethical principle that relates to fair, equitable, and appropriate distribution of goods and services. Critics argue that utilitarianism sacrifices the rights of individuals in favor of the overall good.

ASK YOURSELF

Is Utilitarianism Useful?

- What useful guidelines does utilitarianism provide in terms of distributing resources?
- To what degree is it permissible to sacrifice the rights of one to provide for the welfare of many?
- To what degree is it permissible to sacrifice the rights of many to provide for the welfare of one?

Even though there are problems inherent in utilitarianism, this ethical theory captures the imagination as an attractive moral philosophy. Its appeal lies in the simple precept of promoting happiness for as many people as possible. It is particularly useful as a method of deciding issues of distributive justice.

Deontology

Deontological theories of ethics are based upon the rationalist view that the rightness or wrongness of an act depends upon the nature of the act, rather than its consequences. The term **deontology** is taken from the Greek word for duty. Occasionally, deontology is called **formalism**; some writers refer to this type of ethical theory as **Kantianism**. Kantianism is based upon the writings of the German philosopher Immanuel Kant, who shaped many deontological formulations. For the purpose of this chapter, the terms *deontology* and *Kantian ethics* are used interchangeably.

Kant was born at Königsberg, Prussia, in 1724. After an uninspiring academic career, he surprised the world with his groundbreaking ethical theory. Late in his life, Kant published volumes of philosophical writings that shook the religious and political systems of his day, and continue to have strong influence on contemporary ethical philosophy. Kant contended that ethical rules are universal, and that humans can derive certain consistent principles to guide action. As Socrates suggested centuries earlier, Kant believed that awareness of moral rules is the product of pure reason, rather than experience, as the naturalists would maintain. Kant asserted that moral rules are absolute and apply to all people, for all times, in all situations. He believed that ethical rules could be known by rational humans. Knowledge of the right course of action in any given situation could be obtained by following a maxim that he called the **categorical imperative**. *Categorical* refers to moral rules that have no exceptions; *imperative* denotes a command that is derived from principle. Kant said there is only one categorical imperative:

> Act only according to that maxim by which you can at the same time will that it should become a universal law. (trans. 1959, p. 39)

In other words, if an action is morally right, it can reasonably be imagined to be a strict universal law. As an example, Kant related a moral problem in which a man needs to borrow money to feed his family. He knows that he will not be able to repay it, but sees that nothing will be loaned to him if he does not promise to repay it at a certain time. In order to satisfy himself that the act of making a false promise to repay the money is morally correct, the man asks himself the question, "Should every person always make promises that they know will not be fulfilled?" Through reasoning the man can see that this could not become a universal law, because no one would ever believe what has been promised. As a consequence, promise making would hold no meaning. Kant gave similar examples of situations related to suicide, squandering of talent, and helping others. Rather than compile a list of specific ethical rules, Kant proposed that each rational person should use the test of the categorical imperative to guide his or her actions.

Following the categorical imperative, Kant also described the **practical imperative**:

> Act so that you treat humanity, whether in your own person or that of another, always as an end and never as a means only. (trans. 1959, p. 47)

To treat another person as an end, according to Kant, is to make his or her ends your own, and to act toward his or her goals as you naturally do toward your own. For example, if a patient's goal is to get well, that should also be the nurse's goal. The nurse should not use this patient simply as a means to a paycheck (a means to an end). Raphael (1994) makes the point that Kant's practical imperative automatically shows that domination of one person over another is morally wrong. Domination makes no allowance for the dominated person's power of decision making. He also notes that acting toward another as you would toward yourself mandates that, whenever possible, you must help people who need help. The practical imperative requires that we must fulfill certain duties owed to others.

When the categorical imperative and the practical imperative are merged, there is a strong implication that each person is a member of a *realm of ends*—a politically organized society. Kant calls this "a systematic union of rational beings through common objective laws" (trans. 1959, p. 51). This requires that we should act as members of a community of equal and autonomous individuals, and that each member should treat all others as moral beings. Each person should have regard for the desires of others, and allow them freedom of decision. In Kantian theory, there is an inherent recognition that all people are equal and equally competent to make universally legislative decisions. Kantian ethics is an ethics of democracy because it requires "liberty, equality, and fraternity" within a politically organized society (Raphael, 1994, p. 57).

Deontology also implies that ethics are derived from fulfilling duties. One must act for the sake of duty or obligation. Kant believed that all *imperatives of duty* can be deduced from his categorical imperative (one should act as if one's actions could become universal law for all people) and must also comply with his practical imperative (treat all people as ends, none as means to an end). He also believed that an action done from duty has its moral worth based upon reverence for the law and for doing one's duty, rather than the results or outcomes of the act (Paton, 1961).

Most professional codes of ethics are based upon Kantian principles. Nurses' codes of ethics stress both the importance of fulfilling duties that are inherently owed to patients and the importance of preserving the dignity and autonomy of each individual patient. For example, section 1.2 of the ANA Code of Ethics for Nurses (Appendix A) notes that, "The nurse establishes relationships and delivers nursing services with respect for patient needs and values, and without prejudice." This statement presumes that the nurse has a duty to respect and care for the patient in terms of the patient's own needs and values. It demonstrates the principles of respect for person, beneficence, and autonomy, which are covered in detail in Chapter 3. These principles are so pervasive in the profession that they often go unnoticed. When you maintain confidentiality, when you advocate for a patient, when you keep your promises, when you tell the truth, and when you practice with expert skill, you are utilizing deontic principles.

Nevertheless there are some acknowledged problems with the practical application of Kantian or deontological ethics. Kantianism is exceptionless and rigid. It does not assist us in choosing among conflicting alternatives or principles and, in fact, may actually present a conflict between two equally compelling duties. In addition, it seems reasonable to speculate that the automatic disregard of the consequences of any given action can occasionally lead to disastrous results.

Like utilitarianism, deontology is an attractive ethical theory. It is, in fact, a most popular foundation for many contemporary beliefs. It provides clear guidelines for judging the rightness or wrongness of action.

Case Presentation

Weighing Rights and Duties in Questions of Justice

Sumiko is the home health nurse for Mrs. "B." Her patient is an 89-year-old widow who lives in the home that she and her husband shared until his death 5 years earlier. She suffers from severe rheumatoid arthritis and has a new colostomy. The colostomy was performed as a last resort for severe ulcerative colitis. Mrs. B. is unable to care for herself because of the advanced state of her arthritis. Her daughter, son-in-law, and two teenage grandchildren moved into her home to take care of her daily needs. After many months, the family feels that caring for the elderly woman has become an unbearable burden. They ask Sumiko to help arrange long-term care in a local nursing home. However, Mrs. B. wants to continue to live in her home.

Think About It

Whose Rights Are More Important?

- *Does Mrs. B. have the right to stay in her home, even if the entire family is made unhappy by her presence?*

- *According to Kantian ethics, what factors must the family consider in deciding?*

- *Kantian ethics is duty-oriented. Assuming that a Kantian basis for ethical decision making is used, to whom does Sumiko owe a duty?*

- *To what degree should the rights of the other family members bear on the decision that Sumiko makes?*

- *How do nursing codes of ethics offer Sumiko guidance as she responds to this situation?*

- *Apply the categorical imperative to Sumiko's decision.*

- *Whose decision is this to make? Why?*

- *What would you do if you were Sumiko? On what basis would you make your decision?*

- *How might cultural factors influence decisions in this situation?*

It recognizes the dignity and autonomy of individuals, and allows all people equal consideration. It serves as a basis for much of the contemporary ethical thinking that guides health care delivery.

Virtue Ethics

Virtue ethics, sometimes called character ethics, represents the idea that individuals' actions are based upon a certain degree of innate moral virtue. First noted in the writings of Plato, Aristotle, and early Christian thinkers, there has been a contemporary resurgence of interest in virtue ethics. Western moralism emerged with the idea of the cardinal virtues of wisdom, courage, temperance, justice, generosity, faith, hope, and charity (Kitwood, 1990). Modern and contemporary writers also include such virtues as honesty, compassion, caring, responsibility, integrity, discernment, trustworthiness, and prudence. Though nearly absent in nursing ethics texts in the past 20 years, virtue ethics is re-emerging as an important framework for examining moral behavior.

The concept of virtue ethics presents a challenge to deontological and utilitarian theories. Deontology and utilitarianism conceive of the demands of morality similarly; ethics provides guidelines that seek the morally correct solution. In contrast, virtue ethics posits that morality rests on the character of persons. There are no principles or rules to follow in virtue ethics. Rather, it is thought that the virtuous person will naturally choose the morally correct action. For example, the reason you should not lie is not because it is against the moral law, nor because it will not maximize well-being, but rather because you know that it is *dishonest* (Crisp & Slote, 1997). Beauchamp (2001) suggests that virtue should not be thought of as a moral requirement, because this confuses it with a principle or rule. Rather, we could say that a *moral* virtue is a character trait, such as truthfulness, kindness, or honesty, that is morally valued. A person with moral virtue has both consistent moral action and a morally appropriate desire.

Plato and Aristotle were the first Western philosophers to write about virtue ethics. Both believed that human well-being is the highest aim of morality and that virtues are necessary character traits for the good person. In fact, the term *ethics* was derived from Aristotle's word *ethika*, which refers to matters having to do with character. Aristotle (384–332 BCE) considered goodness of character to be produced by the practice of virtuous behavior, rather than virtuous acts being the end result of a good character. According to Aristotle, virtues are tendencies to act, feel, and judge that are developed from a natural capacity by proper training and exercise. He believed that practice creates a habit of acting in a virtuous way, and that virtue can be learned and improved. Virtue, according to Aristotle, is equal to excellence of character and depends on motivation, deliberation, clear judgment, self-control, and practice (Aristotle, trans. 2000). He considered virtue to be the fruit of intelligent pursuit—the achievement of wise and mature experience in the fully developed person. Aristotle believed that virtue could only be achieved by training and habituation—thus a virtuous character is created by repeatedly acting in a virtuous manner. Aristotle's traits of a virtuous character provided three criteria:

1. Virtuous acts must be chosen for their own sake.

2. Choice must proceed from a firm and unchangeable character.

3. Virtue is a disposition to choose the mean.

The *golden mean* of virtuous behavior, for Aristotle, meant practicing moderation: avoiding both excess and deficiency. Aristotle did not list a number of moral principles. For him, the basic moral question is not "what should one do" but rather "what should one be" (Aristotle, trans. 1953).

Phillipa Foot, one of the founders of contemporary virtue ethics, added another perspective to Aristotle's concept of a virtuous person. Foot proposed that virtue lies not only in engaging in virtuous acts, but also in will. She defined will as "that which is wished for as well as what is sought." According to Foot, a positive or moral will is sometimes the necessary ingredient in success. She wrote,

> Sometimes one man succeeds where another fails not because there is some specific difference in their previous conduct but rather because his heart lies in a different place; and the disposition of the heart is part of virtue. What this suggests is that a man's virtue may be judged by his innermost desires as well as by his intentions and this fits with our idea that a virtue such as generosity lies as much in someone's attitudes as in his actions. (1997, p. 166)

According to Foot, virtue is not like a skill or an art. It cannot merely be a practiced and perfected act: it must actually engage the will. In other words, an act, for example, although apparently kind or generous, cannot be considered to be virtuous if the intention is not good. Although Aristotle's idea of virtue is one of hope (everyone has the capacity to learn virtuous action), Foot makes the road to virtuous character less easily traveled.

Focal Virtues

In the discussion of virtue as related to biomedical ethics, Beauchamp and Childress (2008) define character as being made up of a set of stable traits that affect a person's judgment and action. Like Aristotle, these authors suggest that although people have different character traits, all have the capacity to learn or cultivate those that are important to morality. Beauchamp and Childress propose that there are four focal virtues that are more pivotal than others in characterizing a virtuous person: compassion, discernment, trustworthiness, and integrity.

Compassion. **Compassion** is the ability to imagine oneself in the situation of another. Beauchamp and Childress (2008) define the term *compassion* in the following manner: a trait combining an attitude of active regard for another's welfare with an awareness and emotional response of deep sympathy and discomfort at the other person's suffering. This virtue embodies the Golden Rule. Compassion is so important that many times the patient's need for a compassionate and caring presence outweighs the need for technical care. We must be careful, however, that compassion does not impede our ability to make objective decisions.

Discernment. The virtue of **discernment** is related to the classical concept of wisdom. Discernment rests on sensitive insight involving acute judgment and understanding, and it results in decisive action (Beauchamp & Childress, 2008). Discernment gives us insight into appropriate actions in given situations. It requires sensitivity and attention attuned to the demands of a particular context. For example, a discerning nurse will recognize when a patient needs comfort and reassurance rather than privacy. Discernment requires that we continually strive to recognize and understand important nuances in human behavior.

Trustworthiness. **Trustworthiness** is another focal virtue for nurses. Trust is a confident belief in the moral character of another person. Trust entails a confidence that another will act with the right motives consistent with moral norms (Beauchamp & Childress, 2008). Trustworthiness is measured by others' recognition of the nurse's consistency and predictability in following moral norms. In practical terms, trustworthiness is accounted for in the reputation we have among coworkers. This virtue is important for us in our relationships with patients, physicians, and other nurses.

Integrity. **Integrity** is perhaps the cardinal virtue. **Moral integrity**, according to Beauchamp and Childress (2008), means soundness, reliability, wholeness, and an integration of moral character. It also refers to our continuing to follow moral norms over time. It is "the character trait of a coherent integration of reasonably stable, justifiable moral values, and active faithfulness to those values in judgment and action." A person with integrity has a consistency of convictions, actions, and emotions and is trustworthy. Integrity is compromised when the nurse acts inconsistently or in a way that is not supported by professed moral beliefs. Deficiencies in moral integrity may include such vices as hypocrisy, insincerity, and bad faith.

Virtue Ethics in Nursing

How does the concept of virtue or character ethics fit with nursing as a principled profession? It is likely that principled behavior, while not the sole domain of a good moral character, is more likely to occur in the presence of one. Certainly Florence Nightingale thought virtue was an important trait of the good nurse. Nightingale learned Greek as a child. She was inspired by Plato and translated parts of *Phaedo, Crito,* and *Apology.* Nightingale was intrigued by Plato's description of elite people with rare gifts who command many kinds of knowledge. The characteristics, or virtues, of these people resonated with Nightingale and were reflected in her writings throughout her life (Dossey, 2000). She believed that one of the aims of philosophy was to cultivate in gifted people their potential intellectual and moral qualities.

The Nightingale Pledge, composed by Lystra Gretter in 1893 and traditionally recited by graduating nurses, implies virtue of character as nurses promise purity, faith, loyalty, devotion, trustworthiness, and temperance. It is reasonable to say that good character is the cornerstone of good nursing, and that the nurse with virtue will act according to principle. If Aristotle was correct in his belief that virtue can be practiced and learned, then we can learn, through practice, those acts that, by their doing, create a virtuous person.

Moral Particularism

Moral particularism utilizes the principles and rules of other moral theories. It is a form of moral theory that embraces the uniqueness of cases, the culturally significant ethical features, and ethical judgment in each particular case (O'Neill, 2001). The moral particularist enters a situation fully aware of the ethical principles and maxims of the profession and appreciates them as illuminators of moral problems (Fletcher, 1966). Particularism would recognize the principles of utilitarianism and deontology, for example, but would view them as generalizations, rather than rules.

Most moral theories are not sensitive to the particulars of each case such as the context, situations, relationships, and individuals. Moral particularists claim that this failure represents a fundamental flaw in these theories. Even in the face of generally accepted moral theory, health professionals' moral decisions are shaped by the practical circumstances of their work (Anspach, 1987). This may be especially true for nurses.

Little (2001) admits that theory is essential to the moral life. Generalizations are useful for teaching and justifying, for understanding the "why." Moral particularism recognizes the need for rules that allow for exceptions in terms of what Aristotle might have meant when he called for "for the most part" generalizations. Little calls these *defeasible* generalizations—ones that are useful, yet capable of being annulled or invalidated in certain situations. Exceptions to these generalizations occur only in situations that deviate from the norm. Following Aristotle's lead, the moral particularist can make explicit what types of actions have a moral nature as well as what sort of conceptual priority, centrality, or evaluative privilege is relevant in particular situations. Because every situation contains unique elements, most of the moral generalizations we make in everyday life turn out to be irreducibly porous, "shot through" with inevitable exceptions. Nevertheless, these generalizations are explanatory and insightful in that they situate particular cases within a framework (Little, 2001).

O'Neill (2001) suggests that there are bona fide practical ethical principles that do not require uniform action; rather, they are indeterminate—constraining but not regimenting action. They are more likely to recommend *types* of action rather than offer detailed instructions for living. The extent of uniformity or differentiation to be stipulated in particular aspects of life is a matter for practical reasoning and judgment—what Aristotle would call *deliberation*. Sensitivity to particulars may originate in perception, intuition, or practical judgment. Because of its sensitivity to the uniqueness of each situation, moral particularism cannot be prescriptive. It must rely on certain

---

ASK YOURSELF

Are You a Moral Particularist?

Moral particularism is seldom discussed, but often used. You will see it practiced every day. In the next chapter you will learn more about ethical principles. One of the principles is autonomy, the principle that demands that we respect people's right to freely make decisions about themselves. Another principle is beneficence, which requires us to "do good." In some situations autonomy and beneficence conflict. A moral particularist will suggest that the "particulars" should determine to what degree we follow these principles. Think about the principles of autonomy and beneficence in the following situations. If you cannot uphold both principles, you might be a moral particularist.

- An 84-year-old patient with Alzheimer's disease was admitted to the hospital yesterday with left lower lobe pneumonia. He is on oxygen and IV antibiotics. He telephones the taxi company for a ride home.

- A 68-year-old hospitalized patient says, "I have taken a Lysol Disinfectant douche every day since I was a new bride. I want to make sure I can get them here every day."

- A 20-year-old woman who is 22 weeks pregnant is admitted to the emergency room following an auto accident. Her liver and spleen are ruptured and she is hemorrhaging. Her blood pressure is 70/30. The fetus is alive, but not viable if delivered today. The woman whispers, "I am a Jehovah's Witness. Do not give me any blood products."

relevant principles, such as those of utilitarianism and deontology, for the starting point of judgment. Always difficult and often not wholly successful, practical judgment is a matter of finding some act that adequately meets many requirements (O'Neill, 2001).

Nurses are involved in patient situations for which caring functions cannot be effectively performed without knowledge of particular individual patients (Donchin, 2001). Nurses' relationships with patients include closeness, touch, and proximity. Criticisms of formal or "formula" ethics include distinctions of "distant" versus "close-up" ethics. Abstract ethical principles and rules are emphasized in distant ethics while close-up ethics attends to the primacy of human relationships and recognizes the importance of feelings, values, and individual and family conscience (Penticuff, 1991).

Nursing's views of what it means to do good for patients accumulate through recognition of the particulars in nurses' stories about caring for patients close-up as they experience illness, recovery, and death. Nurses attend to the concrete details of everyday experience. Nurses' perspectives on doing what is good for the patient originate from the unique viewpoints of the nurse and patient within arm's length of each other (Penticuff, 1997). This within-arm's-length type of relationship is necessary because human touch and close scrutiny of patients' responses are integral to nursing care. According to Donchin (2001), within this relationship, the nurse and patient share a common goal unique to the circumstances and choices of the patient, recognizing that the individual cannot be abstracted from an "entwinement in particulars."

SUMMARY

Ethical theory helps us understand the origin and process of ethical and moral thinking and behavior. Two important theories are particularly important to nursing ethics. The ethical theory of utilitarianism was developed in part by Jeremy Bentham, and later refined by John Stuart Mill. Utilitarianism suggests that ethical decisions should be made in regard to the outcome or end result. Accordingly, no action in itself is inherently right or wrong. This theory also provides for the greatest good for the greatest number. Utilitarianism is particularly useful in situations of distributive justice but tends to ignore the rights of the minority or the individual.

Deontology, or Kantian ethics, was initially developed by Immanuel Kant. This theory, through the use of the categorical imperative, assists one in making ethical decisions. The categorical imperative demands that the person ask the question, can this action be a law for all people in all circumstances? Additionally, the theory presents the practical imperative, which requires that we treat all individuals as if they were ends only, rather than means. Kantian ethics provides clear guidelines for making ethical decisions, but does not provide for making decisions when there are conflicting duties or obligations.

Virtue, or character, ethics, as described by Aristotle, describes each person as capable of practicing and learning virtue through repetition of virtuous acts. Thus, the virtuous person is one in whom virtue is habituated. Virtue ethics complements other ethical theories, and can be used to nurture or predict character in individuals. Ethical theories can help us understand ethical decision-making models, and assist in developing a cohesive and logical system for making individual decisions.

Particularism utilizes the principles and rules of other moral theories. It is a form of moral theory that embraces the uniqueness of cases, their culturally significant ethical features, and ethical judgment in each particular case. Because of its sensitivity to the uniqueness of each situation, moral particularism cannot be prescriptive. It must rely on certain relevant principles, such as those of utilitarianism and deontology, for the starting point of judgment.

CHAPTER HIGHLIGHTS

- Philosophy is the intense and critical examination of beliefs and assumptions.
- Moral philosophy is the philosophical discussion of what is considered to be good or bad, right or wrong.
- Ethics is a formal process for making logical and consistent decisions, based upon moral philosophy.
- As the morally central health care profession, nursing requires astuteness in moral and ethical issues.
- Ethical theories explain values and behavior related to cultural and moral norms.
- Utilitarianism holds that the right action is that which has the greatest utility or usefulness, and that no action is in itself either good or bad.
- Deontology is based upon the rationalist view that the rightness or wrongness of an act depends upon the nature of the act, rather than the consequences that occur as a result of it.
- Kantianism is a particular deontological theory developed by Immanuel Kant.
- The categorical imperative is the Kantian maxim requiring that no action can be judged as right that cannot reasonably become a law by which every person should always abide.

- The practical imperative is the Kantian maxim requiring that one always treat others as ends and never as a means.
- Virtue ethics, usually attributed to Aristotle, represents the idea that individuals' actions are based upon innate moral virtue.
- Moral particularism takes into account the unique aspects of each case and utilizes appropriate generalizable moral principles.

DISCUSSION QUESTIONS AND ACTIVITIES

1. Go to the Kennedy Institute of Ethics website at bioethics.georgetown .edu. Do a literature search for recent articles on ethical theory. Report your findings to the class.
2. Describe the differences in beliefs about the origin of ethical rules.
3. Describe a hypothetical situation in which an ethical dilemma exists, and discuss solutions to the dilemma in terms of act-utilitarianism and rule-utilitarianism.
4. Identify specific health care funding policies, and discuss them in terms of utilitarian theory.
5. Identify different ethical codes, including professional codes, that are based upon Kantian or deontological ethics.
6. Describe a real or hypothetical situation in which there is an ethical dilemma. Use the rule of the categorical imperative to solve the dilemma.
7. List and describe the virtues that you feel are important for nurses.
8. Consider the following situation: Two nursing students are discovered to have cheated on several assignments. After being questioned by the instructor, both students deny having cheated, even though the evidence is irrefutable. Discuss these students in terms of virtue ethics and Kantian ethics. Do these students have integrity? Do these students have the character to become good nurses? How would you apply the categorical imperative?

REFERENCES

Anspach, R. R. (1987). Prognostic conflict in life-and-death decisions: The organization as an ecology of knowledge. *Journal of Health a Human Behavior, 28,* 215–231.

Aristotle. (Trans. 1953). *Ethics.* (J. A. K. Thompson, Trans.). Londc Penguin.

Aristotle. (Trans. 2000). *Nicomachean ethics* (R. Crisp, Ed. & Trans.). New York: Cambridge University Press.

Beauchamp, T. L. (2001). *Philosophical ethics* (3rd ed.). Boston: McGraw-Hill.

Beauchamp, T. L., & Childress, J. (2012). *Principles of biomedical ethics* (6th ed.). New York: Oxford University Press.

Bentham, J. (1948). *An introduction to the principles of moral legislation.* New York: Hafner Press.

Buber, M. (1965). *The knowledge of man: A philosophy of the interhuman.* New York: Harper & Row.

Bullock, M., & Sangeeta, P. (2003). Ethics for all: Differences across scientific society codes. *Science and Engineering Ethics, 9*(2), 159–170.

Crisp, R., & Slote, M. (Eds.). (1997). *Oxford readings in philosophy: Virtue ethics.* New York: Oxford University Press.

Donchin, A. (2001). Understanding autonomy relationally: Toward a reconfiguration of bioethical principles. *Journal of Medicine and Philosophy, 26*(4), 365–386.

Dossey, B. M. (2000). *Florence Nightingale: Mystic, visionary, healer.* Springhouse, PA: Springhouse Corporation.

Fletcher, J. (1966). *Situation ethics: The new morality.* Philadelphia: Westminster Press.

Foot, P. (1997). Virtues and vices. In R. Crisp & M. Slote (Eds.), *Virtue ethics* (pp. 163–177). New York: Oxford University Press. (Reprinted from P. Foot, *Virtues and vices*, Berkley, CA: University of California Press.)

Hesse, H. (1971). *Siddhartha.* New York: Bantam.

Jameton, A. (1984). *Nursing practice: The ethical issues.* Englewood Cliffs, NJ: Prentice-Hall.

Kant, I. (Trans. 1959). *Foundations of the metaphysics of morals* (L. W. Beck, Trans.). Indianapolis, IN: Bobbs-Merrill.

Kitwood, T. (1990). *Concern for others: A new psychology of conscience and morality.* London: Routledge.

Kneller, G. F. (1971). *Introduction to the philosophy of education* (2nd ed.). New York: John Wiley & Sons.

Little, M. O. (2001). On knowing the "why": Particularism and moral theory. *The Hastings Center Report, 31*(4), 32–40.

Mill, J. S. (1910). *Utilitarianism.* London: Dent & Sons.

O'Neill, O. (2001). Practical principles and practical judgment. *The Hastings Center Report, 31*(4), 15–24.

Patillo, M. (2005). UT School of Nursing response to Hurricane Katrina. University of Texas at Austin. Retrieved March 14, 2006, from http://www.utexas.edu/katrina/nursing.html

Paton, H. J. (Ed. & Trans.). (1961). *The moral law.* London: Hutchinson.

Penticuff, J. H. (1991). Conceptual issues in nursing ethics research. *Journal of Medicine and Philosophy, 16,* 235–258.

Penticuff, J. H. (1997). Nursing Perspectives in Bioethics. In K. Hoshino (Ed.), *Japanese and Western bioethics* (pp. 49–60). Norwell, MA: Kluwer.

Pipes, R. B., Holstein, J. E., & Aguirre, M. G. (2005). Examining the personal-professional distinction: Ethics codes and the difficulty of drawing a boundary. *American Psychologist, 60*(4), 325–334.

Rand, A. (1982). *Philosophy: Who needs it?* New York: Bobbs-Merrill.

Raphael, D. D. (1994). *Moral philosophy* (2nd ed.). New York: Oxford University Press.

Smart, J. J. C. (1997). Utilitarianism. In C. Sommers & F. Sommers (Eds.), *Vice and virtue in everyday life: Introductory readings in ethics* (4th ed., pp. 110–123). Fort Worth, TX: Harcourt Brace College. (Reprinted from *Utilitarianism: For and against,* by J. J. C. Smart & B. Williams (Eds.), 1973, New York: Cambridge University Press.)

Van der Arend, A. (2003). Content and use of codes of ethics in nursing. *Nursing Ethics, 10* (1), 97–98.

Vankawala, H. (2005). A doctor's message from Katrina's front lines. *NPR.org.* Retrieved March 14, 2006, from http://www.npr.org/templates/story/story.php?storyId=4836926

Chapter

3

ETHICAL PRINCIPLES

The quality of mercy is not strain'd
It droppeth as the gentle rain from heaven
Upon the place beneath. It is twice blest:
It blesseth him that gives, and him that takes.
(William Shakespeare, *The Merchant of Venice***)**

OBJECTIVES

After completing this chapter, the reader should be able to:

1. Discuss the principle of respect for autonomy in terms of patients' rights, informed consent, advocacy, and noncompliance.

2. Discuss the principle of beneficence as it relates to nursing practice.

3. Define the principle of nonmaleficence, and weigh actions in terms of harm and benefit.

4. Relate the principle of veracity to nursing practice.

5. Examine the principle of confidentiality in nursing practice, recognizing legal implications and reasonable limits to confidentiality.

6. Discuss the principle of justice as it relates to the delivery of health care goods and services.

7. Relate the principle of fidelity to nursing's promise to society.

8. Discuss situations in which there is a conflict between two or more ethical principles.

INTRODUCTION

Ethical issues are commonly examined in terms of a number of **ethical principles** Ethical principles are basic and obvious moral truths that guide deliberation and action. Major ethical theories utilize many of the same principles, though either the emphasis or meaning may be somewhat different in each. For example, respect for autonomy is a dominant principle in deontological theory but is less important in utilitarian theory. It is vital for nurses to understand ethical principles and be adept at applying them in a meaningful and consistent manner. (See Figure 3–1.) It is the authors' contention that consistent attention to principle is an important basis for ethical practice in nursing. This chapter examines the following ethical principles: respect for autonomy, beneficence, nonmaleficence, veracity, confidentiality, justice, and fidelity.

Respect for Persons

All of the principles discussed in this chapter presuppose that nurses have respect for the value and uniqueness of persons. Occasionally viewed as an ethical principle in its own right, **respect for persons** implies that 1 considers others to be worthy of high regard. Certainly, genuine regard and respect for others is the moving force behind all caring professions. Codes of nursing ethics explicitly state that respect for persons is a cornerstone of professional ethics. Discussion of the ethical principles in this chapter is based upon the belief that nurses value the principle of respect for persons.

RESPECT FOR AUTONOMY

As you would expect, the ethical principle of **respect for autonomy** denotes the ethical obligation to honor the autonomy of other persons. The word **autonomy** literally means self-governing. *Autonomy* denotes having

Autonomy
Beneficence
Nonmaleficence
Veracity
Confidentiality
Justice
Fidelity

FIGURE 3–1   Principles of Ethics

the freedom to make choices about issues that affect one's life, free from lies, restraint, or coercion. Respect for autonomy is closely linked to the notion of respect for persons, and is an important principle in cultures where all individuals are considered unique and valuable members of society.

Implied in the concept of autonomy are four basic elements. First, the autonomous person is respected. It is logical that those choosing the nursing profession would inherently value and respect the unique humanness of others. This element is essential to assuring autonomy. Second, the autonomous person must be able to determine personal goals. These goals may be explicit and of a global nature, or may be less well defined. For example, the patient with an ankle injury may have a goal to return to athletic play within 2 weeks of the injury, or may simply wish to be pain free. In either case the patient develops personally chosen goals that are consistent with a particular lifestyle. Third, the autonomous person has the capacity to decide on a plan of action. The person must be able to understand the meaning of the choice to be made and also deliberate on the various options, while understanding the implications of possible outcomes. Imagine, for example, ordering from a restaurant menu written in a language you do not understand. You have the freedom and responsibility to make a choice, but cannot make a meaningful choice without an understanding of the various foods offered. When we believe that a patient is not able to comprehend the meaning of choices, goals, or outcomes, we say that the person is incompetent to make decisions, or lacks decision-making capacity. There are certain groups of patients that are generally thought of as unable to make informed choices. Children, fetuses, and those with mental impairments are among these groups. Fourth, the autonomous person has the freedom to act upon the choices. In situations where persons are capable of formulating goals, understanding various options, and making decisions, yet are not free to implement their plans, autonomy is either limited or absent. Autonomy may also be limited in situations where the means to accomplish autonomously devised plans do not exist. An example is seen in the case of the indigent person who has no health care insurance. This person may choose to have, for example, a pancreas transplant in lieu of insulin injections, but has no financial means to meet this goal. In order to assure autonomy, each of the four elements must be present to a reasonable degree.

A number of factors may threaten patient autonomy. The patient's role is a dependent one. The patient seeks health care assistance because of a real or perceived need and, as a result, can be perceived as dependent upon the health care provider. The role of the health care professional, on the other hand, is one of power. This power is based upon knowledge

ASK YOURSELF

Is the Patient Role a Dependent One?

- Describe a time when you or a family member experienced the role of hospitalized patient.
- How did you or your family member feel when interacting with members of the health care team, who were dressed, while you or your family member were in pajamas or a hospital gown or, worse yet, naked?
- Describe the degree to which you or your family member were able to maintain dignity and autonomy.

and authority and is inherent in the role. This complementary relationship, while a necessary one, can lead to violations of patient autonomy because the patient may not have the strength of will to exert his or her own autonomy.

Health care professionals are often insensitive to the ways in which the health care industry systematically dehumanizes and erodes the autonomy of consumers. Patients are forced to comply with rules that require them to be and act dependent. Immediately upon admission to a hospital, patients are disrobed, asked questions about personal and private matters, forced to relinquish money and belongings, and expected to remain in a bed, emphasizing the dependency of the patient role. We place patients in rooms with doors that are seldom closed and ask them to wear bed clothing. Workers who are strangers to patients freely enter and leave the patients' rooms, making privacy impossible. Regardless of patients' personal habits or knowledge of their own health care, they are forced to bathe at certain times, eat at certain times, and take medications at certain times, and are often prohibited from practicing self-care measures that may have been their habits for many years. Patients are expected to follow each plan that is made. Otherwise, they will be labeled difficult or *noncompliant.* For all the lip service given the importance of autonomy, health care professionals are often guilty of creating a climate of dependency for patients—of coercing otherwise autonomous, intelligent, and independent adults into essentially a very dependent role.

In cultures that do not regard all people as being of equal worth and in cultures that respect social structure above individual rights, autonomy is less important. Where slavery exists, where women are expected to be subservient to men, where minority races are not respected, or where children are exploited, the notion of autonomy is meaningless. Autonomy cannot thrive in a climate that does not allow for either the independent planning of personal goals or the privilege of examining and choosing options to meet goals.

Recognizing Violations of Patient Autonomy

Often, nurses and other health care workers fail to recognize subtle violations of patient autonomy. This especially occurs when nurses perceive choices to be self-evident. At least four factors are related to this failure. First, nurses may falsely assume that patients have the same values and goals as themselves. This state of mind compels some nurses to believe that the only reasonable course of action is the one that is consistent with their own values. This leads to faulty conclusions. For example, if an elderly person chooses to stay in her own home, even though to others she seems incapable of caring for herself, her choice might be viewed as unreasonable and might become grounds to believe the patient is incompetent to make decisions. In other words, "If you don't make the choices that seem correct to me, you must be incompetent to make decisions." In truth, the elderly person may recognize that life is drawing to a close and may want to remain in familiar surroundings, maintain dignity, remain independent, and prevent needless depletion of her life savings. The decision is based upon her thoughtful consideration of the consequences of staying home versus the consequences of living in a long-term care facility. There are some who would insist that she should be allowed to stay at home, even if she places herself at considerable danger, as long as she does not jeopardize the autonomy of others.

The second cause of failure to recognize subtle violations of patient autonomy lies in our failure to recognize that individuals' thought processes are different. Discounting a particular decision as incorrect may not take into consideration the fact that people process information in different ways. For example, there are those whose thought processes are very logical and methodical, and there are others who think in ways that are creative and free-flowing. It is particularly important to recognize these types of differences when several people are working together to come to a common decision. What is obvious to one will not be obvious to all—not necessarily because of a difference in values, knowledge base, or intellect, but because of different backgrounds and styles of thinking (Harrison & Bramson, 1982). This is an important consideration when collaborating with patients, families, and other professionals.

The third cause of failure to recognize subtle violations of patient autonomy lies in our assumptions about patients' knowledge bases. It is easy for us to forget that we have gained a specialized body of knowledge through nursing education and work experience. Knowledge about basic anatomy and physiology, disease process, the mechanism of action of drugs, and so forth is so ingrained in our minds that it is easy to presume everyone has at least some of the same type of knowledge. We often assume patients have more knowledge than is reasonable for them to have. Consequently, we may discount or criticize patients' decisions, even though flaws lie in the patients' level of knowledge, rather than the appropriateness of decisions. Recall that an understanding of the choices, outcomes, and implications is inherently necessary for autonomous decision making. The nurse must accurately assess the patient's level of understanding in order to assure autonomy.

Most people accept the concept of autonomy, but few are prepared to accept total autonomy for every person in every situation. The ethical principle of respect for autonomy does not require you to respect all autonomous actions no matter how irrational the decision or horrible the results might be. Although you value the principle of respect for autonomy, you must simultaneously uphold responsibilities to yourself and to other people who could be harmed by a patient's choices. This can be a difficult distinction to make. To the extent that it is unreasonable accept the autonomous decisions and actions of all people in all circumstances, we are called to respect the principle of autonomy, rather than each autonomous action (Gillon, 1985).

The fourth cause of our failure to recognize subtle violations of patient autonomy lies in the unfortunate fact that in some instances the "work" of nursing becomes the major focus. This produces a climate of industrious habit. As we go about our work—doing procedures, giving medications, writing care plans, and trying to keep up a frantic pace—attentiveness to patient autonomy is sometimes neglected. In today's climate of advanced technology, fiscal uncertainty, staffing reductions, and bottom-line management, we should guard against focusing on work rather than caring.

Case Presentation

Noncompliance Versus Autonomy

Cora is a 45-year-old woman who looks years older than her stated age. She has very limited monthly income and no health insurance. Cora smokes two and one-half packs of cigarettes per day. She has severe COPD with constant dyspnea and frequent exacerbations. The nurse who sees her at a local free clinic is interested in at least preventing further problems, and speaks to Cora often about the importance of quitting smoking. The situation becomes very frustrating for all involved when Cora returns repeatedly for increasingly severe problems, having failed to quit smoking. Cora, of course, becomes labeled as noncompliant. During a particularly severe exacerbation, the nurse says to Cora, "You know you are committing suicide by continuing to smoke." Cora's reply is, "You don't understand. I live alone. I have no money, no friends, no family, and will never be able to work. I know the damage I'm doing, but smoking is the only pleasure I have in life."

Think About It

Do Nurses Coerce Patients?

- *In attempting to persuade Cora to stop smoking, to what degree is the nurse violating Cora's right to autonomy?*

- *Does Cora have the right to choose to continue smoking?*

- *If rights and responsibilities are correlative, how should the clinic respond to Cora's continuing to smoke? Would you suggest that the clinic continue to serve Cora, even though she is not following the plan of care?*

- *To what degree is coercion employed in situations such as Cora's? Is coercion an appropriate strategy?*

- *What would you do if you were the nurse?*

Autonomy for patients is more frequently discussed in terms of larger issues, such as informed consent, paternalism, advocacy, compliance, and self-determination. Let us review this principle as related to these and other recurrent themes.

Informed Consent

Informed consent is a term used to describe the process by which competent patients give voluntary consent for medical or surgical treatments or biomedical research after receiving disclosure about potential risks and benefits. Informed consent is the practical application of the principle of respect for autonomy. It demonstrates legal protection of a patient's right to personal autonomy in regard to specific treatments and procedures. The concept of informed consent is one that has come to mean that patients are given the opportunity to autonomously choose a course of action in regard to plans for medical care. This is usually discussed in relation to surgery, complex medical procedures, and research.

Our contemporary practice of informed consent is a direct outcome of past research atrocities. Although research focusing on the human body, illness, and injury has its roots in the ancient world, it was not until after World War II that organizations and governments began to create policies to protect human subjects of medical research. World War II created a perfect storm in which ethical research violations seemed to occur on a large scale in many countries. Voluntary and non-voluntary medical experiments to improve medical practice included infecting participants with pathogens; inflicting mortal wounds; and exposing subjects to high-altitude, freezing conditions, radiation, and biological and chemical agents (Harris, 1999; United States Holocaust Memorial Museum, 2010; Weindling, 1996). Highly publicized accounts of atrocious human rights violations spurred the development of policies that now affect every aspect of health care delivery.

When Nazi physicians were charged with war crimes, there were no established guidelines for ethical conduct in research. Therefore, in the course of the trial, the judges developed a set of 10 ethics guidelines by which to compare the conduct of the Nazi physicians (Nuremberg Military Tribunal, October 1946–April 1949; Shuster, 1997; Weyers, 2007). The first and most prominent guideline established that research must be voluntary, as follows:

> The voluntary consent of the human subject is absolutely essential. This means that the person involved should have legal capacity to give consent; should be so situated as to be able to exercise free power of choice, without the intervention of any element of force, fraud, deceit, duress, over-reaching, or other ulterior form of constraint or coercion; and should have sufficient knowledge and comprehension of the elements of the subject matter involved as to enable him to make an understanding and enlightened decision. This latter element requires that before the acceptance of an affirmative decision by the experimental subject there should be made known to him the nature, duration, and purpose of the experiment; the method and means by which it is to be conducted; all inconveniences and hazards reasonably to be expected; and the effects upon his health or person which may possibly come from his participation in the experiment. (Nuremberg Military Tribunal, October 1946–April 1949, pp. 181–182)

Following the Nuremberg trials, international government and professional bodies began to institute policies and guidelines for informed consent that spilled over from research into medical and surgical care. These policies include many ethical and legal requirements. Nurses must understand the process and the legal requirements for each step. More specific details about informed consent are found in Chapters 11 and 12.

Paternalism

Paternalism is a gender-biased term that literally means acting in a *fatherly* manner. The traditional view of paternal actions includes such role behaviors as leadership, benevolent decision making, protection, and discipline. As commonly used in nursing, however, the term *paternalism* carries negative connotations, particularly related to implied dominant male versus submissive female roles. For example, before the age of informed consent, physicians advocated a "fatherly" role that allowed them to make decisions regarding the best form of treatment. An early leader in medical ethics, Dr. Thomas Percival, advocated this fatherly and authoritative role when he wrote, "Physicians should study, also, in their deportment, so to unite tenderness with steadiness, and condescension with authority, as to inspire the minds of their patients with gratitude, respect, and confidence (Percival, 1803, p. 27). Apparently not an advocate of informed consent, he also advocated withholding information from the patient when he wrote, "As misapprehension may magnify real evils or create imaginary ones, no discussion concerning the nature of the case should be entered into before patients. . . ." (p. 29). As viewed today, this gender-biased concept of paternalism has negative connotations.

The term *paternalism* generally evokes negative sentiments among nurses. This is due in part to recognition that in the past the autonomy of patients was frequently violated in the name of beneficence. Professionals sometimes make the dangerous assumptions that they are uniquely qualified to make health care decisions by virtue of their professional knowledge and, further, that professional knowledge is the only knowledge needed to make decisions for patients. This kind of thinking allows us to ignore multiple factors that might be unrelated to physical outcomes, yet affect the whole person. These factors include, among others, economic considerations, lifestyle, values, role, culture, and spiritual beliefs. In making decisions, all possible factors must be taken into consideration. This dictates that the patient must be autonomously engaged in the decision-making process.

It is interesting to compare discussions of the concept of paternalism in both the nursing and medical literature. Nursing literature generally describes paternalism in a negative way. Nurses often think of paternalism as behavior that precludes autonomy. Medical literature, as noted previously in the writings of Thomas Percival, discusses paternalism as a benevolent quality. The following passage that supports paternalism illustrates this point (note the pronoun "she"):

> In its strong version, the principle of paternalism justifies restricting someone's autonomy if by doing so we can benefit her. In such a case, our concern is not only with preventing the person from harming herself, but also with promoting her good in a positive way. The principle might be appealed to even in cases in which our actions go against the other's known wishes. (Munson, 1992, p. 43)

Advocacy

Advocacy is the act of speaking or pleading on another's behalf. Patient advocacy is central to nursing and is implicitly or explicitly included in nursing codes of ethics. It honors patients' autonomy. The act of advocacy in nursing is generally an informal, implicit function of the nurse-patient relationship. The goal of nursing advocacy is to ensure the welfare of the patient. Differing from paternalism, advocacy seeks goals that are determined by the patient or that the nurse believes the patient would have chosen. Virginia Henderson was one of the first nursing scholars to describe the advocacy role of nurses. She described advocacy as nurses helping patients do what they would ordinarily do for themselves when they lack the strength, will, or knowledge to care for themselves (Henderson, 1966).

Nursing advocacy occurs in many different types of situations. The nurse who communicates the patient's wishes in a staff meeting and the one who supports the patient in decision making are both advocates. Nurses can be advocates when in the presence of patients, when patients are not present to express their own wishes, or when patients have diminished decision-making capacity.

Advocacy is especially appropriate when a patient has diminished decision-making capacity or is unable to communicate. The nurse is often in the best position to know the patient's wishes. As advocates, we choose for the patient what we believe the patient would have chosen for his-or herself, if that were possible. For example, we assume that a person would choose to be protected from injury. Within that context, when we believe an elderly, agitated patient is incompetent, we might employ means to eliminate falls or wandering. This type of advocacy should not be evoked simply because the nurse senses a risk of harm. Ironically, Virginia Henderson, the well-known nursing leader who first defined nursing advocacy, recounts her experience as a hospitalized patient:

> I was in the room with another patient, and I couldn't stand being in bed any longer, and I would sit in a chair. This nurse came in and saw me sitting in the chair, and she said "Ms. Henderson if you keep doing that, we are going to have to tie you down"... I thought, You just try it.... (Goldsmith, 1992, p. 4)

Even though Ms. Henderson was 94 years old at the time of her hospitalization, she was certainly competent to make decisions for herself. Patients who are competent must be allowed to act autonomously—even if the choices can be predicted to cause them harm or render them incompetent. The exception can be made that even competent persons cannot be allowed to act in a way that would cause harm to others. Advocacy combines genuine concern for the patient with a well-founded belief that the patient is unable to make autonomous decisions.

ASK YOURSELF

Who Should Make Decisions?

- How do you feel when someone else makes a decision about you without your input?

- Since nurses and doctors know more about the science of health care, when, if ever, is it appropriate for them to make decisions about the health care regimen without participation of the patient?

Especially when patients are unable to communicate or have diminished decision-making capacity, there can be a thin line between advocacy and paternalism (Zomorodi & Foley, 2009). We suggest that the difference lies in the locus of power. Paternalism places power in the hands of the person who is making the decision for the patient. It implies that the decision maker knows what is best. With true advocacy, the patient retains the power. Advocacy expresses respect for the patient's autonomy because it aims to act according to the patient's own values. Zomorodi and Foley (2009) warn that nurses may not know the patient's wishes and may not have access to family members who can act as surrogates. In this situation, it is possible for nurses to act in what they think are the best interests of the patient, but they can unwittingly move toward medical paternalism. Therefore, nurses must constantly evaluate their actions to enhance the advocacy role and avoid paternalism.

Noncompliance

The term **noncompliance** is generally thought of as denoting an unwillingness of the patient to participate in health care activities. This commonly entails lack of participation in a regimen that has been planned by the health care professional but must be carried out by the patient. Examples of such activities include taking medication as scheduled, maintaining a therapeutic or weight-loss diet, exercising regularly, and quitting smoking. Use of the term *noncompliance* is just as likely to represent failure of the nurse as it represents failure of the patient. Discussions about noncompliance and care of the noncompliant patient center around two basic factors. First, the autonomous participation of the patient in the health care plan is essential to success. When patients are fully aware of the choices in health care therapies and the consequences of non-treatment, and are encouraged to make health care decisions, they are more likely to assume ownership of them and, as a result, to participate in their own care. Often nurses formulate plans of care that are consistent with a scientific base of knowledge but seem unreasonable to the patient. The nurse is remiss if the patient is not an autonomous participant in the formulation of the plan. Second, nurses and other health care professionals must assess patients' abilities to follow plans of care. Patients may be unable to comply with plans for a variety of reasons, including lack of resources, lack of knowledge, lack of support from family members, psychological factors, and cultural beliefs that are not consistent with proposed plans of care. An example of patients' inability to comply with a plan of care is seen every day in physicians' offices and emergency departments. Often patients are given prescriptions for medications that are prohibitively expensive. When they return with the same symptoms, not having taken the prescribed medication, they are invariably labeled as noncompliant. The problem is not one of compliance, but rather the health care professionals' negligence in assessing their patients' ability to follow a plan of care.

What are we to do when patients are well informed and apparently able to follow plans of care, yet do not? One hears stories of physicians who dismiss patients who do not comply with instructions—smoking cessation, for example. In a climate of limited resources, this is a question worthy of contemplation. Codes of ethics for nurses universally support respect for individuals and individual choice, and are not restricted by considerations of social or economic status (American Nurses Association [ANA], 2001; International Council of Nurses [ICN], 2006; Canadian Nurses Association [CNA], 2008). Further, the nurse must not be affected by patients' individual differences in backgrounds, customs, attitudes, and beliefs. Because health care practices are an integral part of patients' backgrounds, customs, and beliefs, refusal to participate in a plan of care, regardless of the outcome, is the prerogative of the patient and must not affect the care given by the nurse. Ultimately, choices about health care practices belong to patients. If allowed to choose, patients should not be labeled in a negative way when nurses do not agree with their choices. It is not appropriate for professionals who express the belief that all competent patients have the right to autonomous choice to make value judgments about the choices made, and subsequently label patients as noncompliant.

BENEFICENCE

The principle of **beneficence** means to do good. It requires nurses to act in ways that benefit patients. Beneficent acts are morally and legally demanded by the professional role (Beauchamp & Walters, 2007). The objective of beneficence provides nursing's context and justification. It lays the groundwork for the trust that society places in the nursing profession, and the trust that individuals place in particular nurses or health care agencies. Perhaps this principle seems straightforward, but it is actually very complex. As we think about beneficence, certain questions arise: How do we define beneficence—what is *good*? Should we determine what is good by subjective, or by objective, means? When people disagree about what is good, whose opinion counts? Is beneficence an absolute obligation and, if so, how far does our obligation extend? Does the trend toward unbridled patient autonomy outweigh obligations of beneficence? Veatch (2002) asks whether the goal is really to promote the total well-being of the patient or to promote only the *medical* well-being of the patient. We must keep these questions in mind as we practice.

The ethical principle of beneficence has three major components: do or promote good, prevent harm, and remove evil or harm. (See Figure 3–2.) Beneficence requires that we do or promote good (Beauchamp & Childress, 2008). Even with the recognition that *good* might be defined in a number of ways, it seems safe to assume that the intention of nurses in general is to do good. Questions arise when those involved in a situation cannot decide what is *good*. For example, consider the case of a patient who is in the process of a lingering, painful, terminal illness. There are those who believe that life is sacred and should be preserved at all costs. Others believe that a natural and peaceful death is preferable to an extended life of pain and dependence. The definition of *good* in any particular case will determine, at least in part, the action that is to be taken.

The principle of beneficence also requires us to prevent or remove harm (Beauchamp & Childress, 2008). In fact, some believe that doing no harm, and preventing or removing harm, is more imperative than doing good. All codes of nursing ethics require us to prevent or remove harm. For example, the International Council of Nurses (ICN) *Code of Ethics for Nurses* (2006) says, "The nurse takes appropriate action to safeguard individuals, families and communities when their care is endangered by a co-worker or any other person." Similarly, the Canadian Nurses Association (CNA) *Code of Ethics for Registered Nurses* (2008) says, "Nurses

Do or Promote Good
Prevent Harm
Remove Evil or Harm

FIGURE 3–2   Beneficence

question and intervene to address unsafe, non-compassionate, unethical or incompetent practice or conditions that interfere with their ability to provide safe, compassionate, competent and ethical care to those to whom they are providing care, and they support those who do the same" (p. 9).

Likewise, the American Nurses Association (ANA) *Code of Ethics for Nurses* (2001) is very clear about the nurse's responsibility in these situations: "As an advocate for the patient, the nurse must be alert to and take appropriate action regarding any instances of incompetent, unethical, illegal or impaired practice by any member of the health care team or the health care system or any action on the part of others that places the rights or best interests of the patient in jeopardy." In regard to removing harm, the ANA *Code of Ethics for Nurses* (2001) is very specific. Steps include the following: expressing concern to the person carrying out the questionable practice, reporting the practice to the appropriate authority within the institution, and if not corrected, reporting the problem to other appropriate authorities, such as practice committees of the pertinent professional organizations or licensing boards.

NONMALEFICENCE

The principle of nonmaleficence is related to beneficence. Whereas beneficence requires us to prevent or remove harm, nonmaleficence requires us to avoid actually causing harm. Included in this principle are deliberate harm, risk of harm, and harm that occurs during the performance of beneficial acts. Most ethicists today tend toward the Hippocratic tradition that says to first do no harm (the principle of nonmaleficence), placing this principle above all others. It is obvious that we must not commit acts that cause deliberate harm. This principle prohibits, for example, experimental research when it is fairly certain that participants will be harmed, and the performance of unnecessary procedures for economic gain or solely as a learning experience.

Nonmaleficence also means avoiding harm as a consequence of doing good. In such cases, the harm must be weighed against the expected benefit. For example, sticking a child with a needle for the purpose of causing pain is always bad—there is no benefit. Giving an immunization, on the other hand, while causing similar pain, results in the benefit of protecting the child from serious disease. The harm caused by the pain of the injection is easily outweighed by the benefit of the vaccine. In day-to-day practice, we encounter many situations in which the distinction is less clear, either because the harm caused may appear to be equal to the benefit gained, because the outcome of a particular therapy cannot be assured, or as a result of conflicting beliefs and values. For example, consider analgesia for patients with painful terminal illness. Narcotic analgesia may be the only type of medication that will relieve very severe pain. This medication, however, may result in dependence and can hasten death when given in amounts required to relieve pain. Cammon and Hackshaw (2000) offer another common example. Orders for patients to have nothing by mouth before procedures and tests are common practice, unquestioned by most nurses. The authors cite examples in which elderly patients were denied food for up to 6 days as tests and procedures were completed. The consequences of starvation in the elderly are unquestionable,

Case Presentation

Beneficence Versus Nonmaleficence

A middle-aged nurse recounts an incident that she believes relates to the principle of nonmaleficence. As a senior nursing student she was responsible for the care of a man who had a shotgun wound to his abdomen. Surgery had been performed, and the surgeon was unable to adequately repair the damage. The man was not expected to survive the day. He was, however, awake and strong, though somewhat confused. He had a fever of 107° Fahrenheit. He was receiving intravenous fluids and had continuous nasogastric suction. The man begged for cold water to drink. The physician ordered nothing by mouth in the belief that electrolytes would be lost through the nasogastric suction if water were introduced into the stomach. The student had been taught to follow the physician's orders. She repeatedly denied the man water to drink. She worked diligently—giving iced alcohol baths, taking vital signs, monitoring the intravenous fluids, and being industrious. He begged for water. She followed orders perfectly. After six terrible hours she turned to find the man quickly drinking the water from one of his ice bags. She left the room, stood in the hallway, and cried. She felt she had failed to do her job. As a result of the gunshot wound, the man died the next morning. Today her view of the situation is different.

Think About It

Weighing Harm Against Benefit

- *Was this patient harmed? Discuss your answer.*
- *What was the benefit of the nothing-by-mouth order?*
- *Discuss whether the harm of thirst or the benefit of maintaining nothing by mouth should take precedence.*
- *What other ethical principles are relevant?*
- *Why did the student experience such extreme distress?*

yet the practice of following NPO orders for long periods of time is seldom questioned. As nurses, we must be alert to situations such as these in which harm may outweigh benefit, taking into account our own values and those of patients.

The Case Presentation on the previous page illustrates the difficulty encountered when attempting to honor the principles of beneficence and nonmaleficence.

VERACITY

The term **veracity** relates to the practice of telling the truth. Truthfulness is widely accepted as a universal virtue. Most of us were taught as children to always tell the truth. Philosophers, in general, favor openness and honesty. The philosophers most frequently cited in nursing literature, Immanuel Kant and John Stuart Mill, agree in favor of truth telling. Nursing literature promotes honesty as a virtue and truth telling as an important function of nurses. However, there are some differences in perspective among health care professionals. Bioethicists disagree on the absolute necessity of truth telling in all instances.

We can support nurses' practice of telling the truth in many ways. Truth telling engenders respect, open communication, trust, and shared responsibility. It is promoted in all professional codes of nursing ethics.

A very general interpretation of the ideas of the philosopher Martin Buber (1965) suggests that true communication between people can take place only when there are no barriers between them. Lying or deception creates a barrier between people and prohibits both meaningful communication and the building of relationships. Recognizing that communication is the cornerstone of the nurse-patient relationship, an argument can be made that nurses must be truthful in order to communicate effectively with patients.

Violating the principle of veracity shows a lack of respect. Telling lies, or avoiding disclosure, implies that the nurse or other person involved assumes prominence over the patient or, at the very least, disrespects the patient's autonomy. Jameton (1984) suggests that manipulating information for the purpose of controlling others is like using coercion to control them. In essence, this keeps them from participating in decisions on an equal basis.

Jameton (1984) also suggests that deceiving others may constitute an unnecessary assumption of responsibility. When unfortunate consequences occur, the one responsible for the deception can also be assumed to be responsible for the consequences. On the other hand, when bad consequences occur after we have reported the truth, we can attribute responsibility to unfortunate circumstances.

Truth telling engenders trust. We can make the argument that truth telling is imperative to assure that patients continue to trust nurses and other health care professionals. It is by virtue of the trust in these relationships that patients are willing to suspend some measure of autonomy and seek help in meeting health care needs. Without this trust the nurse-patient relationship would be destroyed.

ASK YOURSELF

Is Truth Telling Always Beneficent?

- What situational variables influence how you feel about giving placebos?
- If your goal is to be beneficent and if the patient would benefit from a placebo, is deception justifiable if it will help the patient?
- What principles are in conflict when giving placebos?

Veracity has been described as desirable by the American Hospital Association (AHA) in the *Statement on a Patient's Bill of Rights* (1973, rev. 1992). According to this document, patients have the right to obtain complete, current information concerning diagnosis, treatment, and prognosis in terms they can be reasonably expected to understand. Though this position relates specifically to physicians' responsibility of disclosure, there are implications for nursing as well. As patient advocates, nurses are responsible for assuring that patients' rights are honored.

As with other principles, there is a dramatic discrepancy between nursing and medical literature in regard to veracity. Recognizing that nearly all health care is an interdisciplinary effort, and that disclosure of information to patients involves both nurses and physicians, it is important for us to understand the medical perspective.

Physicians often make the claim that patients do not want bad news, and that truthful information has the potential to harm them. In the name of beneficence, some physicians proceed with either nondisclosure or outright lies. Lipkin (1991) argues that physicians should sometimes deceive their patients or withhold information from them. It is his view that patients do not have sufficient information about how their bodies function to interpret medical information accurately, and sometimes they do not want to know the truth about their illness. Joseph Ellin (1991) discusses special considerations that have been posed by the medical profession in relation to truth telling. He suggests that it does not seem beneficent to adopt an ethic of absolute veracity in which it is an obligation to cause avoidable anguish to someone who is already ill, especially when hope and positive outlook may promote healing and help prolong life. He writes, "One could hope to avoid this dilemma by holding that the duty of veracity, though not absolute, is to be given very great weight, and may be overridden only in the gravest cases…" (p. 82). Ellin draws a distinction between lying and deception: lying is the purposeful telling of untruths, whereas deception is usually accomplished through nondisclosure. He argues that there is an absolute duty to avoid lying to patients; however, there is no duty not to deceive. Examples he gives include withholding information about a poor prognosis or giving placebo medication. Consider the following situation: A mother of four is admitted to the emergency department after an automobile accident in which two of her children are killed. Recognizing that she is in very serious condition, it would be appropriate, according to Ellin, to avoid telling her of the death of her children. If, however, she asks about their condition, she must be told the truth.

ASK YOURSELF

Is the Truth Sometimes Harmful?

- Do you think it is acceptable to deceive a patient in order to prevent unnecessary suffering?

- How would you feel if you were a patient and the health care team and your family conspired to deceive you—if, for example, you were ill and you had a bleak prognosis?

- Do you think it is acceptable to tell an Alzheimer's patient "little white lies" in order to decrease agitation?

Bok (1991) examines the practice of physicians deceiving patients in the name of beneficence. Although many would classify deceiving patients as paternalism, Bok writes that lying to patients has historically been seen as an excusable act. "Some would argue that doctors, and only doctors, should be granted the right to manipulate the truth in ways so undesirable for politicians, lawyers, and others" (p. 75). In fact, truth telling has never been a principle that was given consideration in physicians' literature. Veracity is absent from virtually all medical oaths, codes, and prayers. Even the Hippocratic Oath makes no mention of truthfulness. The 1847 version of the American Medical Association Code of Ethics endorses some forms of deception by stating that the physician has a sacred duty to avoid "all things which have a tendency to discourage the patient and to depress his spirits" (Bok, 1994, p. 1683).

Nursing and medicine view veracity from two different perspectives. It is clear that physicians have traditionally seen disclosure or nondisclosure to be a facet of care within their control that can have implications for patient welfare. Physicians often consider withholding bad news to be a beneficent act if they think disclosing the information will harm the patient. Nursing, on the other hand, upholds veracity as supporting individual rights, respect for persons, and the principle of respect for autonomy. To collaborate successfully, however, one must recognize the viewpoints of others. Chapter 4 discusses methods of making decisions about ethical problems when there are differences of perspective among those involved.

Confidentiality

The terms *confidentiality* and *privacy* are interrelated. **Privacy** refers to the right of an individual to control the personal information or secrets that are disclosed to others. Privacy is a fundamental right of individuals (O'Keefe, 2001). The ethical principle of **confidentiality** demands nondisclosure of private or secret information about another person with which one is entrusted. That is, confidentiality requires that one maintain the privacy of another. When the nurse learns private information about a patient, the nurse must keep that information confidential, sharing only that information necessary to provide patient care (ANA, 2001). Codes and oaths of nursing and medicine dating back many centuries support the principle of confidentiality. Nursing codes of ethics require that we maintain the confidentiality of patient information. According to the ICN *Code of Ethics for Nurses* (2006), "The nurse holds in confidence personal information and uses judgement in sharing this information." Similarly, the ANA *Code of Ethics for Nurses* (2001) and the CNA *Code of Ethics for Registered Nurses* (2008) direct nurses to maintain confidentiality. Confidentiality is the only facet of patient care mentioned in the Nightingale Pledge. This oath has been recited for decades by graduating nurses: "I will do all in my power to elevate the standard of my profession and will hold in confidence all personal matters committed to my keeping and all family affairs coming to my knowledge in the practice of my profession." Physicians do not escape the promise of confidentiality. The Hippocratic Oath is very clear: "Whatever, in connection with my professional practice, or not in connection with it, I see or hear, in the life of men, which ought not to be spoken of abroad, I will not divulge, as reckoning that all such should be kept secret." Although there are compelling arguments in favor of maintaining confidentiality, there is disagreement about the absolute requirement of confidentiality in all situations.

The ability to maintain privacy in one's life is an expression of autonomy. The capacity to choose what others know about us, particularly intimate personal details, is important because it enables us to maintain dignity and preserve a measure of control over our own lives. Markus and Lockwood discuss the importance of privacy:

> Privacy is thus a value closely related to, and perhaps ultimately grounded on, the value of personal autonomy. To take this value of privacy seriously is to subscribe to a number of familiar precepts. It means that we should be reluctant to pry, that we should respect personal confidences, and that when we enter into relationships with others that render us privy to sensitive or intimate personal information, we should be [careful] about passing this information on, even in the absence of any specific request not to do so. (1991, p. 349)

Thus, maintaining confidentiality of patients is an expression of respect for persons and, in many ways, is essential to the nurse-patient relationship. Consider the following Case Presentation.

There are at least two basic ethical arguments in favor of maintaining confidentiality. The first of these is the individual's right to control personal information and protect privacy. The second argument is one of utility.

This right to privacy flows from respect for persons and their autonomy. On one level, patients have the right to expect that personal and private information will not be shared unnecessarily among health care providers. Patient information is not an appropriate topic for elevator or dinner conversation. It is most likely that violations of this nature were what authors

Case Presentation

Making the Best Choice

Lora is a 17-year-old cheerleader. She comes to the local family planning clinic requesting birth control pills. Lora is a very attractive, neat, and pleasant patient. In the process of completing the initial physical examination, the nurse practitioner finds evidence of physical abuse, including a recent traumatic perforated eardrum. Lora hesitantly and tearfully admits that her biological father slapped her across her left ear prior to her coming to the clinic. She reports that she recently moved into his home after living most of her life with her mother and stepfather. She tearfully reports that her stepfather was sexually abusive to her and that she wishes to remain with her biological father. She says that she can tolerate being slapped around occasionally, and she does not want to get her biological father in trouble or be forced to move back to her stepfather's home. State law requires that the nurse report any suspicion of child abuse. Both codes of ethics and federal law require that the nurse maintain confidentiality.

Think About It

To Tell or Not to Tell

- *What are the principles involved?*
- *Does the nurse's obligation to report the incident of child abuse supersede the obligation to maintain confidentiality—particularly considering that the patient requested confidentiality? What if Lora were 14 years old?*
- *What are the options for the nurse?*
- *What are the possible outcomes of the different options?*
- *Does Lora's autonomy outweigh the nurse's responsibility to report the abusive situation?*

had in mind when writing early creeds and oaths that promise confidentiality. Nurses and other professionals often casually discuss private patient matters. On another level, nurses must keep in mind the number of people who have legitimate access to patient records. In a hospital situation, patient charts are accessible to many personnel. Nurses, physicians, dieticians, respiratory therapists, utilization review staff, financial officers, students, secretaries, physical therapists, and others have legitimate reason to view patient records. Information of a sensitive and private nature that the patient intends for the nurse alone can become widely known in a large health care facility. Care must be taken in choosing information to be recorded in patients' charts. Special care must be taken to avoid inadvertent breaches of confidentiality (Erlen, 1998), including those involved with electronic records (Muldoon, 1996). It is important for nurses to be aware of the many threats to patient confidentiality.

Confidentiality is particularly important when revelation of intimate and sensitive information has the potential to harm the patient. Harm can take various forms, such as embarrassment, ridicule, discrimination, deprivation of rights, physical or emotional harm, and loss of roles or relationships. Consider the plight of many AIDS victims whose diagnoses have become public knowledge. Confidentiality is also particularly important when dealing with vulnerable populations (Winston, 1988).

The second argument is one of utility. If patients suspect that health care providers reveal sensitive and personal information indiscriminately, they may be reluctant to seek care. Government policy makers recognize this problem. Because of the intimate and private nature of reproductive health issues, confidentiality of those seeking family planning services, for example, is mandated. Those caring for AIDS patients also recognize the need to maintain confidentiality. According to Winston (1988), many who work with AIDS patients find such arguments particularly compelling, believing that disclosure of patients' antibody status or a diagnosis of AIDS would have a "chilling effect," discouraging those in high-risk groups from seeking care. There are other diagnoses, such as mental illness, alcoholism, and drug addiction, that, if revealed, could lead to public scorn and subsequently discourage others from seeking care.

Limits of Confidentiality

Should the principle of confidentiality be honored in all instances? There are arguments that favor questioning the absolute obligation of confidentiality in certain situations. These arguments include theories related to the principles of harm and vulnerability (Winston, 1988). The harm principle can be applied when the nurse or other professional recognizes that maintaining confidentiality will result in preventable wrongful harm to innocent others. Mandatory premarital testing for syphilis, for example, is intended to prevent the spread of a serious communicable disease to innocent babies and spouses. In this instance, society chooses to override the privacy of the individual to protect the health of the innocent. Though directing nurses to maintain confidentiality, the ANA *Code of Ethics for Nurses* (2001) recognizes that duties of confidentiality are not absolute and may need to be modified to protect the patient, other innocent people, and, in cases of mandatory disclosure, for public safety.

In rare instances, case law supports the harm principle. In July of 1976, the California Supreme Court ruled that a psychologist, Dr. Lawrence Moore; his superior, Dr. Harvey Powelson; and the agency for which they worked were liable in the wrongful death of Tatiana Tarasoff. Prosenjit Poddar killed Tatiana Tarasoff in October of 1969. According to Tatiana's parents, 2 months earlier Poddar had confided his intention to kill Tatiana to his psychologist, Dr. Moore. Though Dr. Moore initially tried to have his patient involuntarily committed, Dr. Powelson intervened and allowed Poddar to return home. Neither Tatiana nor her parents were informed of the patient's threats. The court found that the defendants were responsible for the wrongful death of Tatiana because they knew in advance of the patient's intentions. The obligation to protect the innocent third party superseded the obligation to maintain confidentiality. According to the majority opinion in this case, the duty to warn arises from a special relation between the patient and the psychologist that imposes a duty to control the patient's conduct (Tobriner, 1991).

Foreseeability is an important consideration in situations in which confidentiality conflicts with the duty to warn. The nurse or other health care professional should be able to reasonably foresee harm or injury to an innocent other in order to violate the principle of confidentiality in favor of a duty to warn. This consideration precludes blanket disclosure of private information that might predict harm to others. The Tarasoff case exemplifies reasonable application of the harm principle. Subsequent court cases support the decision in the Tarasoff case. Courts have found that privacy is not absolute and is subordinate to the state's fundamental right to enact laws that promote public health.

The harm principle is strengthened when one considers the vulnerability of the innocent (Haggarty, 2000). The duty to protect others from harm is stronger when the third party is dependent on others or is in some way especially vulnerable. This duty is called the vulnerability principle. Vulnerability implies risk or susceptibility to harm when vulnerable individuals have a relative inability to protect themselves (Winston, 1988). For example, nurses have an absolute duty to report child abuse. Because children are dependent and vulnerable, they are at greater risk of harm. Coupling of the harm principle with the vulnerability principle produces a rather strong argument for abandoning the principle of confidentiality in certain instances.

Actions that are considered ethical are not always found to be legal. Though there is an ethical basis for subsuming the principle of confidentiality in special circumstances, and there is some legal precedent for doing so, there is legal risk to disclosing sensitive information. There is dynamic tension between the patient's right to confidentiality and the duty to warn innocent others. Nurses need to recognize that careful consideration of the ethical implications of actions will not always be supported in bureaucratic and legal systems.

U.S. federal legislation made the delicate balance between ethical principles more complex when confidentiality of patient information

Think About It

Can Nurses Violate Confidentiality?

- *How do you think confidentiality and the harm and vulnerability principles can be reconciled?*

- *How would you feel if a relative contracted HIV from a source who public health officials knew was infected, and had reason to believe would infect your relative, but neglected to warn?*

- *How would you feel if you were HIV infected and your health care provider violated your right to confidentiality?*

became a legal mandate. In 1996, Congress enacted Public Health Law 104–199, the Health Insurance Portability and Accountability Act (HIPAA). In response to public concerns related to a more mobile society, the need for health insurance, and the rising administrative costs of health care (Erlen, 2004), federal legislators set out to create and protect a universal databank of medical information using standardized coding systems (Deshefy-Longhi, Dixon, Olson, & Grey, 2004). Because of a growing number of criminal violations of electronic records, Congress inserted a provision that enjoined the U.S. Department of Health and Human Services to create medical privacy rules. Even though the original intent of HIPAA was never realized, the privacy guidelines went into effect in 2003 (Department of Health and Human Services [HIPAA], 2002, rev. 2003). Known widely as HIPAA, these privacy rules made confidentiality a legal requirement. Whereas other ethical principles do not carry the weight of law, *per se*, confidentiality stands alone. Today, a breach of confidentiality may result in criminal conviction or other penalties.

JUSTICE

Justice is the ethical principle that relates to fair, equitable, and appropriate treatment in light of what is due or owed to persons, recognizing that giving things to some will deny receipt to others who might otherwise have received those things. Within the context of health care ethics, the most relevant application of the principle focuses on distribution of goods and services. This application is called **distributive justice**. Unfortunately, there is a finite supply of goods and services, and it is impossible for all people to have everything they might want or need. One of the primary purposes of governing systems is to formulate and enforce policies that deal with fair and equitable distribution of scarce resources.

Decisions about distributive justice are made on a variety of levels. The government is responsible for deciding policy about broad public health access issues, such as children's immunization and Medicare for the elderly. Hospitals and other organizations formulate policy on an institutional level and deal with issues such as how decisions will be made concerning who will occupy intensive care beds and which types of patients will be accepted in emergency rooms. Nurses and other health care providers frequently make decisions of distributive justice on an individual basis. For example, having assessed the needs of patients, nurses decide how best to allocate their time (a scarce resource).

There are three basic areas of health care that are relevant to questions of distributive justice. First, what percentage of our resources is it reasonable to spend on health care? Second, recognizing that health care resources are limited, which aspects of health care should receive the most resources? Third, which patients should have access to the limited health care staff, equipment, and so forth (Jameton, 1984)?

In making decisions of distributive justice, one must ask the question, "Who is entitled to these goods or services?" Philosophers have suggested a number of different ways to choose among people. Figure 3–3 lists some of the ways that people have historically made these types of decisions.

There are those who believe that all should receive equally regardless of need. On the surface, nationalized health care systems would seem to meet this criterion, since all citizens are eligible for the same services. However, because some citizens would necessarily require more health care services than others, nationalized systems also meet the criterion of need. The German philosopher Friedrich Nietzsche had a different perspective. He believed that there are superior individuals, and that society's goal should be to enhance these "supermen." For Nietzsche, the choice of distribution was a clear one—to each according to his present or future social contribution (Durant, 1926). To each according to that person's rights indicates a libertarian viewpoint, and to each as he or she would wish to be treated is a reflection of the Golden Rule. The idea that each should receive according to effort is a common belief in our culture and indicates the traditional "work ethic." Entitlement programs in the United States generally award benefits based upon a combination of need and the greatest good that can be accomplished for the greatest number of people. Chapter 15 discusses the application of the principle of distributive justice in greater detail.

To each equally
To each according to need
To each according to merit
To each according to social contribution
To each according to the person's rights
To each according to individual effort
To each as you would be done by
To each according to the greatest good to the greatest number

FIGURE 3–3 **Distributive Justice**

Case Presentation

The Case of H1N1

The H1N1 influenza pandemic of 2009–2010 provides a dramatic example of distributive justice in health care. In April 2009 a new strain of an old virus emerged. Venters for Disease Control and Prevention (CDC) officials were required to distribute resources during this period of crisis and to make morally pertinent decisions about how to ration the scarce vaccine. Some have criticized the CDC's 2009–2010 response to H1N1. When discussing the ethics of distributive justice, it is important to examine all factors. We will review two previous outbreaks and try to understand their impact on the 2009 public health response.

In 1918, an estimated 500 million people worldwide were infected with the "swine flu" virus. The strain of the disease was exceptionally severe, with total deaths estimated to be 50 million (Taubenberger & Morens, 2006). The virulent, highly contagious virus produced three pandemic waves in rapid succession. Before the pandemic receded, one-third of the world's population had been infected.

In 1976, U.S. public health officials identified a handful of swine flu cases. With the 1918 pandemic hovering in the background and a consensus that a vaccine came too late for a 1956 Hong Kong flu pandemic, CDC officials called for rapid mass immunizations. The first shots were given on October 1, 1976. Within 2 months it became clear that those who were vaccinated had an 11 times greater chance of developing Guillain-Barré Syndrome. By the time the mass immunizations were suspended in December 1976, 40 million Americans had already received the vaccine. The predicted pandemic never materialized and those who were infected experienced low morbidity and almost no mortality. The vaccine appeared to have been more dangerous than the disease. The 1976 swine flu vaccine program was "overwhelmingly recalled as a true 'fiasco,' a 'disaster,' and a 'tragedy,'" (Neustadt & Fineberg, 2005).

When the first case of H1N1 emerged on April 15, 2009, the CDC quickly became involved. The CDC initially referred to the new influenza as "swine origin influenza" virus. Officials quickly moved forward with awareness that the potential death toll could mimic that of the 1918 pandemic, yet they recalled the harm that was caused by the poorly tested 1976 vaccine. Decision makers knew they must balance consideration of the potential harms of these two competing scenarios. Within 6 days, the CDC began simultaneously pursuing multiple high-yield methods of developing a vaccine. Since this was a new virus strain, no stored vaccine existed. On April 22, the CDC activated its Emergency Operations Center that focused on virus gene sequencing, surveillance, laboratory issues, communications, at-risk populations, antiviral medications, vaccines, and traveler's health issues (U.S. Centers for Disease Control and Prevention, 2010). At this point, the CDC recognized the potential for rapid spread of the disease, high morbidity and mortality, unusual morbidity age distribution, and multiple pandemic waves. Officials were also aware of the high morbidity and mortality associated with the 1976 rapid administration of the poorly tested swine flu vaccine. Beginning in October 2009, millions of doses of antiviral medications were distributed, the necessarily slow process of vaccine development was given high priority, and a media campaign focused on ways to minimize exposure. The first available vaccines were distributed to high-risk groups and health care workers beginning on October 5, 2009. Production and distribution seemed to be a slow process

(continued)

that continued through mid-2010 in anticipation of multiple waves of pandemic. No one had a crystal ball. If the new virus had been highly contagious and virulent (like the 1918 outbreak), the public health response would probably have been viewed as heroic. As it turned out, the 2009 H1N1 virus was not as virulent as anticipated and the dollar cost of the CDC campaign was tremendous. It is impossible to know how many lives were actually saved by the mass campaign. Balancing potential harm against potential benefit is like a juggling act done in the dark.

Think About It

Judge the CDC Response

- *What potential large-scale harms and benefits were inherent in this situation?*

- *What factors would you have taken into consideration if you were making the decision about the 2009 H1N1 public health response?*

- *Health care workers and people at known high risk were given first access to the 2009 H1N1 vaccine. How would you describe this distributive justice decision? Was it fair?*

- *Would you have done anything differently in order to protect large numbers of people?*

FIDELITY

The ethical principle of **fidelity** relates to the concept of faithfulness and the practice of keeping promises. Society has granted nurses the right to practice nursing through the processes of licensure and certification. "The authority for the practice of nursing is based on a social contract that acknowledges professional rights and responsibilities as well as mechanisms for public accountability" (ANA, 1995, p. 3). The process of licensure is one that ensures no other group can practice within the domain of nursing as defined by society and the profession. Thus, to accept licensure and become legitimate members of the profession mandates that nurses uphold the responsibilities inherent in the contract with society. Members are called to be faithful to the society that grants the right to practice—to keep the promise of upholding the profession's code of ethics, to practice within the established scope of practice and definition of nursing, to remain competent in practice, to abide by the policies of employing institutions, and to keep promises to individual patients. To *be* a nurse is to *make these promises.* In fulfilling this contract with society, nurses are responsible to faithfully and consistently adhere to these basic principles.

On another level, the principle of fidelity relates to loyalty within the nurse-patient relationship. It gives rise to an independent duty to keep promises or contracts (Veatch, 2002) and is a basic premise of the nurse-patient relationship. Problems sometimes arise when there is a conflict between promises that have been made and the potential consequences of those promises in cases in which carrying them out will cause harm in other ways. Though fidelity is the cornerstone of a trusting nurse-patient relationship, most ethicists think there are no absolute, exceptionless duties to keep promises—that, in every case, the harmful consequences of the promised action should be weighed against the benefits of keeping the promise.

SUMMARY

As we participate in meeting the health care needs of society, we must be constantly aware of the ethical implications inherent in many situations. Each nurse must develop a philosophically consistent framework from which to base contemplation, decision, and action. It is this framework that gives shape to our concept of various ethical principles. The principles discussed in this chapter presuppose nurses' innate respect for persons. Ethical principles include respect for autonomy, beneficence, nonmaleficence, veracity, confidentiality, justice, and fidelity.

CHAPTER HIGHLIGHTS

- Ethical principles are basic and obvious moral truths that guide deliberation and action.
- All ethical principles presuppose a basic respect for persons.
- Respect for autonomy denotes respecting another person's freedom to make choices about issues that affect his or her life.
- Various intrinsic and extrinsic factors threaten patient autonomy.
- The principle of beneficence maintains that one ought to do or promote good, prevent evil or harm, and remove evil or harm.
- The principle of nonmaleficence requires one to avoid causing harm, including deliberate harm, risk of harm, and harm that occurs during the performance of beneficial acts.
- The principle of veracity relates to the universal virtue of truth telling.
- Confidentiality is the ethical principle that requires nondisclosure of private or secret information with which one is entrusted.
- Justice is the ethical principle that relates to fair, equitable, and appropriate treatment in light of what is due or owed to persons,

recognizing that giving to some will deny receipt to others who might otherwise have received these things.

- Fidelity is the ethical principle that relates to faithfulness and promise keeping.

DISCUSSION QUESTIONS AND ACTIVITIES

1. Read the ANA *Code of Ethics for Nurses* (Appendix A) and discuss how the various statements relate to the principles discussed in this chapter.

2. Read the following hypothetical situation and answer the questions that follow:

    An elderly gentleman presents himself to the emergency department of a small community hospital. The patient has contractures and paralysis of his left hand; he apparently has complete expressive and at least partial receptive aphasia. Upon questioning, the man takes off his right shoe and points to his right great toe and grimaces, apparently indicating a problem in that area. The nurse is unable to gather any further information from him because of his difficulty in communicating. In attempting to help him, she asks if he has a neighbor or friend accompanying him. He shakes his head, indicating that he is alone. Curious, the nurse asks him how he came to the hospital. The patient smiles and proudly produces a driver's license from his shirt pocket. Subsequently, the nurse leaves the room and returns a few minutes later to find that the patient left the hospital, having received no care. The nurse suspects that because of his current physical condition the man is unsafe to drive a motor vehicle.

    - What are the ethical implications in this situation?
    - What ethical principles are involved?
    - Should the nurse pursue avenues to locate the patient and ensure that he is not endangering himself or others by driving? Would this be a breach of confidentiality? Autonomy?
    - How does the nurse express fidelity in this situation?
    - What is the beneficent action?

3. Describe situations you have witnessed in which decisions were made for patients in a paternalistic manner. Discuss your perception of the difference between paternalism and advocacy. Give examples.

4. Read the following hypothetical case and answer the questions that follow:

    Martha is a 75-year-old woman who has terminal cancer of the bladder. During the course of her therapy, she sustains third-degree radiation burns to her lower abdomen and pelvic area. Her wounds are extensive and deep, involving her abdominal wall, bladder, and vagina. The physician orders frequent medicinal douches and wound irrigations. These treatments are very painful, and the patient wants the treatments discontinued but is too timid to actually refuse them. The physician will not change the order.

- Discuss the situation in terms of beneficence and nonmaleficence.
- How does this patient express her autonomy?
- What is the nurse's responsibility in assisting the patient to maintain autonomy?
- How does the nurse deal with conflicting loyalties and principles?

5. Do you think health care professionals should disclose information to patients related, for example, to a poor prognosis, even though the information may cause distress? Discuss your views in depth.

6. Jameton (1984) says that for nurses to be less than competent is unethical. Discuss this statement in terms of fidelity.

7. Read the following hypothetical case and answer the questions that follow:

Nels Gruder is a 40 year-old disabled truck driver. He was injured several years ago in a trucking accident. He subsequently has had back surgery but continues to have severe pain. He has been seen by every local neurosurgeon and, for one reason or another, is not pleased with the care he has gotten. Because of the seriousness of his initial injuries, there is little doubt that Mr. Gruder has chronic back pain. Even though the local emergency room policy of not prescribing narcotic analgesics for chronic pain is clearly stated on signs in the waiting area, Mr. Gruder comes there frequently complaining of severe back pain. He reports a history of gastric ulcers and allergy to nonsteroidal anti-inflammatory drugs (NSAIDs). The nurse practitioner who sees Mr. Gruder is faced with a man who is in obvious pain. She wishes to help him relieve the pain he is experiencing. At the same time she realizes that narcotic analgesia is not appropriate for this type of problem, and is unable to prescribe NSAIDs because of his reports of gastric ulcers and allergy. He says he has tried exercises and a local pain clinic, neither of which was effective. He is aware of the emergency room policy regarding narcotic analgesics for chronic pain, but he comes there in desperation. He insists that his pain is relieved only by narcotic analgesia.

- What ethical principles are involved?
- Does the benefit of pain relief outweigh the harm potentially caused by long-term narcotic analgesic use for this patient?

- Should Mr. Gruder's perceived need for narcotic pain medications be honored even though the nurse practitioner feels he has a problem with drug dependence?
- How does the nurse do what she thinks is right and yet respect Mr. Gruder's autonomy?
- Is it important whether or not the nurse's actions please the patient?

REFERENCES

American Hospital Association. (1973, rev. 1992). *Statement on a patient's bill of rights.* Chicago: Author.

American Nurses Association. (1995). *Nursing's social policy statement.* Washington, DC: Author.

American Nurses Association. (2001). *Code of ethics for nurses.* Washington, DC: Author.

Beauchamp, T. L., & Childress, J. (2008). *Principles of biomedical ethics* (6th ed.). New York: Oxford University Press.

Beauchamp, T. L., & Walters, L. (2007). *Contemporary issues in bioethics* (6th ed.). Belmont, CA: Wadsworth.

Bok, S. (1991). Lies to the sick and dying. In T. A. Mappes & J. S. Zembaty (Eds.), *Biomedical ethics* (pp. 74–81). New York: McGraw-Hill.

Bok, S. (1994). Truth telling. In W. Reich (Ed.), *Encyclopedia of bioethics* (pp. 1682–1686). New York: Macmillan.

Buber, M. (1965). *The knowledge of man: A philosophy of the interhuman.* New York: Harper & Row.

Cammon, S. A., & Hackshaw, H. S. (2000). Are we starving our patients? *American Journal of Nursing, 100*(5), 43–46.

Canadian Nurses Association. (2008). *Code of ethics for registered nurses.* Ottowa, Canada: Author.

Department of Health and Human Services. (2002, rev. 2003). *General overview of standards for privacy of individually identifiable health information.* [45 CFR Part 160 and Subparts A and E of Part 164]. Retrieved March 17, 2006, from http://www.hhs.gov/ocr/hipaa/finalreg.html

Deshefy-Longhi, T., Dixon, J. K., Olson, D., & Grey, M. (2004). Privacy and confidentiality issues in primary care: Views of advanced practice nurses and their patients [Electronic version]. *Nursing Ethics, 11,* 378–393.

Durant, W. (1926). *The story of philosophy.* New York: Washington Square Press.

Ellin, J. S. (1991). Lying and deception: The solution to a dilemma in medical ethics. In T. A. Mappes & J. S. Zembaty (Eds.), *Biomedical ethics* (pp. 81–87). New York: McGraw-Hill.

Erlen, J. A. (1998). The inadvertent breach of confidentiality. *Orthopaedic Nursing, 17*(2), 47–50.

Erlen, J. A. (2004). HIPAA: Clinical and ethical considerations for nurses [Electronic version]. *Orthopaedic Nursing, 23,* 401–403.

Gillon, R. (1985). Autonomy and the principle of respect for autonomy. *British Medical Journal, 290,* pp. 1806–1808.

Goldsmith, J. (Ed.). (1992). Virginia Henderson, RN: Humanitarian and scholar. *Reflections, 18*(1), 4–5.

Haggarty, L. A. (2000). Informed consent and the limits of confidentiality. *Western Journal of Nursing Research, 22*(4), 508–514.

Harris, S. H. (1999). Japanese medical atrocities in World War II: Unit 731 was not an isolated aberration. Paper presented at the International Citizens Forum on War Carimes and Redress, Tokyo, Japan. Retrieved from http://www.vcn.bc.ca/alpha/speech/Harris.htm

Harrison, A. F., & Bramson, R. M. (1982). *Styles of thinking.* New York: Doubleday.

Henderson, V. (1966). *The nature of nursing: A definition and its implications for practice, research, and education.* New York: MacMillan.

International Council of Nurses. (2006). *The ICN code of ethics for nurses.* Geneva, Switzerland: Author. Retrieved from http://icn.ch/icncode.pdf

Jameton, A. (1984). *Nursing practice: The ethical issues.* Englewood Cliffs, NJ: Prentice-Hall.

Lipkin, M. (1991). On lying to patients. In T. A. Mappes & J. S. Zembaty (Eds.), *Biomedical ethics* (pp. 72–73). New York: McGraw-Hill.

Markus, A., & Lockwood, M. (1991). Is it permissible to edit medical records? *British Medical Journal, 303,* 349–351.

Muldoon, J. D. (1996). Confidentiality, privacy and restriction for computer-based patient records. *Hospital Topics, 74*(3), 32–37.

Munson, R. (1992). Major moral principles. In *Intervention and reflection: Basic issues in medical ethics* (4th ed., pp. 31–45). Belmont, CA: Wadsworth.

Neustadt, R. E., & Fineberg, H. V. (2005). *The swine flu affair: Decision-making on a slippery disease.* Honolulu, HI: University Press of the Pacific.

Nuremberg Military Tribunal. (October 1946–April 1949). *Trials of War Criminals Before the Nuremberg Military Tribunals* (Vol. 2, pp. 181–182).

Washington, DC: U.S. Government Printing Office. Retrieved from http://www.loc.gov/rr/frd/Military_Law/NTs_war-criminals.html

O'Keefe, M. H. (2001). *Nursing practice and the law: Avoiding malpractice and other legal risks.* Philadelphia: F. A. Davis.

Percival, T. (1803). *Medical ethics: A code of institutes and precepts adapted to the professional conduct of physicians and surgeons* (3rd ed.). Oxford: Shrimpton.

Shuster, E. (1997). Fifty years later: The significance of the Nuremberg Code. *New England Journal of Medicine 337.*, 1436–1440. Retrieved from http://www.nejm.org/doi/full/10.1056/NEJM199711133372006

Taubenberger, J.K., & Morens, D. M. (2006). 1918 influenza: The mother of all pandemics. *Emerging Infectious Diseases.* Retrieved from http://www.cdc.gov/ncidod/EID/vol12no01/05-0979.htm

Tobriner, M. O. (1991). *Majority opinion in Tarasoff v. Regents of the University of California.* In T. A. Mappes & J. S. Zembaty (Eds.), *Biomedical ethics* (pp. 165–169). New York: McGraw-Hill.

United States Holocaust Memorial Museum. (2010). The doctors trial: The medical case of the subsequent Nuremberg proceedings. Retrieved November 4, 2010, from http://www.ushmm.org/research/doctors/

U.S. Centers for Disease Control and Prevention. (2010). The 2010 H1N1 pandemic: Summary highlights, April 2009–April 2010. Retrieved from http://www.cdc.gov/h1n1flu/cdcresponse.htm

Veatch, R. (2002). *The basics of bioethics* (2nd ed.). Upper Saddle River, NJ: Prentice Hall.

Weindling, P. (1996). Human guinea pigs and the ethics of experimentation: The *BMJ's* correspondent at the Nuremberg medical trial. *British Medical Journal, 313*(1), 1467–1470.

Weyers, W. (2007). *The abuse of man: An illustrated history of medical experimentation.* New York: Ardor Scribendi.

Winston, M. E. (1988). AIDS, confidentiality, and the right to know. *Public Affairs Quarterly, 2*, 91–104.

Zomorodi, M., & Foley, B. J. (2009) The nature of advocacy vs. paternalism in nursing: Clarifying the "thin line." *Journal of Advanced Nursing, 65*(8), 1746–1752.

DEVELOPING PRINCIPLED BEHAVIOR

Recognizing that values and beliefs are culturally relative, Part II describes theories related to moral development and values clarification. This section examines the process of ethical decision making and its application to clinical situations. Because personal values and moral development influence perceptions and decisions, readers are encouraged to become aware of their own values and to examine personal levels of moral development in light of the different theories presented in Part I. Benefiting from this knowledge, readers can begin to be more sensitive to the perspectives, decision-making abilities, and tendencies of other people, and to acknowledge the influence of their own values and moral development on various decision-making processes.

Chapter 4

VALUES CLARIFICATION

As your actions are informed by your awareness of values, your thinking and your ideas are shaped and changed by your experiences with those actions.

(Chinn, *2004*)

OBJECTIVES

After completing this chapter, the reader should be able to:

1. Define and differentiate personal values, societal values, professional values, organizational values, and moral values.

2. Discuss how values are acquired.

3. Discuss self-awareness as a tool for living an ethical life.

4. Explain the place of values clarification in nursing.

5. Explain the valuing process.

6. Describe values conflict and its implications for nursing care.

7. Describe the interaction between personal and institutional values.

8. Discuss the importance of attending to both personal values and patient values.

INTRODUCTION

Principled behavior flows from personal values that guide and inform our responses, behaviors, and decisions in all areas of our lives. Ethical decision making requires self-awareness and knowledge of ethical theories and principles. Such awareness of self includes knowing what we value or consider important. The branch of philosophy that studies the nature and types of values is called **axiology**, a word that comes from the Greek for worth or worthy. Axiology includes the study of values in art, known as aesthetics; in human relations and conduct, known as ethics; and in relation to beliefs regarding relationship with the Divine, known as religion. This chapter discusses the importance of being aware of personal values and how these values influence the way we relate to self and others within personal and professional arenas.

WHAT ARE VALUES?

Values are ideals, beliefs, customs, modes of conduct, qualities, or goals that are highly prized or preferred by individuals, groups, or society. They are abstract concepts that reflect what is meaningful and important to us. Values are learned in both conscious and unconscious ways and become part of a person's makeup. They manifest as subjective preferences or dispositions that motivate and guide behavior and decisions. Values become "real" or actualized when they are expressed through the ways we behave and the choices we make in the context of daily life. When we are faced with choices, our preferences and the hierarchical nature of values become evident. For example, if both comfort and appearance are valued in how we dress, the hierarchy becomes evident when a woman chooses to wear the more restrictive suit rather than the more relaxed dress for a professional interview. Our values influence choices and behavior whether or not we are conscious that the values are guiding the choices. Values provide direction and meaning to life and a frame of reference for integrating, explaining, and evaluating new experiences, thoughts, and relationships. Values may be expressed overtly, as espoused behaviors or verbalized standards, or they may manifest in an indirect way through verbal and nonverbal behavior.

Moral Values

As discussed in Chapter 2, individual cognitive evaluation of right and wrong, good and bad, is reflective of **moral thought**. Flowing from this, preferences or dispositions in human behavior reflective of right or wrong, should or should not, are considered **moral values** (Omery, 1989). Moral values constitute a special case of values because the particular circumstances that call them forth deal with ethical issues or dilemmas. These values may be acquired within contexts such as the family, through our religious or philosophical orientation, or through our profession.

ACQUIRING VALUES

Personal ethical behavior flows from values held by an individual that develop over time. Cultural, ethnic, familial, environmental, educational, and other experiences of living help to shape our values. We begin to learn and incorporate values into our beings at an early age and continue the process throughout our lives. As noted previously, values are acquired in both conscious and unconscious ways. Values may be learned in a conscious way through instruction by parents, teachers, religious leaders and educators, and professional and social group leaders. Many values are formally adopted by groups and are written in professional codes of ethics, religious doctrines, societal laws, and statements of an organization's philosophy. Socialization and role modeling, which are other ways in which values are acquired, lead to more subconscious learning. Some values stay with us for much of our lives, and others may change or be altered in response to personal development and experiences. Freely choosing those values that we most cherish and relinquishing those that have little meaning is an important step in values formation (Lewis, 2007; Smith, 2001).

Because values become a part of who we are, they often enter into our decision making in less-than-conscious ways. We constantly make judgments that reflect our values, though not always realizing that we

---

ASK YOURSELF

How Have Your Values Developed?

Think of three ideals or beliefs that you prize in your personal life. Try to trace each belief or ideal back to the earliest time in your life when you were aware of its importance or presence.

- When and how did you learn to view each belief or ideal as important?

- How have they changed or evolved over time?

- Where do you find your support for them?

- How prevalent do you think these beliefs or ideals are among other people?

- What do you think of people who hold different beliefs or ideals?

- Think of a time in your life when one of these beliefs or ideals had been challenged. How did you feel? How did you react?

have a given set of values or that these values are affecting our decisions (Engebretson, 2013; Simon, Howe, & Kirschenbaum, 1995). Becoming more aware of one's values is an important step in being able to make clear and thoughtful decisions. In the area of ethical decision making, knowing one's own values in a conscious way and being able to help others to name their values clearly are particularly important.

SELF-AWARENESS

Ethical relationships with others begin with self-knowledge and the willingness to honestly and appropriately express that awareness to others. Self-knowledge is an ongoing, evolving process that requires us to make a commitment to know the truth about ourselves. This is not an easy commitment to make. Although the truth can be painful at times, paradoxically, it can also set us free. Remember that what we believe to be the truth is always colored by our perceptions and can change over time (Covey, 2004). Keep in mind that most situations are not black or white. All sides are present in each situation. Like the aperture of a camera, what we see in any situation depends upon the lens we are using, how close or far we are standing, and the angle from which we are looking. From this perspective, there can be many views of a situation, depending upon how many people are picturing it. Awareness of the particular lens through which we view the world enables us to identify and better understand our own responses in a situation. Understanding that there can be different views and openly sharing individual perspectives helps us to appreciate the truth inherent in each perspective.

The term **values clarification** refers to the process of becoming more conscious of and naming what we value or consider worthy. It is an ongoing process that is grounded in our capacity for reflective, intelligent, self-directed behavior (Burkhardt & Keegan, 2013; Hoalt & Hoalt, 2005; Lewis, 2007). By focusing time, energy, and attention to reflecting on our values, we shed light on our personal perspective and discover our own answers to many concerns and questions. One approach to values clarification is the process for developing a personal value portrait described by Gibson (2008). This process, which focuses on delineating personal and professional values, begins with writing down characteristics one admires in self and others, characteristics one respects in others, and characteristics one considers undesirable in others. The next part of the process is to rank the values on each list in order of importance, and, after reflection on these lists, to develop a brief statement or description of personal values. The process continues with identifying and rank ordering personal and professional responsibilities, obligations, and loyalties in relation to the identified personal values. After reflection, these are combined into a statement that provides a personal value portrait.

Developing insight into our values improves our ability to make value decisions. No one set of values is appropriate for everyone; we must appreciate that values clarification may lead to different insights for different people (Engebretson, 2013; Gibson, 2008). Engaging in values clarification promotes a closer fit between our words and actions, enabling us to more clearly "walk our talk," thus enhancing personal integrity. As noted in Chapter 2, **integrity** refers to adherence to moral norms that is sustained over time. Trustworthiness and a consistency of convictions, actions, and emotions are implicit in integrity. It is only to the extent that we appreciate our own values that we can truly understand the values of another.

Since values include dimensions of knowing and of feeling, the process of becoming clearer about what we treasure addresses both the cognitive and the affective domains. By becoming more conscious of our own behavior and feelings, we learn to discern whether our choices flow from chosen values or are the result of preconditioning. Assessment of personal values requires a readiness and willingness to take an honest look at our ideals and behaviors; at our words, actions, and motivation; and at the congruencies and incongruencies among them. An important goal of the process is to be aware of and choose our own values rather than to merely act out prior conditioning.

Enhancing Self-Awareness

Self-awareness is the ultimate tool for living a personally ethical life. Values clarification and **self-awareness** go hand in hand. The first and most important step in awareness of the self is the conscious intention to be aware. Being conscious of our thoughts, feelings, physical and emotional responses, and insights in various situations can promote appreciation of our values. Conversely, by identifying and analyzing personal values, we become more self-aware (Burkhardt & Nagai-Jacobson, 2002; Reich & Levin, 2013). We can enhance insight by developing the ability to step back and see what is going on in any situation, being aware of self and aware of our reactions in the present moment. Self-awareness can begin with as simple an act as tuning in to our breathing—noting its rate, rhythm, depth, and other characteristics without any effort to change it. It is a way of becoming conscious of an act that usually occurs quite unconsciously. Another way to become more aware is to pay attention to how we are feeling physically and emotionally in any given situation—to name the feelings without judging them. We might ask, "What do I think I am reacting to here, and can I identify where that reaction comes from?" For example, when you see a beautiful sunset, you might note a feeling of peace, exhilaration, or relaxation, and realize you are responding to beauty, with an ensuing memory that your mother was always one to be observant of beauty in her world. You thus recognize that you learned this value, at least in part, from your mother. Introspection, observation, reflection, meditation, journaling, art, writing, therapy, reading, discussion groups, and feedback assist us in expanding self-awareness.

Individual reflection and discussion with another person or in small groups help us both to become more aware of and to analyze our values. Group discussion enables us to react and to hear the reactions of others. Such processes may lead us to see more clearly those values we have accepted because of conditioning and to articulate better those values we have chosen for ourselves. These processes may also lead us to modify our perspective based on the insights of others. Other tools that open our perspective include taking the other side of a debate, interviewing people with differing opinions, walking in another's shoes and defending their position, and asking for feedback on our own positions. Another way to look at values is to ask general questions such as "If I knew I would die in 6 weeks, what would I be doing today?" or "If I had to leave my house and could only take three things with me, what would they be?" or "Where would I like to be 5, 10, or 20 years from now?"

The valuing process includes three areas (Simon et al., 1995). (1) *Prizing and cherishing* one's beliefs and behaviors includes knowing what one does and does not support and communicating this to others. (2) *Choosing* one's beliefs and behaviors by evaluating values received from others includes examining alternatives and their consequences and then deciding what is one's own. (3) *Acting* on these beliefs with a consistent pattern reinforces actions supportive of the values. The intent of values clarification is to help us become more aware of our own values and the valuing process in our lives; there is no intention to impose particular values on us or others.

Journaling

Journals are personal records or notes that may include thoughts, feelings, experiences, ideas, reactions, dreams, drawings, and other expressions related to what is going on in one's life. They may be kept on a regular or periodic basis, may be structured or unstructured, and may include art as well as words. For many people, keeping a diary or journal of experiences and personal reactions to situations is a useful tool in developing awareness. Many books are available to guide someone new to journaling, and readers are encouraged to explore these resources. Figure 4–1 offers guidelines that may help students utilize the journaling process to gain insight into personal values. When writing in a journal, let your thoughts flow as freely as possible without censoring or judging what you are writing. Allow yourself time and privacy when you are journaling, and keep the journal in a place where you feel comfortable that you can control who has access to it. Commit to journaling on a regular basis. Recognize that journaling is a personal process, so go with your own style. If a format such as that suggested in Figure 4–1 helps you, go for it! If not, write as the thoughts flow from you.

- Describe a situation in your personal or professional experience in which you felt uncomfortable or felt that your beliefs or values were being challenged, or in which you felt your values were different from those of others involved.
- As you record the situation, include how you felt physically and emotionally at the time you experienced the situation.
- Write down your feelings as you remember the situation. Are your reactions now any different from when you were actually in this situation?
- What personal values do you identify in the situation? Try to remember where and from whom you learned these values. Do you totally agree with the values, or is there anything about them that you question or wonder about their validity?
- What values do you think were being expressed by others involved? Where are they similar to or different from your values?
- What do you think you reacted to in the situation?
- Can you remember having similar reactions in other situations? If yes, how were the situations similar or different?
- How do you feel about your response to the situation? Is there anything you would change if you could repeat the scene? Rewrite the scene with the changes. What might be the consequences of these changes?
- How do you feel with the new scenario?
- What do you need to do to reinforce behaviors, ideals, beliefs, or qualities that you have identified as personal values in this situation? When and how can you do this?

FIGURE 4–1 Journaling for Values Awareness

VALUES IN PROFESSIONAL SITUATIONS

Values clarification is important to nurses in several ways. A fundamental aspect of ethical behavior is being conscious of our motives. Thus, knowing and appreciating our own value system provides a basis for understanding how and why we react and respond in decision-making situations. Knowing our own values enables us to acknowledge similarities and differences in values when interacting with others. This ultimately promotes more effective communication and care. Commitment to developing more awareness of personal values enables us to be more effective in facilitating the process with others. In the professional realm, these others may be staff, patients, families, or institutions.

Values Conflict

When personal values are at odds with those of patients, colleagues, or the institution, internal or interpersonal conflict may result. This can subsequently affect patient care. Dealing in an effective way with **values conflict** requires conscious awareness of our own values, as well as awareness of the perceived values of the others involved. Such awareness enables nurses to be more alert to situations in which they are judging the behaviors of others according to their own values, or in which their personal values are being imposed upon another. When differences in values are identified, the nurse can choose to respond to the other's viewpoint in a way that seeks understanding and common ground, rather than reacting in a "knee-jerk" fashion. In this way the integrity of the caring relationship can be maintained.

The following case presentation provides an example of values conflict. As you read the case, think about the values that are evident in the situation. Put yourself in the position of each of the participants and ask yourself what you might do if you were in their shoes.

Impact of Institutional Values

Nurses need to be conscious of both the spoken and unspoken values in their work settings. Values of individual institutions and organized health care systems that are explicitly communicated through philosophy and policy statements are called **overt values**. Values may also be implicit in expectations that are not in writing. Implicit or **covert values** are often identified only through participation in or controversies within the setting (Maedel, 2011; Omery, 1989). When seeking employment, nurses should identify congruencies or incongruencies between their personal values and those of the institution, because accepting employment implies committing to the value system of the organization. Consider, for example, Anton, a nurse who accepts a position at a health center because the center publicizes a commitment to providing quality care to all patients. Within 2 months he notices that patients with Medicaid cards are kept waiting longer than those with private insurance, and are treated rudely by many of the staff. When he initiates teaching with the Medicaid patients, he is told not to waste his time because "those people won't change their ways." Overtly, the health center is committed to quality care for all patients; however, the

Case Presentation

A Conflict of Values

Nine-year-old Benton is a patient on the pediatric unit with a diagnosis of terminal-stage Ewing's sarcoma. He has three sisters, age 7, 6, and 3, who are presently being cared for by a grandmother. His father is self-employed and works long hours. His mother has never worked outside the home. Both parents have high school educations, and their primary activities outside of family are church-related. They belong to a small nondenominational rural church and state that they hold fast to what is taught in the Bible and put their faith in the word of God.

(continued)

Prior to his illness, Benton, a healthy child, had been brought to the clinic only for acute health concerns. The family does not have health insurance. Shortly after entering second grade 2 years ago, he began limping. The family attributed the limp to a playground injury. When he continued to complain of pain and the limp persisted after 3 months, his mother took him to a local health clinic. Above-the-knee amputation followed diagnosis, but metastasis was evident in 9 months. Chemotherapy has only been palliative.

The physician has discussed Benton's poor prognosis with the parents, recommending comfort care. The parents say they want everything possible to be done for him, and the father conducts nightly prayer sessions at Benton's bedside, affirming that God is healing Benton. Although Benton has asked whether he is going to die, his father refuses to allow staff to speak with him regarding fears or concerns about his condition. When asked what Benton has been told, the father responds, "He knows God is trying us and we must have faith." The mother, who appears less confident of a healing, is there 24 hours a day. She supervises Benton's care relentlessly, at times irritating staff with questions and demands. She keeps a notebook record of her son's care, including medication, times of care, intake and output, and personal assessments. Although Benton used to talk to staff, he now appears frightened and remains quiet, sleeping off and on.

Think About It

Dealing with Values Conflict

Respond to these questions from the vantage point of the nurse in the preceding Case Presentation:

* *What is your first personal reaction to this situation? Identify your values relative to the situation.*
* *What do you perceive to be the values of the others involved?*
* *Identify value incongruencies that might lead to conflict. Give specific examples of how such a conflict can potentially affect patient care.*
* *Describe specific nursing interventions aimed at managing the conflict in a professional manner, and give examples of how nursing codes would guide such actions.*
* *Describe your own strengths and limitations as you consider dealing with this situation.*

covert values reflect different attitudes toward and levels of care for those on public assistance. Anton's values of providing quality care for all may prompt a variety of responses in this situation. He may compromise his values if he wants to get along with other staff and do well in the job, he may expend much energy challenging the covert value system, or he may decide that he cannot continue to work in this system.

What one believes and how one thinks about a job are important and have a direct impact on job performance (Demarest & Schoof, 2011). Such internal belief systems tend to shape people's thinking and direct them to do what they think is right, regardless of the employer's philosophy. These authors suggest that it is better to identify that which is valued by employers, that is, where they stand and what they pay attention to and reward, and then to decide whether one can work in that environment. In health care settings, for example, there are three primary ways to approach patient care: focus on meeting patient needs (intrinsic care), focus on doing all the tasks (extrinsic care), and focus on following the rules (systemic care). If there is a conflict between our values regarding patient care and the values of the institution, physician, and family, we may experience moral distress. **Moral distress** is the reaction to a situation in which there are moral problems that seem to have clear solutions, yet we are unable to follow our moral beliefs because of external restraints. This distress is often evidenced in anger, dissatisfaction, frustration, and poor performance in the work setting.

Gingerich and Ondeck (1993) describe one process for defining and making organizational values more explicit. This process includes determining what is valued by staff, board members, management, and physicians regarding the elements of the organization's philosophy, and identifying specific expectations for each group. Exercises focused on self-awareness, clinical priorities, and opinions about value-laden issues are conducted within each of the groups to develop awareness of and consensus around the values. This allows all involved to have an investment in the value system.

The Hartman Value Profile is another approach to looking at values within an organization (Demarest & Schoof, 2011). The process involves having the institution select a number of employees representing two groups within the organization: those considered to be the *shining stars*

ASK YOURSELF

How Should Values Influence Job Selection?

Maria, a recently divorced mother of three, desperately needs to return to work, but nursing jobs in her area are scarce. There is one opening at a women's health clinic that performs abortions. The job, which has excellent salary and benefits, including on-site child care, looks great to Maria, except that abortions are against her religious and personal beliefs. A friend who works at the clinic said that, unless they are short staffed, Maria would not have to assist with abortions if she had objections.

- What dilemmas are evident in this situation?

- What are the value incongruencies?

- What are your values related to this situation?

- What factors should Maria consider in deciding whether to take the job?

Case Presentation

Differences in Personal and Organizational Values

Joan has been the nurse manager of her unit for the past 10 years and is highly regarded by the hospital's administration. For the past several months, however, she has been feeling more frustrated and less satisfied with her work because of staffing cuts and other institutional decisions related to patient care priorities. Attending to patient needs has always been the most rewarding part of her job. However, recently she feels that she has been forced to overlook these needs and attend more to the needs of the organization. She considers leaving, but she has seniority, good benefits, and two children to support. She is also aware that her distress at work is affecting her family, because she carries a lot of the frustration home with her.

Think About It

How Values Affect Choices

- *Identify values evident in this situation. Which of these reflect your personal values?*
- *What conflicts might arise from these values?*
- *What do you think Joan should do?*
- *If you were in Joan's position, what beliefs, ideals, or goals would guide you in making a decision to stay or leave? Identify potential consequences of each choice.*

and those considered least satisfactory. Those identified complete the profile, which is a forced ranking ranging from best to worst or most despicable, of 18 items relating to how these employees perceive the world around them and 18 items related to how they perceive their inner selves. Patterns are identified by analyzing the participants' responses utilizing a computerized mathematical system that identifies how each item compares with the others that are ranked. The resulting information provides a profile of the underlying values within the organization. Decision makers can use this information to examine how prevailing belief systems are influencing performance, and to seek potential employees whose values are most consistent with those of the organization.

Clarifying Values with Patients

Values of both nurses and patients influence patient care situations. Since patients are the recipients and consumers of health care, it is good to know

ASK YOURSELF

What Would You Do?

- You are busy and two call lights go on at the same time. What factors enter into deciding which one you respond to first?

- Consider that in the above situation one patient is in serious condition and has been verbally abusive to staff, while the other is not quite as serious and is someone you really enjoy being with. Whom would you respond to first and why?

- Your patients let you know how much they appreciate the extra care and time you give them compared to the other nurses. At the same time, your evaluation is coming up and your supervisor has indicated that you need to be more efficient with your time. What would you do in this situation and why?

what they expect or value. Patient and provider perceptions of what constitutes quality of care can be quite different. Great discrepancies in these perceptions may lead to patient dissatisfaction. This can have a variety of consequences, including affecting a patient's attitude and decisions regarding following recommendations for care and treatment (which may affect recovery), marring the reputation of the agency, and potentiating malpractice litigation. Consider the potential conflict of values and resulting dissatisfaction when patients expect nurses to spend time with them and the institution puts more emphasis on getting the tasks done, or when patients need to share their stories and nurses are focused on entering standard history data into the computer.

When working with patients regarding health care decisions, nurses need to be aware of personal values and patients' values pertaining to health. When the health values of the nurse and those of the patient are different, the patient may become labeled as uncooperative, self-destructive, noncompliant, ignorant, or unwilling to take responsibility for her or his own health. Attentiveness to cultural and religious values is especially important in this regard. Refer to Chapter 18 for discussion of transcultural and spiritual issues.

Nurse theorist Dr. Nola Pender (1987, 1996) discusses the role of values in health promotion. She notes that knowing personal values is important, as is the need to avoid imposing our values on patients. Consider, for example, an obese patient with terminal lung cancer and a prognosis of 3 to 6 months to live, who continues to smoke and is a confirmed agnostic. If priorities on the care plan include weight loss, smoking cessation, and facilitating the patient's making peace with God, we must consider whether nursing values are being imposed on the patient.

With self-awareness, the nurse can be more effective in helping patients to identify their own values. Assisting patients to clearly articulate their values is important because a lack of clarity about values may result in inconsistency, confusion, misunderstanding, and inadequate decision making. The ability to make informed choices, including the process of informed consent, is enhanced by having clarity about our values. "Assisting clients to clarify values; understand the personal and social consequences of acting on current values; achieve greater consistency among values, attitudes, and behaviors; and plan health-related experiences that may result in self-initiated changes in value hierarchies" are key nursing actions (Pender, 1987, p. 161).

Many instruments and processes are available to facilitate exploring values in general and health values in particular. One example is a process that asks people to rank a list of 10 health values from most important to least important. The list includes a comfortable life, an exciting life, a sense of accomplishment, freedom, happiness, health, inner harmony, pleasure, self-respect, and social recognition (Pender, 1987, p. 165). Pender notes that if health appears within the top four on the list, the person places a high value on health. However, definitions of health will vary, since each person defines health according to personal beliefs and values.

Another approach to analyzing health values described by Doyle (1994) asks people to identify, from a list of 10 health-related behaviors, what they do and why they do it. Behaviors include activities such as exercising a minimum of three times per week, talking to a close friend or relative about worries, and practicing sex without using a condom. Doyle notes that the response to why a behavior is practiced provides insight into values surrounding the behavior, such as choosing not to exercise in order to have more time, or choosing to exercise because it helps in weight control.

SUMMARY

This chapter has discussed the importance of self-awareness regarding values and the valuing process. Values are learned and change in response to life situations as a person develops. The process of values clarification enables persons to begin to identify and choose their own values rather than merely act according to prior conditioning. The interaction between personal values and those of patients and organizations can affect job satisfaction and patient care. The reader is encouraged to explore various processes that facilitate values clarification, both those presented in this chapter and those found in other resources.

CHAPTER HIGHLIGHTS

- Values are highly prized ideals, behaviors, beliefs, or qualities that are shaped by culture, ethnicity, family, environment, and education and are acquired in both conscious and unconscious ways.

- The process of incorporating values begins at an early age and continues throughout life. Some values remain consistent while others change in response to growth and life experiences.

- Awareness of personal values undergirds the ability to make clear and thoughtful decisions and enables us to acknowledge similarities and differences in values when interacting with others, thus promoting more effective communication, care, and facilitation of values clarification with others.

- Values clarification is not intended to instill values; rather, the aim is to facilitate awareness of personal values and the valuing process in order to move toward the point of choosing our own values rather than merely reacting from prior conditioning.

- The valuing process includes prizing and cherishing, choosing, and acting on beliefs and behaviors.

- Dealing effectively with values conflict requires attention to personal values, the perceived values of others, and the ability to recognize both overt and covert expression of values in a situation.

- Congruence between personal values and those of an institution is an important consideration for a nurse seeking employment.

- Assisting patients to articulate their values and beliefs is an important part of nursing care and may help prevent confusion and misunderstanding when there are differences in values between patients and providers.

DISCUSSION QUESTIONS AND ACTIVITIES

1. A non-nursing classmate asks you what studying values has to do with nursing. How would you respond? Incorporate your understanding of the nature of values and how they become part of us into your response.

2. What values guide your personal life? How did you learn these values? Select something that you consider important in professional nursing practice and trace how you learned this value.

3. Discuss why values clarification is important both personally and professionally.

4. Identify the overt values of your health care agency and identify overt and covert values of nurses and others within the agency. Explain the importance of knowing about both.

5. Describe a situation in which you experienced someone (it could be you) reacting from values that were not conscious at the time. How did this affect the interaction?

6. Determine the health values of three patients or people you do not know well and discuss why nurses need to be attentive to what others, particularly patients, value.

7. Describe a situation in which you experienced values conflict and how you dealt with the conflict.

8. Find current examples of public or professional figures whose personal values seem at odds with their professional or public trust. Discuss your reaction to the discrepancy in values that you identify and the interplay between personal values and professional integrity.

9. Use values clarification exercises to help you reflect on your own values. Examples of these exercises can be found in many self-help books and online at websites such as:

> http://faculty.weber.edu/molpin/healthclasses/1110/bookchapters/valueschapter.htm

> http://www.itp.edu/resources/crc/pdf/values.pdf http://hrweb.mit.edu/system/files/Value+Clarification+Exercise.pdf

REFERENCES

Burkhardt, M. A., & Keegan, L. (2013). Holistic ethics. In B. M. Dossey & L. Keegan (Eds.), *Holistic nursing: A handbook for practice* (6th ed., pp. 129–142). Boston: Jones & Bartlett.

Burkhardt, M. A., & Nagai-Jacobson, M. G. (2002). *Spirituality: Living our connectedness.* Clifton Park, NY: Delmar.

Chinn, P. L. (2004). *Peace and power: Building communities for the future* (6th ed.). Boston: Jones & Bartlett.

Covey, S. R. (2004). *The seven habits of highly effective people.* New York: Simon & Schuster.

Demarest, P. D., & Schoof, H. J. (2011). *Answering the central question: How science reveals the keys to success in life, love, and leadership.* Philadelphia, PA: HeartLead Publications.

Doyle, E. I. (1994). Recognizing the value–health behavior connection: "What I do and why I do it." *Journal of Health Education, 25,* 116–118.

Engebretson, J. C. (2013). Cultural diversity and care. In B. M. Dossey, L. Keegan, & C. E. Guzzetta (Eds.), *Holistic nursing: A handbook for practice* (6th ed., pp. 677–702). Boston: Jones & Bartlett.

Gibson, P. A. (2008). Teaching ethical decision making: Designing a personal value portrait to ignite creativity and promote engagement in case method analysis. *Ethics & Behavior, 18,* 340–352.

Gingerich, B. S., & Ondeck, D. A. (1993). Values incorporation throughout the organization. *Caring Magazine, 12,* 18–23.

Hoalt, K., & Hoalt, P. (2005). Teaching techniques: Charting your course using a sea bag philosophy. *Journal of School Health, 74,* 145–146.

Lewis, H. (2007). *A question of values: Six ways we make the personal choices that shape our lives* (Rev. ed.). Edinburg, VA: Axios Press.

Maedel, C. (2011, February 28). HR's role in adding value to corporate values. *Canadian HR Reporter: The National Journal Of Human Resource Management.* Retrieved from http://www.hrreporter.com

Omery, A. (1989). Values, moral reasoning, and ethics. *Nursing Clinics of North America, 24,* 499–507.

Pender, N. J. (1987). *Health promotion in nursing practice* (2nd ed.). Norwalk, CT: Appleton & Lange.

Pender, N. J. (1996). *Health promotion in nursing practice* (3rd ed.). Norwalk, CT: Appleton & Lange.

Reich, J. L., & Levin, J. D. (2013). Self-reflection: Consulting the truth within. In B. M. Dossey & L. Keegan (Eds.), *Holistic nursing: A handbook for practice* (6th ed., pp. 247–260). Boston: Jones & Bartlett.

Simon, S. B., Howe, L. W., & Kirschenbaum, H. (1995). *Values clarification: A handbook of practical strategies for teachers and students.* New York: Hart.

Smith, H. W. (2001). *What matters most: The power of living your values.* New York: Fireside.

Chapter

5

VALUES DEVELOPMENT

What is firmly established cannot be uprooted.
What is firmly grasped cannot slip away.
It will be honored from generation to generation.

(**Lao Tsu,** *Tao Te Ching*, **trans. 1972**)

OBJECTIVES

After completing this chapter, the reader should be able to:

1. Discuss influences of culture on values development.

2. Contrast theoretical approaches to moral development.

3. Describe and differentiate the ethic of care and the ethic of justice.

4. Evaluate the personal phase of moral development.

5. Discuss gender bias and cultural bias regarding theories of moral development.

INTRODUCTION

Nurses frequently encounter situations that present ethical dilemmas. In some situations the "right" choice seems quite evident, while in other circumstances a considerable lack of clarity about what is "right" may exist. How do we come to know what is right or how to respond in a principled way in a given situation? This chapter addresses the question of how, over time, a person comes to have certain values, and reviews factors that influence values formation, theoretical perspectives related to stages of values development, and considerations for nursing regarding moral development.

TRANSCULTURAL CONSIDERATIONS IN VALUES DEVELOPMENT

The world view, or **cosmology**, that is characteristic of a particular culture is rooted in the culture's shared story. Cosmology is an organizing way of looking at the nature of the universe as a whole and the role of the human in it that incorporates both the physical plane and the interconnected, multidimensional universe. It is a set of assumptions about perceived reality that guide, support, and empower members of the culture. Beginning with the culture's origin story, the shared story provides a context for ascribing meaning to and determining relationships with all aspects of human experience. It is the big picture that explains how and why things are and helps people understand how they can live in the world and deal with the various experiences and events of life. The world view reflected in a culture's cosmic story influences roles and relationships among its members, between its members and other humans, and between its members and the natural and supernatural worlds. Cosmology is the way people of all cultures address the big questions of life: Where did we come from? Where are we going? What is the meaning of life? What is right and wrong? What is good and bad?

Human values development, often referred to as **moral development**, is a product of the sociocultural environment in which we live and develop. The sociocultural environment includes cultural, historical, familial, social, and institutional influences through which we process deep experiences and acquire insights and tools that help us develop an ethical stance (Maldonado, Efinger, & Lacey, 2003; Tappan, 2006). We learn what is considered right and wrong within the culture in formal ways such as by precept and admonition, through informal processes such as role modeling, and by technical learning in a teacher-to-student process (Hall, 1973). Norms for etiquette and ethical behavior that are "known" within the culture may be acquired by an outsider through technical learning; however, they are often appreciated by a neophyte only when a transgression has occurred and corrections to, or sanctions for, the behavior have been imposed. There is an innate human capacity for developing an ethical stance to life congruent with the sociocultural world in which one lives that emerges through this process.

In approaching values development from a sociocultural perspective, we understand that an individual's level of development is profoundly influenced by the values and level of moral development in the society as a whole. Transcultural nurses speak of culture in terms of values, beliefs, customs, and behaviors that are learned within and shared by a group of interacting persons (Leininger, 1984; Ray, 2010; Spector, 2009). Because values are *learned* within the context of a particular culture, moral values need to be viewed within a cultural perspective. This suggests that a value such as individual autonomy may be regarded highly in a culture that prizes independence and individualism. However, the same value may be considered contrary to the norm in a society in which persons are defined by their relation to others. Fowler (1981) notes that "we are formed in social communities and that our ways of seeing the world are profoundly shaped by the shared images and constructions of our group or class" (p. 105). Understandings of principles such as justice and care may vary in different cultures. In the ensuing discussion regarding stages of values development, it is important to be aware that the norms described have been derived primarily from Anglo-American and Anglo-European populations. Although significant work has been done, there is a need for further exploration of values development within a transcultural context.

ASK YOURSELF

How Did I Learn My Values?

Think about a professional or personal situation in which you were faced with an ethical dilemma.

- What made it a dilemma for you?
- How did you decide the best course of action?
- What factors did you consider in making your decision?
- What values or principles guided you in this process?
- When and how did you learn these values or principles?
- Are these values and principles congruent with the sociocultural world in which you grew up? In which you now live?

BELIEFS AND VALUES

The question that this chapter poses is this: Over time, how does a person come to have certain values? In Chapter 4 we defined values as ideals, customs, modes of conduct, qualities, or goals that are highly prized or preferred by individuals, groups, or society. A person's values are the internalized ideas about the worthiness or desirability of something. Our view of life shapes what we value. Values derive from beliefs—ideas that one holds to be fact. Beliefs may flow from empirical observation, logic, tradition, faith, or other sources. Beliefs form one's conception of the world and the framework within which perceptions occur. Together with other mental states, beliefs function as reasons for action.

How does one develop beliefs, and why does one hold onto beliefs that may seem to be illogical to other people? Plato's famous cave metaphor gives us the opportunity to think about how people begin to imagine meaning and derive beliefs, even when based upon falsehoods. In *The Republic*, Socrates makes the point that people have a tendency to hold onto beliefs even when they have no facts to back them up. People tend to attach meaning when none exists and tend to continue to believe regardless of contradictory evidence. In Plato's "Cave" analogy, Socrates envisions a dreadful scene in which some humans have lived their entire lives underground in a cave. The entrance is high up in the cave and open to the daylight. The prisoners have been chained there since childhood, restrained in one place with their arms and legs tied. They cannot turn their heads and can only see the cave wall in front of them. There is a fire burning far up and behind them, and there are other people walking upward toward the cave opening carrying large items. The prisoners who are tied cannot see the other people or the fire, but they can see flickering shadows of the people and the items they are carrying on the wall in front of them. Socrates asks us to imagine, if the prisoners could talk to one another, wouldn't they start to create names for the things they see on the wall and wouldn't they start to imagine the meanings of the shadows and noises? They would become convinced that their beliefs were "truth." Socrates also asks what would happen if the prisoners were released and able to see the actual items being carried upward. Wouldn't they resist changing their beliefs (Plato, trans. 1997)?

What does this metaphor mean? For Socrates, the light at the opening of the cave represents truth. The people chained at the bottom of the cave are located far from truth. Endlessly sitting there, they begin to interpret random clues and to attach meaning and value to them. Given enough time, they would develop beliefs, based upon these fabricated meanings. The other people in the cave are climbing to the opening, moving toward knowledge of the truth. Coming out of the cave, or even moving toward the opening, the people who have been moving forward can see what is true—not a flickering shadow obscured by smoke, but objects as they really exist. Plato thus suggests that anyone who seeks knowledge must strive and move forward. He also implies that one must be careful about establishing and holding onto beliefs based primarily upon imagination or tradition.

Values are derived from belief, and belief drives action. With this in mind, it is helpful to examine ideas about the origin and development of beliefs. Charles Sanders Peirce, a prolific American philosopher who was introduced in Chapter 1, proposed that doubt and belief are two states of mind that feel entirely different: belief is satisfactory and doubt is unsatisfactory. Peirce suggested that self-assurance and absolute belief (even in the presence of total ignorance) may be a satisfying mode of living to which one clings tenaciously (Houser & Kloesel, 1992). On the other hand, the state of doubt is intolerable. It forces a person to action until belief is attained. Peirce identified "truth" as the goal of all human inquiry. Yet, the only condition that produces inquiry is one that begins when a person really questions something. Real inquiry begins with genuine doubt and ends when belief is established. Peirce proposed four basic methods of fixing belief: tenacity, authority, *a priori*, and reasoning.

The *tenacity* method of fixing belief is one in which the person obstinately adheres to beliefs already held. "The instinctive dislike of an undecided state of mind, exaggerated into a vague dread of doubt, makes [people] cling spasmodically to the views they already take" and further that "the pleasure he [or she] derives from his calm faith overbalances any inconveniences resulting from its deceptive character" (Houser & Kloesel, 1992, p. 116). The person believes what was previously believed, does not question it, and does not recognize the validity of others' beliefs.

Peirce's second method of fixing belief is the *authority* method. This method occurs when some institution forces its doctrines on the people by repeating them perpetually and teaching them to the young. This method has been one of the chief means of upholding doctrines. Theological or political institutions sometimes have the power to prevent contrary doctrines from being taught, advocated, or expressed. This method is often accompanied by atrocities and forces people "to adopt one belief, to massacre all who dissent from it and burn their books" (Kloesel, 1986, p. 16).

Peirce calls the third method of fixing belief the *a priori* method. This method occurs when one sees that other people, communities, or countries have totally different beliefs. One may then begin to think about his or her own view in terms of a higher value (Houser & Kloesel, 1992). A wider sort of social feeling and understanding is generated in which previous beliefs are questioned. The willful adherence to beliefs forced by authority is given up. People talk with each other and gradually develop beliefs consistent with what Peirce calls "natural causes" (Houser & Kloesel, 1992). When the *a priori* method of fixing belief does not work, Peirce believes there is a tendency for people to begin inquiry based upon true induction and thus begin to practice reasoning.

Reasoning is based on discovering what is *real:* it seeks *truth.* Peirce proposes that reasoning is the only method that presents a distinction of a right and a wrong way, and it fixes belief more surely than the other three methods (Kloesel, 1986). According to Peirce, truth is the conclusion that would be reached by every person who would pursue the same method of reasoning if taken far enough. This reasoning process is one way that moral development occurs.

THEORETICAL PERSPECTIVES OF VALUES DEVELOPMENT

Discussions of moral development found in current literature flow primarily from frameworks developed by Kohlberg (1981) and Gilligan (1982). An overview of the work of each of these scholars is presented in this section, followed by discussion of how they contribute to understanding moral reasoning within nursing. Fowler's (1981) work on faith development is briefly discussed regarding insights relative to values development. Kohlberg's theory, which suggests that cognitive development is necessary though not sufficient for moral development, draws upon Piaget's (1963) work on cognitive development in children. Thus, a brief review of Piaget's theory is included here. As you review the models highlighted in this section, remember that a **theory** is a proposed explanation for a class of phenomena. A given theory is not necessarily truth or reality, but it does shed light on truth. Engage critical thinking and intuitive knowing as you read, being attentive to what rings true in your own experience.

Piaget's Stages of Cognitive Development

Piaget's (1963) description of stages of cognitive development addresses how the mind works, that is, the development of intellectual capacities through the time of childhood, from birth to about 15 years of age. He notes that cognitive development progresses through four stages, provided there is an intact neurological system and appropriate environmental interaction and stimuli. Although Piaget suggests specific ages for each stage, there may be variation due to environmental factors or innate intellectual capacities. Piaget's stages are:

- Sensorimotor (birth to 24 months), including six substages;

- Preoperational (age 2–7), including the preconceptual and intuitive stages;

- Concrete operations (age 7–11); and

- Formal operations (age 11–15).

Piaget believes that there are no further quantifiable changes in cognitive abilities after age 15. According to his theory, cognitive development progresses from thought dominated by motor activity and reflex, through development and use of symbolic representations such as language, to logical thought applied to concrete and then to abstract situations.

Kohlberg's Theory of Moral Development

Kohlberg's (1981) theory of moral development was derived initially from interviews conducted with boys distributed in age from early childhood to late adolescence. In these interviews he asked participants to respond to hypothetical ethical dilemmas, such as a man considering stealing a drug to save his dying wife because he cannot afford the drug and has exhausted other possibilities of paying for it. The pattern of the responses that he observed, coupled with inferences about the reasoning behind the responses, suggested a progression in moral reasoning spanning three levels, each of which includes two stages. These levels and stages are summarized as follows.

Level I

The Preconventional Level has an egocentric focus and includes two stages. In Stage 1, *The Stage of Punishment and Obedience,* rules are obeyed in order to avoid punishment. In Stage 2, *The Stage of Individual Instrumental Purpose and Exchange,* conformity to rules is viewed to be in our own interest because it provides for rewards. Fear of punishment is a major motivator at this level.

Level II

The Conventional Level is focused more on social conformity and includes two stages. In Stage 3, *The Stage of Mutual Interpersonal Expectations, Relationships, and Conformity,* concern about the reactions of others is a basis for decisions and behavior, and being good in order to maintain relations is important. In Stage 4, *The Stage of Social System and Conscience Maintenance,* we conform to laws and to those in authority because of duty, both out of respect for them and in order to avoid censure. For persons in this level, fulfilling our role in society and living up to expectations of others are important, and guilt is more of a motivator than the fear of punishment noted in Level I.

There is a transitional phase between Stages 4 and 5 in which emotions begin to be recognized as a component of moral reasoning. This transition includes an awareness of personal subjectivity in moral decision making and a recognition that social rules can be arbitrary and relative.

Level III

The Postconventional and Principled Level has universal moral principles as its focus. It includes two stages. In Stage 5, *The Stage of Prior Rights and Social Contract or Utility,* the relativity of some societal values is recognized, and moral decisions derive from principles that support individual rights and transcend particular societal rules such as equality, liberty, and justice. In Stage 6, *The Stage of Universal Ethical Principles,* internalized rules and conscience reflecting abstract principles of human dignity, mutual respect, and trust guide decisions and behaviors. Persons at this level make judgments based on impartial universal moral principles, even when these conflict with societal standards.

This model proposes a linear movement through hierarchical stages, whereby each stage presupposes having completed the prior stage and is the basis for the subsequent stage. It is the pattern of a person's utilization of a particular level of reasoning that determines the stage, noting that each successive stage requires more advanced levels of moral reasoning. Research utilizing this framework indicates that not everyone moves through all the stages, and that few people actually progress to the postconventional level (Colby & Kohlberg, 1987). Within this framework, women seem to plateau in Stage 3, and most men never move beyond Stage 4. Kohlberg's model is generally considered an **ethic of justice**, because it is an approach to ethical decision making based on objective rules and principles in which choices are made from a stance of separateness.

Gilligan's Study of the Psychological Development of Women

Gilligan (1982, 1987; Gilligan, Ward, & Taylor, 1994) studied the psychological development of women, arguing that women approach moral decision making from a different perspective than men. In contrast to the justice ethic described by Kohlberg, in which personal liberty and rights are prime, Gilligan noted that women utilize an **ethic of caring**, in which the moral imperative is grounded in relationship with and responsibility for one another. "Women's construction of the moral problem as a problem of care and responsibility in relationship rather than of rights and rules ties the development of their moral thinking to changes in their understanding of responsibility and relationship, just as the conception of morality as justice ties development to the logic of equality and reciprocity" (Gilligan, 1982, p. 73). Gilligan's research did not say that most women think in the care perspective, while most men think in the justice perspective. Rather, as Little (2000) points out, Gilligan identified the default perspective that women use, the perspective that they feel most comfortable with and that they would turn to first. She noted that many women think in the justice perspective, about one-third of the adult population are mixed between them, and, when pressed, all people can shift to the other perspective. However, the primary group who start off from the care perspective are women, so if you leave women out of the study, you leave out the care perspective.

Gilligan's research suggests a progression of moral thinking through three phases, each of which reflects greater depth in understanding the relationship between self and others, and two transitions that involve critical reevaluation of the conflict between responsibility and selfishness. The sequence described proceeds from an initial concern with survival, to focusing on goodness, to reflectively understanding care as the most adequate guide for resolving moral dilemmas.

Phase 1

In this phase, *the concern for survival,* the focus is on what is best for the self, and includes selfishness and dependence on others. The *transition* to Phase 2 involves an appreciation of connectedness, and that responsible choices take into account the effect they have on others.

Phase 2

The phase of *focusing on goodness* includes a sense of goodness as self-sacrifice, in which the needs of others are often put ahead of self, and there is a sense of being responsible for others, so that one is regarded positively. This focus on goodness reflects an awareness of relationship with others and may be used to manipulate others through a "see how good I have been to you" attitude. In the *transition* to Phase 3 there is a shifting from concern about the reactions of others to greater honesty about personal motivation and the consequences of choices and actions. Responsibility to self is taken into account, along with responding to the needs of others.

Phase 3

The phase of *the imperative of care* reflects a deep appreciation of connectedness, including responsibility to self and others as moral equals, and a clear imperative to harm no one. We take responsibility for choices, in which projected consequences and personal intention are the motivation for actions, rather than concern for the reactions of others.

Although Gilligan does not clearly associate particular ages with each phase of development, she suggests a linear process moving from one phase to the next through the transitions. This process may be associated with cognitive and emotional development as they interface with experiences of connectedness. Gilligan's model is generally considered an ethic of care.

Fowler's Stages of Faith Development

Fowler's (1981) discussion of faith development incorporates reflections on the development of values. His insights offer another perspective on the process of moral development. Fowler refers to **faith** as "a generic feature of the human struggle to find and maintain meaning . . . a dynamic existential stance, a way of leaning into and finding or giving meaning to the conditions of our lives" (pp. 91–92). He notes that faith is not synonymous with religion and that it may or may not find religious expression. He suggests that faith development flows from an integration of ways of knowing and valuing. This perspective is different from the work of Piaget and Kohlberg, who conceptually separate cognition or knowing from emotion or affection, suggesting that logical knowing is separate from other important modalities of knowing. Fowler writes that "in moral judgments the valuations of actions and their consequences as well as evaluations of self in relation to the expectations of the self and others are difficult to conceive, even in formal and structural terms, apart from inherent affective or emotive elements of knowing" (1981, p. 102).

Fowler (1981) proposes six stages of faith, beginning with an intuitive faith in early childhood and progressing to universalizing faith. He notes that movement through the stages may not be limited to a linear pattern, recognizing that spiraling back to earlier stages may occur in response to various life experiences.

Stage 1

Occurring after the undifferentiated faith of infancy, *Intuitive Projective* faith is image and fantasy filled. The child's understandings and feelings toward the ultimate conditions of life are intuitive and shaped by the stories, actions, moods, and examples of those around them.

Stage 2

Mythic-Literal faith reflects beliefs and moral rules and attitudes that symbolize belonging within a community or family and that are taken on with literal interpretations. Story provides a major source of meaning, and a world view based on reciprocity and fairness is developed.

Stage 3

Synthetic-Conventional faith reflects a movement into a world beyond the family in which values and beliefs derive from experiences in interpersonal relationships. Expectations and judgments of significant others are very influential in determining the values one holds. Although a personal clustering of values and beliefs is emerging in this stage, reliance on those in traditional authority roles or on the consensus of a valued group for validation of beliefs and actions is common. Fowler notes that although this stage arises in adolescence, many adults remain in this stage.

Stage 4

In the stage of *Individuative-Reflective* faith, persons must begin to take responsibility for their own beliefs, values, and commitments, differentiating personal identity and world view from that of others. In this way one's own values become recognized as factors in judgments on and reactions to the actions and decisions of self and others.

Stage 5

Conjunctive faith requires an opening to our inner depths in which we are able to recognize values, beliefs, and myths developed within our particular cultural, social, or religious tradition that separate one from others. This stage requires an attitude of openness to that which formerly might have been perceived as threatening, different, and *other*, appreciating that although our own values provide a framework for ascribing meaning, they are only relative and partial apprehensions of transcendent reality.

Stage 6

With *Universalizing* faith, the imperatives of absolute love and justice become prime, and we focus energy on transforming the present reality toward a transcendent actuality inclusive of all beings. Fowler notes that persons in Stage 6 are quite rare, frequently being honored more after death than in life.

Kohlberg and Gilligan suggest that values development moves from a focus on self and survival, through responding to external forces such as perceived authority or opinions of others, toward being motivated and guided by universal considerations. They also note that it is more common to find adults functioning in the middle phases of relying on external authority as guideposts for moral decisions than to find adults who base their actions and decisions on internalized universal guides that transcend codified rules. Fowler's model acknowledges that both reason and emotional response are factors in moral decision making, and includes the suggestion that development may follow a pattern more spiral than linear. Within this pattern it is conceivable that, in response to life-changing experiences, persons may spiral back to an earlier stage and move through the stages again from a renewed perspective.

Because we develop values within a sociocultural context, it is important to incorporate cultural sensitivity into the study and evaluation of values development. Cultural sensitivity includes considering sociocultural factors that support and encourage movement from one phase or stage of moral development to another. The theorists discussed previously note that people with the highest level of moral development demonstrate actions that move beyond moral behavior based on social conformity and the reaction of others to actions prompted by internalized universal guides. With this in mind, where do you see evidence in the world today of role models from different backgrounds who demonstrate a high level of moral development?

ASK YOURSELF

Where Are You in Your Values Development?

- Where do you think you fit in each of the frameworks discussed?

- Where would you place your parents? Classmates? Friends? Government officials? People like Gandhi, Mother Teresa of Calcutta, or Martin Luther King, Jr.? Where would you place the overall society in which you live?

- Based on your critical thinking and intuitive knowing, which framework rings most true for you?

- What is the sociocultural context from which your values have developed?

Case Presentation

Three Nursing Students

Pat, Tanya, and Kuan are discussing experiences they had in clinical today. Tanya describes her distress about her dying patient who wanted to see her 6-year-old granddaughter. Tanya thought this would be very therapeutic, but her preceptor said absolutely not because there were strict rules against children under 12 visiting that unit. Pat notes that she did not even have time to change her patient's bed, but that the sheets were clean so she just straightened them out and the instructor did not even notice. She said the nurses on that unit do that sometimes when they are busy, so it was okay. Kuan says she had gotten behind too, but decided she had better get everything done the right way so she would get a good grade and not get into trouble.

Think About It

Indicators of Values Development

- *What insights into the values of each of these students can you glean from this discussion?*

- *How do you think the theorists noted previously would describe the level of development of each of the students?*

- *How do you think you would have responded in the situations described by the students? What values would guide your response?*

SOME NURSING CONSIDERATIONS

Gilligan (1982, 1987) and others (Gilligan et al., 1994; Larrabee, 1993; Little, 2000; Noddings, 1984) have suggested that there are gender differences in approaching moral decision making: Women tend to utilize a care or relational perspective, whereas men more frequently use the justice perspective. These authors note that Kohlberg's perspective on moral development tends to portray women's choices as deficiencies in moral capacities. Many authors claim that research related to differences in ethical decision making based on gender is inconclusive and that the justice perspective is used by both women and men (Colby & Kohlberg, 1987; Duckett et al., 1992; Walker, 1993). When considering developmental norms for moral development, nurses must be alert for gender and cultural factors, norms, and bias in order to avoid erroneously classifying particular groups as lacking in moral capabilities.

The literature offers an ongoing deliberation about the ethic of care versus the ethic of justice. A comparison of the two perspectives reveals that the justice framework suggests that choices are made primarily from a stance of separateness, based on objective rules and principles. The care perspective arises from natural relatedness with particular others in which the choice is contextually bound and requires responding to others in their terms, developing strategies that maintain connections when possible, and striving to hurt no one. Moral concern within the ethic of justice is with rights and responsibilities; in the ethic of care the concern is with competing needs and responsibilities in relationships. Fowler's model suggests that both are important factors in making moral decisions. Although much of the discussion in the literature focuses on the dichotomy between the two, we recognize that, rather than negating each other, the perspectives of justice and care offer different foci from which to examine problems. Offering balance to each other, these perspectives broaden the view from which to see the situation as a whole, and collectively constitute a more comprehensive moral perspective (Botes, 2000a, 2000b; Cooper, 1989; Little, 2000). As Hekman noted in 1995, there continues to be a need for a paradigm shift that requires a reconceptualization of morality and moral language away from the notion of universal morality toward recognition of a plurality of moral voices.

Because of nursing's concern for relational caring, an ethic of care may more faithfully reflect nursing's experience than a primary focus on justice (Bowden, 2000; Cooper, 1989). One of the lessons the ethic of care offers to health care professionals is the directive to meet the needs of *particular* others, recognizing that these needs are not always clear (Little, 2000; Watson, 2005). This means caring about persons as individuals and developing processes to help them figure out what they need. Part of this process is developing a caring heart, recognizing that emotions are a constitutive part of the moral life. Considering the politics of caring, these authors speak to the need to restructure our health care systems to value caring through supporting and justly compensating those who do the sometimes emotional and taxing work of caring.

Research supports an understanding that ethical decision making is a socially and culturally mediated process that involves emotion as well as reason. Findings from a study by Larin, Geddes, and Eva (2009) indicate that using instruments based on a Western developmental cognitive paradigm of moral development to measure moral judgment in different cultures may not provide an accurate measure of moral development. Outcomes of this study suggest that transcultural assessment of moral development needs to include examples of moral dilemmas and principles that are culturally specific and to include factors that influence moral judgment such as religion and culture.

Findings of a study that explored the meaning of ethics for both nursing students and practicing nurses highlighted that ethical nursing practice is a personal and socially mediated process that is lived within the complexity of professional role expectations (Doane, Pauley, Brown, & McPherson, 2004). A study exploring whether nurses deal with moral decisions using the justice or the care perspective found that both perspectives were utilized, with care being predominant overall (Chally, 1992). In this study, older nurses with more professional experience were more likely to utilize the care perspective than younger nurses with less experience. Several authors propose a possible developmental process through which growth in experience leads from a reliance on rules to guide one's choices to a focus on the needs of patients and families, which is reflective of the care perspective (Begley, 2006; Chally, 1992; Lemonidou, Papthanassoglou, Giannakopoulou, Patiraki, & Papadatou, 2004).

In their research exploring holistic ethics, Victoria Slater and colleagues (personal communication, November 13, 2000) discovered that holistic nurses blend the justice and care ethics. She notes that the pure justice ethic is about autonomy, whereas the pure care ethic is about relationships and nonviolence. The way holistic nurses blended them is seen in their sense that violating a person's autonomy (justice) means doing violence to that person. The concern about the person reflects the care perspective. They came to their ethical decision based on experience and intuition. They fit their ethical decision to the situation with a focus of maintaining the patient's autonomy, which, for these nurses, was a form of nonviolence.

We need to understand that there are different perspectives from which moral decisions are made, so that we can better appreciate our own and our patients' approaches to ethical dilemmas. We need to honestly identify our own phases of values development and ethical perspective in order to better understand personal responses to situations and to recognize more effectively how our approaches may differ from those of colleagues or patients. Acknowledging differences and similarities may prevent making inappropriate judgments about another's moral capabilities, and thus make possible better communication and collaboration in care.

Case Presentation

A Difficult Decision

Reba's 82-year-old father has been hospitalized with a stroke that has left him severely incapacitated, requiring total care. She has been informed that her father is ready for discharge, and the physician is suggesting that he go to a nursing home. Reba feels that she should take him home with her because her faith and culture direct her to care for her parents, but the house is small and would need a bathroom added to the first floor. She also has concerns about performing her father's care because she works full time and has three small children. She has considered quitting her job, but the family needs her income because her husband's work is seasonal. When visiting her father, she tells the nurse, Moira, that she does not know what is best for him, noting that her sister in another state told her it is her duty to care for their father, but her husband, who comes from a different cultural background, says it is too much to take on with all her other family responsibilities. She asks Moira what she should do.

Think About It

Justice or Care—Is One Way Better?

- *What factors and forces do you think weigh most heavily in this situation?*
- *How would you respond if you were Moira?*
- *How would you approach this situation from the perspective of justice? From the perspective of care? Do you think one approach is better than the other? Explain.*
- *How would you describe Reba's phase of moral development? Her husband's? Her sister's?*
- *What sociocultural factors are evident here?*

SUMMARY

This chapter has presented an overview of theoretical perspectives related to values development, the importance of recognizing that values and beliefs are culturally relative, and nursing considerations related to moral development. Students are encouraged to explore and critique each model of values development in order to formulate a personal knowledge base to guide their own processes of development. Each perspective provides insight into what is true.

CHAPTER HIGHLIGHTS

- Human values development, which is a product of our sociocultural environment, reflects the content and process of learning what is considered right and wrong within the culture.
- Values development moves from a focus on self, through responding to external forces, toward being guided by universal considerations.
- Moral values need to be viewed within a cultural perspective.
- Current models of values development need further transcultural and transgender validation.
- Kohlberg's model, often referred to as an ethic of justice, suggests that choices are based on objective rules and principles and are made from a stance of separateness.
- In Gilligan's model, often referred to as an ethic of care, the moral imperative is grounded in relationship and mutual responsibility. Choices are contextually bound, requiring strategies that maintain connections and a striving to hurt no one.
- The notion of a plurality of moral voices, which recognizes that perspectives of both justice and care are factors in moral decision making, is an important consideration for nursing.
- Understanding varying perspectives from which moral decisions are made enables nurses to appreciate their own and their patients' approaches to ethical dilemmas and to avoid making inappropriate judgments about another's moral capabilities.

DISCUSSION QUESTIONS AND ACTIVITIES

1. What does it mean to say that moral values need to be viewed within a cultural perspective?
2. What factors would you consider in determining a person's phase of moral development? What about a society's phase of moral development?
3. Explore in more depth the model that you think most accurately describes the process of values development. Discuss it with classmates, giving a rationale for your choice.
4. Describe what you perceive to be the stages of values development of three patients of different ages.
5. Compare and contrast the ethic of care and the ethic of justice, and discuss this topic with classmates. Which perspective do you think is most appropriate for nursing? Why?

6. Why is it useful for nurses to be aware of phases of values development for themselves, patients, and colleagues?

7. Identify two contemporary individuals or groups that you believe base their moral actions and decisions on internalized universal guides. Support with specific examples.

REFERENCES

Begley, M. A. (2006). Facilitating the development of moral insight in practice: Teaching ethics and teaching virtue. *Nursing Philosophy, 7*, 257–265.

Botes, A. (2000a). A comparison between the ethics of justice and the ethics of care. *Journal of Advanced Nursing, 32*(5), 1071–1075.

Botes, A. (2000b). An integrated approach to ethical decision-making in the health team. *Journal of Advanced Nursing, 32*(5), 1076–1082.

Bowden, P. (2000). An "ethic of care" in clinical settings encompassing feminine and feminist perspectives. *Nursing Philosophy, 1*(1), 36–49.

Chally, P. S. (1992). Moral decision making in neonatal intensive care. *Journal of Obstetrics, Gynecology, and Neonatal Nursing, 21*(6), 475–482.

Colby, A., & Kohlberg, L. (1987). *The measurement of moral judgment: Theoretical foundations and research validation* (Vol. I). Cambridge, MA: Cambridge University Press.

Cooper, M. C. (1989). Gilligan's different voice: A perspective for nursing. *Journal of Professional Nursing, 5*(1), 10–16.

Doane, G., Pauley, B., Brown, H., & McPherson, G. (2004). Exploring the heart of ethical nursing practice: Implications for ethics education. *Nursing Ethics, 11*(3), 250–253.

Duckett, L., Rowan-Boyer, M., Ryden, M. B., Crisham, P., Savik, K., & Rest, J. R. (1992). Challenging misperceptions about nurses' moral reasoning. *Nursing Research, 41*(6), 324–331.

Fowler, J. W. (1981). *Stages of faith: The psychology of human development and the quest for meaning.* San Francisco: Harper & Row.

Gilligan, C. (1982). *In a different voice: Psychological theory and women's development.* Cambridge, MA: Harvard University Press.

Gilligan, C. (1987). Moral orientation and moral development. In E. F. Kittay & D. T. Meyers (Eds.), *Women and moral theory* (pp. 19–33). Savage, MD: Rowman & Littlefield.

Gilligan, C., Ward, J. V., & Taylor, J. M. (Eds.). (1994). *Mapping the moral domain.* Cambridge, MA: Harvard University Press.

Hall, E. T. (1973). *The silent language.* Garden City, NY: Anchor Press.

Hekman, S. J. (1995). *Moral voices, moral selves.* University Park: Pennsylvania State University Press.

Houser, N., & Kloesel, C. (Eds.). (1992). *The essential Peirce: Selected philosophical writings* (Vol. 1). Bloomington: Indiana University Press.

Kloesel, C. J. W. (Ed.). (1986). *Writings of Charles S. Peirce: A chronological edition.* Bloomington: Indiana University Press.

Kohlberg, L. (1981). *The philosophy of moral development.* New York: Harper & Row.

Lao Tsu. (1972). *Tao Te Ching* (Gia-fu Feng & Jane English, Trans.). New York: Vintage Books.

Larin, H. M., Geddes, E. L., & Eva, K. W. (2009). Measuring moral judgment in physical therapy students from different cultures: A dilemma. *Learning in Health and Social Care, 8*(2), 103–113.

Larrabee, M. J. (Ed.). (1993). *An ethic of care.* New York: Routledge.

Leininger, M. (1984). *Transcultural care diversity and universality: A theory of nursing.* Thorofare, NJ: Slack.

Lemonidou, C., Papthanassoglou, E., Giannakopoulou, M. Patiraki, E., & Papadatou, D. (2004). Moral professional personhood: Ethical reflections during initial clinical encounters in nursing education. *Nursing Ethics, 11*(2), 122–137.

Little, M. (2000). Introduction to the ethics of care. Presentation at New Century, New Challenges: Intensive Bioethics Course XXVI, Kennedy Institute of Ethics, Georgetown University, Washington, DC.

Maldonado, N., Efinger, J., & Lacey, C. H. (2003). Shared perceptions of personal moral development: An inquiry in social research. *International Journal of Human Caring, 7*(1), 8–19.

Noddings, N. (1984). *Caring: A feminine approach to ethics and moral education.* Berkeley, CA: University of California Press.

Piaget, J. (1963). *The origins of intelligence in children* (M. Cook, Trans.). New York: Norton.

Plato. (Trans. 1997). *The republic* (G. M. A. Grube, C. D. C. Reeve, Trans.). In M. Cooper & D. Hutchinson (Eds.), *Plato: Complete works.* Indianapolis, IN: Hackett.

Ray, M. A. (2010). *Transcultural caring dynamics in nursing and health care.* Philadelphia: F. A. Davis.

Spector, R. (2009). *Cultural diversity in health and illness* (7th ed.). Upper Saddle River, NJ: Prentice Hall.

Tappan, M. B. (2006). Moral functioning as mediated action. *Journal of Moral Education, 35*(1), 1–18.

Walker, L. J. (1993). Sex differences in the development of moral reasoning: A critical review. In M. J. Larrabee (Ed.), *An ethic of care* (pp. 157–176). New York: Routledge.

Watson, J. (2005). *Caring science as sacred science.* Philadelphia: F. A. Davis.

Chapter

6

ETHICS AND PROFESSIONAL NURSING

[A]s we stand on the threshold of a historic event in nursing, let us repeat that we join to accomplish for nursing those objectives impossible to do so singularly. We are living in a very complicated world and with the pressures of science, technology, and societal demands, nursing must foster its image, determine its goals, and plan its direction, or the outside forces will indeed obliterate this profession.

(Zschoche, *1983)*

OBJECTIVES

After completing this chapter, the reader should be able to:

1. Describe the evolution of professional nursing ethics.

2. Discuss the meaning of the term *professional*, including traits commonly associated with professional status and the historical debate regarding the professional status of nursing.

3. Discuss contemporary codes of nursing ethics.

4. Discuss the importance of caring to the profession of nursing.

5. Discuss the relationships among the concepts of expertise, ethics, and professional status.

6. Discuss autonomy in terms of both the individual nurse and the profession of nursing.

7. Discuss the relationship between professional autonomy and ethics.

8. Discuss the concept of *accountability,* including various mechanisms of nursing accountability.

9. Explain the relationship between accountability and professional status.

10. Define the concept of *authority,* differentiating between professional and personal authority.

11. Discuss the concept of *unity* and its relationship to professional status in nursing.

INTRODUCTION

Nursing codes of ethics reflect prevailing moral values and perceptions about nursing at the time in which they are developed. The historical evolution of formal nursing codes of ethics has been a century-long process correlating with other social movements of the times. Modern views about the nature of nursing evolved from the nineteenth century, when nursing was considered a vocation of servitude, through the mid-twentieth century, when nursing strived to attain professional status. Today, views about the nature of nursing may be changing yet again. However, an examination of current codes of ethics in nursing inevitably leads us back to an examination of early efforts to establish nursing as a profession. It was through the discipline's twentieth-century struggles to be recognized as a profession that organized nursing seriously began to develop codes of ethics. This chapter examines the struggle of nursing to define itself as a profession; the historical context of nursing ethics; contemporary codes of nursing ethics; and the selected ethical ideals of caring, expertise, autonomy, accountability, authority, and unity in nursing.

The fierce debate about the professional status of nursing has now subsided. Contemporary nurses propose new perspectives from which to view the discipline. Some propose that nursing is a discipline or practice rather than a profession, and some have even suggested that nursing be viewed simply as work. Each view carries with it certain implications for nursing, but to understand the evolution of nursing ethics, it is necessary to examine the debate about nursing's professional status.

PROFESSIONAL STATUS

Historically, law, medicine, and the clergy were considered true professions, although in the late nineteenth century, nursing seemed to have gained professional status. Perhaps due to strong leaders such as Isabel Hampton Robb, American nurses were secure in their identity as professionals. Even physicians and the judicial system recognized nursing as a profession. In 1915, however, everything changed.

Abraham Flexner, an American educator, evaluated the professional status of medical schools. In 1910, he published the *Flexner Report*, which reformed medical education in the United States. Flexner developed a list of traits that he observed in the established professions of medicine, law, and the clergy. He proposed that an occupation must meet all of these criteria in order to be recognized as a profession. Flexner proposed the following:

1. Professional activities are essentially intellectual and autonomous operations.

2. Professionals derive their raw materials from science and learning.

3. The purpose of professional learning is its practical application.

4. Professions possess orderly and highly specialized education. Professionals tend to self-organize around a democratic, professional nucleus.

5. Professions are more likely than other groups to be responsive to public interest. (Flexner, 1915)

Unsolicited by the nursing community, Flexner later evaluated nursing according to his criteria and declared that nursing was not a profession. In 1915, he presented a paper to the Congress of Charities and Corrections in which he referred to nursing alternately as a "vocation" and an "occupation." He described the nurse as "another arm of the physician or surgeon" (Covert, 1917). Optimistically, Flexner proposed that occupations can alter their status by developing the traits described in his report.

Subsequently, in 1945 and 1959, two educators, Genevieve and Roy Bixler, published landmark articles evaluating the professional status of nursing. These articles utilized criteria similar to those proposed by Flexner. They listed the following seven criteria of a profession:

1. A profession utilizes in its practice a well-defined and well-organized body of specialized knowledge that is on the intellectual level of the higher learning;

2. A profession constantly enlarges the body of knowledge it uses and improves its techniques of education and service by the use of the scientific method;

3. A profession entrusts the education of its practitioners to institutions of higher education;

4. A profession applies its body of knowledge in practical services that are vital to human and social welfare;

5. A profession functions autonomously in the formulation of professional policy and in the control of professional activity, thereby;

6. A profession attracts individuals of intellectual and personal qualities who exalt service above personal gain and who recognize their chosen occupation as a life work; and

7. A profession strives to compensate its practitioners by providing freedom of action, opportunity for continuous professional growth, and economic security. (Bixler & Bixler, 1959, pp. 1142–1147)

Predictably, the Bixlers came to the same conclusion as Flexner—nursing was not a true profession.

Following the *Flexner Report* and the subsequent Bixler articles, nurses began to question their own status as professionals (Parsons, 1986). Like sixteenth-century women who came to believe the myth that women were intrinsically evil, many nurses accepted the idea that nursing was not a true profession (Newman, 1990; Sleicher, 1981). The process of examining and evaluating, though, resulted in many positive changes for nursing. Striving to meet the criteria set by Flexner and the Bixlers, nurses began to conduct research in order to create a unique body of knowledge for nursing, to move "professional" nursing education to the university setting, to become politically involved, to increase the autonomy of nursing, to extend practice boundaries, and to establish a code of ethics.

The tumult surrounding the debate about the professional status has subsided, but the discussion continues to be relevant to twenty-first-century nursing. The struggle to be identified as a profession has led to the development of a substantial body of work that attempts to describe nursing, define its boundaries, clarify the ethical parameters, and distinguish the discipline within society.

Professions have been described in a number of ways, most of which can be related back to the *Flexner Report*. Gruending (1985) describes a **profession** as a complex, organized occupation preceded by a long training program. Professional education is geared toward the acquisition of exclusive knowledge necessary to provide a service that is either essential or desired by society. These attributes lead to a monopoly that provides autonomy, public recognition, prestige, power, and authority for the practitioner. Many other distinguishing attributes of professions have been proposed over the years. These include, among others, expertise, accountability, the presence of systematic theory, ethical codes, a professional culture, an altruistic service orientation, competence testing, licensure, high income, credentialing, the description of a scope of practice, and the establishment of standards.

Professions are exclusive groups that exist to meet the needs of society. *Exclusive* means that professional groups have strict criteria for membership—they exclude all people who do not meet the criteria. Professionals are connected to each other by common experiences, language, and body of knowledge. Nurses are connected to each other and set apart from others by virtue of the prestige and mystique offered members of a profession, and by the knowledge that comes from personal and spiritual experiences surrounding the intimacies of human suffering and the beginning and the end of life.

Professions are formed through a social process. The larger society determines its own needs, and authorizes certain people to meet those needs. There is a uniform process by which professionals develop the values that lead to a type of social responsibility and a desire to meet the needs of society (Aydelotte, 1990). Professionals contract with society by promising to meet a set of identified needs better than any other group of people. In turn, society grants the profession a monopoly over these particular services. Historically, professions have attempted to instill in their members a somber recognition of the profound nature of their responsibility through the recitation of pledges and oaths, such as the Hippocratic Oath for physicians and the Nightingale Pledge for nurses.

Nurses as Professionals

Many authors have attempted to describe what it means to be a professional. Beletz describes a professional as "one bound by values and standards other

---

ASK YOURSELF

Is Nursing a Profession?

In years past, most nursing programs had course content geared toward identifying the professional status of nursing through the use of identified traits or functions.

- Have you been involved in discussions about the professional status of nursing? If so, what do you recall from those discussions?

- What (or whose) criteria were used to judge professional status?

- Based upon what you recall, would you identify nursing as a profession, an emerging profession, a quasi-profession, or an occupation struggling to become a profession?

than those of his or her employing organization, setting one's own rules, seeking to promote standards of excellence, and being evaluated and looking for approval from one's own professional peers" (1990, p. 18). Jameton further suggests that being a professional is similar to having a calling. He describes a calling as "something one feels called upon to do, perhaps by God, by some need in one's being, or by the demands of historical circumstance. A calling is central to one's life and gives it meaning" (1984, p. 18). M ng the discussion further, Reed proposes that nursing is a spiritual discipl e. She argues that regarding a discipline as spiritual enhances the meaning of a profession. Reed writes that there is a pragmatic and normative call to action that is freely chosen by its members—one in which the person is said to be "called" or "launched outward to others" (2000, p. 132).

Codes of Nursing Ethics

A **code of nursing ethics** is an explicit, written articulation of the primary goals and values of the profession. Nearly universally accepted as one criterion of a profession, a code of ethics is a means by which a discipline articulates the values that regulate the conduct of members. Like other professions, nursing has developed and enforces specific obligations to ensure that nurses are competent and trustworthy. These obligations correlate with the rights of individual patients and society as a whole. Upon entrance into the profession, nurses make an implicit moral commitment to uphold the values and moral obligations expressed in their code. Codes of ethics direct nurses to base professional judgment upon consideration of consequences and the universal moral principles of respect for persons, autonomy, beneficence, nonmaleficence, veracity, confidentiality, fidelity, and justice.

Establishment of codes of nursing ethics is a relatively modern development. In the late nineteenth and early to mid-twentieth centuries, many disciplines were struggling to develop professional codes of ethics. For nurses, this was a long struggle. Florence Nightingale set the stage for the later development of codes of ethics for nurses. In the early nineteenth century there were no formal training schools and a nurse was simply a person in charge of the personal health of another (Nightingale, 1859). Hospitals that employed nurses served largely to house the dying poor. Hospital nurses were reputed to be prone to drunkenness and nurses from religious orders were more likely to focus on spiritual matters than on healing of the body. Nightingale was the first to publically encourage nurses to be caring, to focus attention on the patient, and to follow the physical principles that promote healing. She founded the first official secular nursing school in 1860. Nursing students there were expected to be virtuous: sober, honest, truthful, and trustworthy. Nightingale's values quickly spread across the Western world.

In the early twentieth century, not everyone agreed that a code of ethics was needed. The first call for a code of ethics for nurses in the United States was documented in 1897 in the founding constitution of what is now the American Nurses Association. Although it was discussed, the association did not develop a code of ethics at that time. Fifteen years later in 1912, Isabel Hampton Robb identified a lack of uniformity among nurses and asserted that the profession needed a code of ethics. Robb authored the first ethics textbook, *Nursing Ethics for Hospital and Private Use* (1912). For many years afterwards, most nursing students used Robb's textbook.

Robb described ethics as the science that treats human actions from a standpoint of right and wrong. She suggested that a formal code of ethics, derived from the full and rich knowledge of experienced nurses, would guide young nurses. Considering the social forces of the times, it is not surprising that Robb viewed nurses' work as a ministry. She believed that nursing should be a Christian service. A contemporary of Abraham Flexner, Robb argued that nursing is a profession, but she respected those who considered nursing a religious calling or vocation (Robb, 1912).

Although the American Nurses Association (ANA) discussed development of a formal code of ethics through the years, the first attempt to write a code in the United States began in 1921. Five years later, an advisory committee suggested a code to the delegates of the ANA convention (Viens, 1989). The suggested code contained a description of the nurse as obedient, trustworthy, loyal, and adept at etiquette. This code was never adopted. Renewed interest in 1940 brought revisions to the suggested code. The 1940 version began to rely more on ethical principles, rather than rules of conduct, but added language about nurses' loyalty to physicians (Viens, 1989). Again, the draft version of the code of ethics was not ratified by members of the organization. It was not until 1950 that the first official ANA code of ethics for nurses was finally adopted. Times were changing. The 1950 official version dropped language about nurses' loyalty to physicians. The International Council of Nurses followed with a code of ethics in 1953 and other countries developed nursing codes of ethics in quick succession.

During the last century, the nursing profession established and refined an international code of ethics and codes of ethics in every Western country. These codes now serve as formal standards that have been ratified by professional nursing organizations. As made explicit by the ANA, nursing codes of ethics are the profession's nonnegotiable ethical standard that nurses are required to follow in every professional situation regardless of other restraints such as employer policy or common practice.

Current codes of nursing ethics from around the Western world are similar in content and purpose. They all reflect a practical combination of concepts from a different ethical theories and traditions. A single code of ethics may include language about duties and responsibilities (deontology); distributive justice (utilitarianism); beneficence, autonomy, and nonmaleficence (deontology or principlism); inherent character traits of nurses (virtue ethics); and other ethical ideas.

The codes of nursing from the World Health Organization (WHO), the United States, Canada, and Europe include 11 strikingly similar common themes. Each code of nursing ethics strongly establishes the following:

1. The nurse should respect the inherent worth, dignity, and rights of every person.

2. The nurse's primary responsibility is to the person seeking care.

3. The nurse has a duty to do good and avoid harm.

4. The nurse is responsible for the ethics of his or her own practice and must carry out daily actions with integrity.

5. The nurse must deliver care that is safe, compassionate, competent, and ethical.

6. The nurse must protect an individual when health is endangered by another person.

7. The nurse is responsible and accountable for individual nursing practice.

8. The nurse promotes justice.

9. The nurse maintains cooperative relationships with others.

10. The nurse participates in advancement of the profession.

11. The nurse is concerned with broader societal issues that affect health.

The ANA adds a caveat that the nurse must also take into consideration duties to self.

Case Presentation

Respect for Persons

Helen is a 24-year-old registered nurse in a federal correctional institution. John is a 21-year-old inmate who is quiet, courteous, and charming, though he often seems depressed. He comes to the prison clinic often for a variety of minor illnesses. Helen knows from media coverage that John was convicted of the brutal rape and murder of a young woman. Whenever she sees John, Helen is torn between her desire to be a good nurse and thoughts of the terrible crimes John was convicted of committing.

Think About It

How Can a Nursing Code of Ethics Guide in This Case?

- *Look at the WHO and ANA codes of nursing ethics. Should Helen demonstrate "respect of persons" in regard to John?*
- *What type of care should Helen deliver to John?*
- *Should Helen's care be related to John's punishment?*
- *How does Helen's situation differ from those of nurses who were forced to care for victims of atrocities in Nazi concentration camps?*

THEMES OF NURSING ETHICS

As you study the various codes of nursing ethics, you will notice the ethical principles discussed in Chapter 3. You will also notice other strong and consistent themes. These themes depict a number of important facets of ethically appropriate nursing care. The following section discusses the themes of caring, expertise, nursing autonomy, accountability, authority, and unity that appear in nursing codes of ethics.

Caring

It has been proposed that care is the root of ethics (May, 1969). The notion of caring developed throughout history in various forms—mythological, religious, philosophical, psychological, theological, and moral (Reich 2003a). We can trace the origins of caring in nursing to the work and writings of Florence Nightingale. However, the connection between nursing and caring strongly emerged during the advent of feminist ethics in the 1980s.

Caring is a major theme in nursing literature and an essential facet of nursing ethics. The first nursing theorist to write about caring was Leininger (1984), who wrote, "care is the essence and the central, unifying, and dominant domain to characterize nursing" (p. 3). Newman, Sime, and Corcoran-Perry (1991) defined nursing as the "study of caring in the human health experience" (p. 298). Watson (2010) contends that caring is a professional and ethical covenant that nursing has with society (p. 15). Leah Curtin (1980) claimed that the distinctiveness of nursing is located in the "moral art of nursing" in which nurses are committed to care for other human beings. Martha Rogers (1966) famously said, "Nursing is the compassionate concern for human beings. It is the heart that understands and the hand that soothes. It is the intellect that synthesizes many learnings into meaningful administrations." Clearly, caring is part of the moral essence of nursing.

In terms of health care ethics, there are two distinctly different aspects of care: "caring about" and "taking care of" (Reich, 2003b). Nursing codes of ethics guide nurses to practice both types of caring. Both caring about and taking care of are integral to ethical nursing care.

Many contend that caring about goes to the heart of nursing. This type of care suggests a virtue of devotion of concern for the other person. Caring about leads a person to *be with* the other person in his or her world (Mayeroff, 1971). It is mindful and reflective, delivered with conscious intentionality (Watson, 2002) and compassionate concern. A nurse who cares about a patient is authentically committed to alleviating vulnerabilities, centering attention and concern on the person, and preserving dignity and humanity (Smith, 1999). Moral virtues and principles come naturally to the nurse who genuinely cares about the patient.

The second type of care, "taking care of," encompasses competence in the technical aspects of delivering care. This type of care focuses more on knowledge of the scientific aspects of health care and on skillful practice. As you will see in the section that follows, giving expert technical nursing care is also a moral imperative.

Expertise

Expertise relates to the characteristic of having a high level of specialized skill and knowledge. It is a composite of knowledge gained through long years of study in an academic setting, and superior skill. Expertise is an essential characteristic of professionals. Professionals must have the knowledge and functional skills required to meet the needs of society and thereby fulfill the purpose of the profession. Expertise also helps to ensure that the nurse's actions are beneficent and nonmaleficent. Expertise allows professions to maintain autonomy because society trusts that professionals are the only ones who fully understand the work of the profession.

Nurses gain expertise in a variety of ways. Extensive educational requirements, intense guided practice, examination for licensure, certification, and mandatory continuing education are ways that we attain, maintain, or assert expertise. Florence Nightingale recognized the importance of an education consisting of depth and breadth of general knowledge, combined with a very specific nursing focus. Today we have a knowledge base that is continually expanded through research. Having completed basic nursing education and successfully demonstrated a minimum level of competence through licensure examination, we are further required (either ethically or legally) to continue the learning process and maintain up-to-date knowledge and technical proficiency. Continuing education programs assist us in this process. Our expertise is also advanced through graduate nursing education, specialty preparation, and the certification process.

Merely claiming expertise is not enough. Through the various mechanisms of accountability, we must prove that we are faithful to the promise the profession makes to the broader society. In response, society grants us the authority to practice with a certain measure of autonomy. Thus, the professional realms of expertise, accountability, autonomy, and authority are interrelated.

Autonomy

Autonomy, as described in Chapter 3, is usually discussed in terms of respect for the autonomy of others, especially our patients. But, to maintain integrity and fully exercise ethical practice, we—as nurses—must also be autonomous. The concept of nursing autonomy can be discussed on two levels: autonomy of the profession and autonomy of the individual practitioner. Self-regulation is the mark of collective professional autonomy. Individual autonomy involves self-determination, responsibility, accountability, independence, and a willingness to take risks. Autonomy is generally considered an important criterion of professional status. People who are considered professionals have the power and authority to control various aspects of their work, including goals toward

ASK YOURSELF

When the Bottom Line Becomes Personal

Imagine that one of your loved ones becomes gravely ill and needs to be hospitalized. Your third-party payer assigns your hospital and provider. Because of your background, you are familiar with the nursing skills and knowledge needed to care adequately for your loved one. The nurses demonstrate poor knowledge and lack of basic skills, potentially leading to threats to the well-being of your family member.

- How would you feel in this circumstance?
- What do you think nurses' responsibilities are regarding their ability to care adequately for your loved one?
- Discuss your beliefs concerning an ethical requirement to maintain expertise in the area of practice.
- Does the profession have an obligation to society in this regard?

which to work, whether to work and with whom, details of how the work is to be done, choice of clientele, and so forth (Jameton, 1984). We continue to debate whether nurses have autonomy.

Since the profession of nursing is self-regulating, it can be said to be autonomous. Unlike in the early years of this century, most state boards of nursing are now predominately made up of nurses. Given the authority granted by statutory law, boards of nursing enforce the individual states' nurse practice acts. This ensures the autonomy of the profession in each state. Among other tasks, boards of nursing oversee the schools of nursing within their states, control licensure, and discipline nurses.

The profession of nursing maintains autonomy through the combination of a claim to maximal competence and a continuing monopoly over nursing work so that other people are prohibited by law from practicing nursing. Credentialing such as licensure, educational requirements, certification, and so forth are the means by which nurses restrict others from doing the same work. This legally sanctioned monopoly helps to establish autonomy.

Nurses are legally and ethically required to practice autonomously. Autonomous practice serves as a safeguard for the patient, nurse, physician, and institution. Nursing codes of ethics support the nurse's autonomous decision making and responsibility. The American Nurses Association (ANA) *Code of Ethics for Nurses* (2001) explicitly calls for nurses to be autonomous, particularly in relation to their responsibility and accountability for nursing judgments and actions that protect the safety of patients. Similarly, the Canadian Nurses Association (CNA) *Code of Ethics for Registered Nurses* (2008) and the International Council of Nurses (ICN) *Code of Ethics for Nurses* (2006) implicitly and explicitly reflect nursing autonomy and responsibility. The purpose of autonomy as described in these codes is to protect the patient from harm and allow for the full benefit of professional nursing care.

Are nurses truly autonomous? We often hear questions about the autonomy of individual nurses. As a nurse, do you really have autonomy? Can you say that you are autonomous, even though you are required to follow physicians' orders? Are you autonomous, even though you cannot get to know the patients because you have too many patients and too much work to do? The argument can be made that nurses are autonomous because they have the authority to make decisions about the care they give that is within the boundaries of nursing practice. Confusion occurs because the work of nurses overlaps the domain of physicians. Some nursing actions require physician authorization and others require no authorization because they fall within the scope of autonomous nursing. This role confusion is a result of business practices.

Hospitals are businesses. They cultivate a population of physicians who bring patients, and thus profits, to their facilities. In order to prosper, they must attract and retain a strong physician staff. So, as a practical necessity, hospitals provide qualified staff to carry out physicians' orders—an essential service. Although we, as nurses, are autonomous professionals, we are also employees. When we accept employment, we implicitly agree to perform the tasks that our employers desire (except those that may be illegal, unethical, or immoral). Even so, ethics and law require us to use autonomous judgment in our practice. Institutions and physicians should welcome independent nursing judgment because of the safeguards it provides. We commonly hear about nurses who refuse to carry out unsafe orders. Such actions protect patients from physician error and thus prevent litigation against nurses, physicians, and institutions. Courts not only recognize but also expect nursing autonomy, ruling against nurses who follow questionable orders or fail to alert the hierarchical chain of command when problems arise.

Autonomy does not mean that we have absolute control of every facet of practice. Although accepted as one of the three prototype professions, medicine, for example, is no longer totally autonomous. Government regulations now guide many facets of medical care such as reimbursement levels and length of hospital stays. Managed care organizations limit expensive procedures, referral networks, and prescription medications. Today, there is far less distinction between the degrees of autonomy of the two professions than there was when Flexner made his comparison in 1915.

ASK YOURSELF

Judgments About Physicians' Orders

Nurses are frequently asked to give medications with which they are not familiar. Unable to quickly determine its appropriateness or safety, a nurse may decide to refuse to administer a particular drug.

- What feelings, emotions, and values are involved in the nurse's decision to refuse to follow a physician's order?
- What are some predictable reactions of the nurse's coworkers, supervisors, and physicians when a nurse refuses to follow a physician's order?
- What ethical principles can be used to guide such decisions?
- How is the nurse empowered in these types of situations?
- How would it affect the nurse if the drug in question is later found to be safe and appropriate? How should this affect future decisions?

Nurses do not always feel autonomous, and, in fact, some may not practice autonomously. Certainly there are nurses who spend each workday following physicians' orders and completing various nonautonomous tasks, never exercising independent nursing functions, making nursing diagnoses, or initiating self-directed treatment. In the truest sense, these nurses are only marginally practicing professional nursing. When we practice in this manner, we fail our ethical duty to make independent nursing judgments.

ACCOUNTABILITY

Accountability means that a person has an obligation to accept responsibility and to account for his or her actions. Accountability in nursing is tied to the moral principles of fidelity and respect for the dignity, worth, and self-determination of patients. Safe, autonomous practice is ensured through various processes of nursing accountability. Because society places trust in nurses (gained through recognition of nurses' expertise), and because society gives the profession the right to regulate practice, individual practitioners and the profession itself must be both responsible and accountable.

Accountability is an inherent part of everyday nursing practice. Each nurse is responsible for all individual actions and omissions. The ANA *Code of Ethics for Nurses* (2001) makes it clear that each nurse has the responsibility to maintain ethical and competent practice regardless of circumstances, stating that "Nurses are accountable for judgments made and actions taken in the course of nursing practice, irrespective of health care organizations' policies or providers' directives." As has been previously noted, the courts consistently support this claim.

Mechanisms of Accountability

Accountability is at the heart of the relationship between nursing and the larger society. The profession of nursing has developed several mechanisms through which this relationship between nursing and society is made explicit. These mechanisms include codes of nursing ethics, standards of nursing practice, nurse practice acts, nursing theory and practice derived from nursing research, educational requirements for practice, advanced certification, and mechanisms for evaluating the effectiveness of nurses' performance of nursing responsibilities. In both a professional and a legal sense, it is necessary that we are familiar with various mechanisms of accountability.

Standards of Nursing Practice

Standards of nursing practice describe the minimum expectations for safe nursing care. Standards may describe in detail specific acts performed by nurses or may outline the expected process of nursing care. Nurses are professionally, legally, and ethically accountable to meet standards. We use standards to guide and evaluate nursing care. Courts use nursing standards to guide deliberations during malpractice cases. Standards may be developed within the profession or within larger organizations.

Some standards of nursing practice are developed within the profession to describe practice and to establish the minimum level of safe practice. They help to ensure that nurses are competent and safe to practice. These documents guide us in giving nursing care, and can be used as a yardstick to measure the practice of individual nurses. They can also be used to determine whether the actions of nurses accused of malpractice are consistent with reasonable minimum expectations. The ANA *Standards of Nursing Practice* is an example of these types of standards. These comprehensive standards utilize the nursing process. They make nurses accountable for ensuring that each step of the process is followed in the delivery of nursing care. Nursing organizations also publish standards of care for nurses in advanced or specialty roles, such as nurse practitioners, clinical nurse specialists, nurse midwives, and nurse anesthetists.

Other standards of nursing practice may be developed by non-nurses, the government, or institutions. These standards describe the specific expectations of agencies or groups that utilize the services of nurses. Examples include the nurse practice acts of each state, Joint Commission guidelines, and formal policies of individual agencies. Nurses are responsible and accountable to know and follow the standards of care for the profession, the specialty (if applicable), the geographic area, and the institution.

While ensuring safe patient care, nursing standards must be practical and reasonable. Nurses in administrative or advisory capacities are often responsible for developing institutional standards. These nurses sometimes develop standards that describe ideal nursing care. This type of standard may actually create a risk by placing both practicing nurses and the employing institution in jeopardy of malpractice litigation. Because standards are used to judge nursing actions, they should reflect reasonable expectations for safe nursing care, rather than optimal or ideal care.

Nurse Practice Acts

Nurse practice acts are considered a form of nursing standards. As the foremost legal statute regulating nursing, the **nurse practice act** of each state protects the public, defines nursing practice, describes the boundaries of practice, establishes standards for nurses, and protects the domain of nursing. Courts use nurse practice acts to determine the appropriateness of accused nurses' actions. Violations can result in civil or criminal prosecution.

Case Presentation

When Standards Are Difficult to Meet

Linda is a registered nurse in charge of a large psychiatric unit. At any given time her unit houses an average of 22 patients with a variety of diagnoses, ranging from drug dependence to acute psychoses. The unit is usually staffed by one registered nurse, two licensed practical nurses, and two attendants. Hospital policy requires that the registered nurse evaluate each patient's physical and mental status at least twice per shift, supervise the administration of all psychotropic medication, participate in group activities, supervise the implementation of each patient's plan of care, and be available to individual patients for one-to-one interaction. There are additional standards that describe the appropriate care for patients who are potentially suicidal: "Patients who are identified as suicidal will be isolated in private rooms and continuously monitored by a registered nurse." On one particular day two of the patients are identified as potentially suicidal, six geriatric patients with dementia need to be fed and ambulated, one patient is exhibiting violent behavior, and all the patients need individual assessment. Linda calls the supervisor for assistance but is told that there is no one available to help her. The reader will no doubt have noticed that in addition to the other duties, Linda is required to simultaneously and continuously monitor two patients in separate rooms—a physical impossibility. Linda tries to meet all of her obligations under these very strict standards, yet while she is answering a question raised by one of her staff members, one of the suicidal patients manages to injure herself attempting to jump out of a window.

Think About It

Problems Posed by Unreasonable Institutional Standards

- *What dilemmas are posed by these standards?*
- *What were Linda's alternatives?*
- *What is the purpose of the standards that Linda is required to follow?*
- *What do you see as the legal liability created by the standards?*
- *Do you think the institution shares the legal blame for the situation?*
- *What is the effect of the standards on Linda's practice?*
- *Is there any way that Linda can meet the standards?*
- *What do you think you would do in similar circumstances?*
- *What are the ethical implications for the institution and for Linda?*

Each of the 50 states independently develops, updates, and interprets its own nurse practice act. Though both the ANA and the National Council of State Boards of Nursing have developed model nurse practice acts in the past, the laws continue to be different in each state. Some nurse practice acts are very general and are somewhat vague in describing the boundaries of the professional role. These laws are considered to be permissive, allowing nursing practice to evolve dynamically. Others list each act that nurses are permitted to perform. As nursing continues to evolve, these very specific nurse practice acts, while originally applauded as recognizing nurses' legitimate authority to perform certain advanced tasks, have become restrictive. With nurses continually expanding the domain of nursing, these very specific and restrictive nurse practice acts have become a barrier to advanced nursing practice.

Because we are legally accountable to follow the standards set by the nurse practice acts within our own states, we must be particularly attentive to the language describing the definition of nursing and the scope of nursing practice. Nurses are accountable to know and follow their states' nurse practice acts. Because legislatures meet and pass laws regularly, nurse practice acts can be changed unexpectedly. We are responsible to know even the most recent changes in our states' nurse practice acts and to implement these changes in practice.

Codes of nursing ethics address the nurse's responsibility to participate in the profession's efforts to implement and improve nursing standards. Recent changes in the health care delivery system, financing mechanisms, and roles of other health care professionals require careful study of existing nurse practice acts and judicious implementation of well-considered changes.

State boards of nursing interpret and carry out the provisions of the various states' nurse practice acts. Their goal is to promote and protect public health, safety, and welfare through ensuring the safe practice of nursing. Boards accomplish this by establishing standards for safe nursing care, issuing licenses to practice nursing, monitoring the practice of nurses, and disciplining nurses as needed. Membership varies from state to state, but commonly includes a mix of registered nurses, licensed practical/vocational nurses, advanced practice registered nurses, and consumers (National Council of Boards of Nursing, 2011).

Nursing Theory and Practice Derived from Research

A frequently cited characteristic of professions is the existence of a unique body of knowledge derived from research. Recall that Genevieve and Roy Bixler's (1959) first two characteristics of a profession relate to a unique body of knowledge. The Bixlers' second characteristic actually calls for professions to constantly enlarge the body of knowledge by use of the scientific method. In the past, authorities debated whether nursing's body of knowledge was unique to the profession or was borrowed from the behavioral and physical sciences and medicine. Responding to arguments that nursing was not a true profession because of this lack of a clearly unique body of knowledge, nurses in academic and clinical settings began gathering data and conducting legitimate research. The process of theory building and research in nursing continues to increase the unique body of nursing knowledge. The benefit of this process is twofold: First, the expanded knowledge base allows nurses to respond more knowledgeably and skillfully to the needs of society. Second, the presence of a clearly unique body of knowledge aids in validating nursing as a true profession.

Authority

The term **authority** means that a person or group has legitimate power and sovereignty. The authority to practice nursing is granted by statute, based upon the contract the profession has with society. The granting of authority acknowledges the professional's rights and responsibilities, and requires mechanisms for public accountability (ANA, 1996). Authority assumes a certain measure of autonomy.

Society acknowledges the authority of a profession by recognizing its existence in statute and granting its members the elite privilege of membership. Thus, like autonomy, authority is two-tiered. State legislatures create laws designed to protect the public's health and safety. The establishment of nurse practice acts is the exercise of this type of power. Nurse practice acts define nursing, describe the scope of practice, and grant the state boards of nursing the power to oversee the licensure of nurses and the practice of nursing in the states. Thus, the state boards of nursing have the legitimate authority to regulate the practice of nursing within each state.

Nurse practice acts empower state boards of nursing to grant individual nurses the authority to practice through the process of examination and licensure. Licensure benefits both the public and the professional. It protects the public from the unqualified, and it protects professionals' job territory by establishing a monopoly. The authority given each nurse to practice is contingent upon the nurse continuing to uphold the established standards of nursing. State boards of nursing have the authority and responsibility to discipline nurses who do not follow established standards or who violate provisions of licensure law.

Unity

There is general agreement that one of the defining characteristics of a profession is a sense of unity among its members. Unity is multifaceted and based on what Aydelotte (1990) calls moral uniformity and class ideology among its practitioners. Unity relates to the ability of nurses to organize for the purpose of fulfilling the profession's promises and the relationships that nurses have with one another.

Unity enables nursing to coherently standardize the professional characteristics of competence, autonomy, authority, and accountability. Through political and policy processes, nurses work together to meet the health care needs of society and to improve the status of the profession. The structural component of a *professional* community is realized through a professional association. The professional association provides a collective identity and serves as the voice of the profession. Unity within the profession helps to standardize the services provided by its members and provides a professional hub for members that assists with the educational and professional needs of members and performs political, advisory, and policy functions. Membership is an expectation within a profession.

Although systematic organization of professional groups is necessary to fulfill the profession's responsibilities, we also need unity among individual members. Unity involves showing sympathy, care, and reciprocity to those with whom one appropriately identifies; working closely with others toward shared goals; keeping promises; making mutual concerns a priority; sacrificing personal interests to the relationship; and attending to these over a period of time (Jameton, 1984). Nurses are members of a special group. They share language, educational background, mysteries of practice, clothing, and other symbols of the profession. Membership in the group is restricted. Nurses are connected with the group and set apart from others.

Though loyalty is a virtue, there are certain risks when we experience an overly strong sense of loyalty to each other. Jameton (1984) warns that nurses must be careful that their loyalty to each other does not supersede loyalty to patients. For example, mistakes that nurses or doctors make should be reported to patients. Because of a sense of loyalty and friendship between coworkers, there is a risk that our duty to patients will be neglected. We are required to examine and prioritize conflicting loyalties closely. Jameton identifies nurses' main priorities as patients, nurses and the nursing profession, physicians, hospitals, other health professions, and society. Questioning which of these priorities should be central and which should be peripheral, he suggests that the best choices for first priority are patient, nursing, and society.

ASK YOURSELF

Are Nurses Loyal to Nursing?

Nurses who are politically active in a particular state nurses' association report an incident that led them to question nurses' loyalty to the profession. At the prompting of hospital and physicians' lobbying groups, a number of nurse administrators participated in writing proposed legislation that would dismantle the all-nurse board of nursing in favor of one composed of hospital administrators and physicians.

- How would you characterize the loyalty of these nurses to the profession and to other nurses?
- What circumstances could justify prioritizing employer loyalty above loyalty to patients or to other nurses?
- What are the ethical implications of the actions of the nurses described in this situation?
- What should the role of nurses' associations be in these situations?

SUMMARY

Codes of nursing ethics are a nonnegotiable guide for nursing action. Because ethics is one criterion proposed to judge the professional status of a discipline, the study of ethics must include a discussion of nursing's professional status. Nursing codes of ethics were partially an outcome of nursing's struggle to meet this criterion. First established in the mid-twentieth century, nursing codes of ethics continue to evolve with sensitivity to the moral standards of society. Current codes of nursing ethics in Western countries are similar. They instruct the nurse to behave in ways that honor traditional ethical principles such as respect of persons, beneficence, nonmaleficence, justice, and fidelity. They contain underlying themes such as caring, expertise, autonomy, accountability, authority, and unity that direct nurses' ethical practice. Codes of nursing ethics serve as a foundation for the practice of nurses.

CHAPTER HIGHLIGHTS

- Acknowledgment of professional status is dependent upon meeting particular criteria that include, but are not restricted to, expertise, autonomy, authority, accountability, and unity.
- Historical and cultural influences have affected the trait definitions commonly used for the term *professional*.
- A system or code of ethics is generally accepted as one trait of professions.

- First established in the mid-twentieth century, nursing codes of ethics continue to evolve with sensitivity to the moral standards of society.
- Codes of nursing practice are nonnegotiable standards.
- Caring is a core value that undergirds nursing ethics.
- Because society allows professionals a monopoly over the services they provide, ethics demands that those services must be provided with expertise.
- Because it is self-regulating, the profession of nursing can be said to be autonomous.
- There are legal and ethical imperatives for individual nurses to practice autonomously.
- Autonomy does not mean full and absolute control over every aspect of practice.
- Grounded in the moral principle of fidelity, accountability refers to being answerable to someone for something one has done.
- Mechanisms of accountability include, but are not restricted to, codes of nursing ethics, standards of nursing practice, nurse practice acts, and nursing theory and practice derived from nursing research.
- Authority for nurses to practice is granted through the legal processes of society.
- Nursing unity relates to the profession's ability to organize for the purpose of fulfilling the promises made to society.

DISCUSSION QUESTIONS AND ACTIVITIES

1. Write your own definition of the term *professional*.
2. List 10 different occupations and compare their common characteristics. Which occupations meet your criteria for professional status?
3. Read two professional codes of ethics found in the appendices of this book. Find concrete examples in the codes related to the ethical principles of autonomy, beneficence, nonmaleficence, justice, and confidentiality. For example, in the ICN *Code of Ethics for Nurses,* the sentence, "The nurse takes appropriate action to safeguard individuals, families, and communities when their health is endangered. . . ." is a practical example of the principle of beneficence.
4. Compare the ICN *Code of Ethics for Nurses* with the ANA *Code of Ethics for Nurses* or the Canadian *Code of Ethics for Registered Nurses.* What are the similarities? What are the differences?

5. Discuss the relationship between historical and cultural influences and Flexner's method of identifying professions.

6. Discuss the relationship between the concepts of fidelity, professionalism, and expertise.

7. Discuss the statement, "To be less than maximally competent is unethical."

8. Find recent examples of case law that relate to autonomy in nursing.

9. Observe a registered nurse at work. List tasks that the nurse performs and categorize them as autonomous or dependent.

10. Visit the National Council of State Boards of Nursing website. Locate your state board of nursing at https://www.ncsbn.org/index.htm. Click on your state board's link and see if you can you locate the law that regulates nursing practice. Is your code vague or restrictive? Visit the websites of at least three states and compare the laws.

11. Discuss how specific language in your state law can be used as a standard of nursing care.

REFERENCES

American Nurses Association. (1996). *Nursing's social policy statement*. Washington, DC: Author.

American Nurses Association. (2001). *Code of ethics for nurses*. Washington, DC: Author. Retrieved from http://www.nursingworld.org/MainMenu Categories/EthicsStandards/CodeofEthicsforNurses/Code-of-Ethics.aspx

Aydelotte, M. (1990). The evolving profession: The role of the professional organization. In N. L. Chaska (Ed.), *The nursing profession: A time to speak* (pp. 16–23). St. Louis, MO: Mosby.

Beletz, E. (1990). Professionalization: A license is not enough. In N. L. Chaska (Ed.), *The nursing profession: Turning points* (pp. 16–23). St. Louis, MO: Mosby.

Bixler, G. K., & Bixler, R. W. (1959). The professional status of nursing. *American Journal of Nursing, 59*(8), 1142–1147.

Canadian Nurses Association. (2008). *Code of ethics for registered nurses*. Retrieved from http://www2.cna-aiic.ca/CNA/documents/pdf/publications/Code_of_Ethics_2008_e.pdf

Covert, E. C. (1917). Is nursing a profession? *American Journal of Nursing, 18*(2), 107–109.

Curtin, L. (1980). Ethical issues in nursing practice and education. In *Ethical issues in nursing and nursing education* (pp. 25–26). New York: National League for Nursing.

Flexner, A. (1910). *Medical education in the United States and Canada: A report to the Carnegie Foundation for the Advancement of Teaching.* Boston: D.B. Updike, The Merrymount Press.

Flexner, A. (1915). Is social work a profession? *School Society, 1*(26), 901–911.

Gruending, D. L. (1985). Nursing theory: A vehicle of professionalization. *Journal of Advanced Nursing, 10,* 553–558.

International Council of Nurses. (2006). *The ICN code of ethics for nurses.* International Council of Nurses, Geneva, Switzerland. Retrieved from http://www.icn.ch/images/stories/documents/about/icncode_english.pdf

Jameton, A. (1984). *Nursing practice: The ethical issues.* Englewood Cliffs, NJ: Prentice-Hall.

Leininger, M. M. (Ed.). (1984). *Care, the essence of nursing and health.* Detroit, MI: Wayne State University Press.

May, R. (1969). *Love and will.* New York: Norton.

Mayeroff, M. (1971). *On caring.* New York: Harper & Row.

National Council of Boards of Nursing. (2011). Retrieved from https://www.ncsbn.org/index.htm

Newman, M. A. (1990). Professionalism: Myth or reality? In N. L. Chaska (Ed.), *The nursing profession: A time to speak* (pp. 49–52). St. Louis, MO: Mosby.

Newman, M. A., Sime, A. M., & Corcoran-Perry, S. A. (1991) The focus of the discipline of nursing. *Advances in Nursing Science, 14*(1), 1–6.

Nightingale, F. (1859). *Notes on nursing: What it is and what it is not.* London: Harrison and Sons.

Parsons, M. (1986). The profession in a class by itself. *Nursing Outlook, 34,* 270–275.

Reed, P. G. (2000). Nursing reformation: Historical reflections and philosophic foundations. *Nursing Science Quarterly, 13*(2), 129–136.

Reich, W. R. (2003a). Care I: Historical traditions of an ethic of care in healthcare. In S. G. Post (Ed.), *Encyclopedia of bioethics* (pp. 349–361). New York: Thomas Gale, Macmillan Reference.

Reich, W. R. (2003b). Care II: Historical traditions of an ethic of care in healthcare. In S. G. Post (Ed.), *Encyclopedia of bioethics* (pp. 361–367). New York: Thomas Gale, Macmillan Reference.

Robb, I. H. (1912). *Nursing ethics: For hospital and private use.* Cleveland, OH: E.C. Koeckert.

Rogers, M. (1966). *The education violet.* New York: New York University.

Sleicher, M. N. (1981, April). Nursing is not a profession. *Nursing & Health Care,* 186–218.

Smith, M. C. (1999). Caring and the science of unitary human beings. *Advances in Nursing Science, 21*(4), 14–28.

Viens, D. C. (1989). A history of nursing's code of ethics. *Nursing Outlook, 37*(1), 45–49.

Watson, J. (2002). Intentionality and caring-healing consciousness: A practice of transpersonal nursing. *Holistic Nursing Practice, 16*(4), 12–19.

Watson, J. (2010). Caring science and the next decade of holistic healing: Transforming self and system from the inside out. *Beginnings, 30*(2), 14–16.

Zschoche, D. (1983). Letter calling for a national nurses' congress. In M. M. Styles, The anatomy of a profession. *Issues in Critical Care, 12,* 570–575. (Original letter December 29, 1972)

Chapter

7

ETHICAL DECISION MAKING

Peace requires that you do what in your heart you know—that your chosen values guide your actions. Peace is the means and the end, the process and the product.

(Chinn, *2004***)**

OBJECTIVES

After completing this chapter, the reader should be able to:

1. Describe and differentiate ethical dilemmas, moral uncertainty, practical dilemmas, moral distress, moral outrage, and moral reckoning.

2. Describe the process of making thoughtful decisions.

3. Discuss similarities between the nursing process and ethical decision making.

4. Describe the role of emotions in ethical decisions.

5. Recognize the moral elements of everyday nursing practice.

6. Examine the process of ethical decision making.

7. Apply the ethical decision-making process to clinical case situations.

INTRODUCTION

Each person makes decisions as part of everyday life. Some decisions seem routine, such as what to have for lunch or what to wear to work. Other decisions, like where to go to college, which job to accept, or whether to marry, call for more deliberation. Moral/ethical decisions such as whether to abort a fetus or when to discontinue life support are even more complex. Nurses constantly make decisions. We make decisions about routine matters such as patient care management and institutional policy. We also participate in decisions about moral/ethical problems. In everyday situations we may not have a conscious awareness of our thought process, but we have an innate sense of knowing what to do. At other times, we grapple with decisions.

Ethical decision making is not as clear cut as decisions made in other areas of life. Moral problems are complex. They may include intricate human relationships among disparate participants who have opposing opinions and power imbalances. They incorporate a mix of values, risks, benefits, and harms. The best solution is often obscure and its ultimate outcome is unknown until the process unfolds.

Nurses are involved in patient care situations imbued with moral implications. Every day, people in the health care system make ethical decisions affecting life and death. Research has shown that as many as 50 percent of nurses leave the bedside because of moral distress. We believe that nurses who are informed, courageous, and involved in ethical decision making are more likely to be satisfied with their work and thus stay at the bedside. Therefore, it is critical that nurses learn the language of ethics and have the courage to participate fully in ethical decision making. This chapter presents a discussion of moral problems, offers a guide for ethical decision making, and suggests approaches to dealing with the personal and professional consequences of difficult decisions.

PROBLEM ANALYSIS

A **problem** is a discrepancy between the current situation and a desired state. Problems are usually unplanned and often unexpected. They may be simple or complex, routine or moral. Before you can begin to solve a problem, you must be able to identify and categorize it. Routine problems may involve how or when to do something, which item to choose, whom to assign to a task, and so forth. When you closely examine a routine problem, you will find that there is a considerable focus on preference, economy, and efficiency. Although sometimes frustrating, you can usually find the resolution to routine problems once you gather the relevant information and resources. Routine problems are important from a personal or business standpoint, but have very little moral focus.

Moral problems differ from routine problems. They are human stories that we describe with value terms such as *good, bad, harm, benefit, should, ought, right, wrong,* and so forth. Moral problems are important, and they seem to defy easy solutions. They are complex and dynamic with elements of uncertainty and conflict. One cannot enter moral decision making capriciously because once made, many decisions cannot be unmade: they are irreversible. Jameton (1984) described different types of moral problems: moral uncertainty, moral dilemmas, practical dilemmas, and moral distress. We discuss the types of moral problems and several intervening factors in the following section and throughout the chapter.

Moral Uncertainty

Moral uncertainty occurs when we sense that there is a moral problem, but are not sure of the morally correct action; when we are unsure which moral principles or values apply; or when we are unable to define the moral problems (Jameton, 1984). This happens to us when we have a sense that something is not quite right. We are uncomfortable with a situation, but can't figure out the problem. Jameton (1984) offers the example of a nurse caring for an older patient who is somewhat neglected, with little attention being given to the patient's problem. The nurse feels dissatisfied with the patient's treatment, but is unable to pinpoint the nature and cause of the inadequacy.

Moral/Ethical Dilemmas

A **dilemma** is a problem that requires a choice between two options that are equally unfavorable and mutually exclusive. A dilemma seems to defy a satisfactory solution. The following is an example of a dilemma: An administrator has only one job opening. There are two candidates. One candidate has been with the organization for many years and is reliable and loyal. His work is consistently satisfactory, but seldom excellent. The second candidate, a new employee, is brilliant, but unproven on the job. The administrator cannot choose both even though each has desirable qualities. Neither choice is patently right or wrong, yet the decision will have important implications in the future for both the organization and the individuals. Since the future is unknown, the administrator will attempt to make the best choice based upon the information at hand.

The previous example describes a routine problem. **An ethical dilemma** occurs when options include conflicting moral claims. Ethical dilemmas present in at least two ways. According to Beauchamp and Childress (2001), a conflict can be experienced when there is evidence to indicate that a certain act is morally right and evidence to indicate that the act is morally wrong, but no evidence is conclusive. An example of this can be seen in the example of a terminally ill patient. While most would think it is morally right to preserve life, many would believe it is morally wrong to prolong suffering. A dilemma may also occur when the agent believes that one or more moral norms exist to support one course of action, and one or more moral norms exist to support another course of action, and the two actions are mutually exclusive. Health care providers face this type of dilemma, for example, when they must decide who gets the critical care bed. Should they make the decision relative to who is most deserving, who arrives first, who can pay, or who has the best chance of survival? Different people perceive or conceptualize conflicts in different ways. Conflicting moral claims can be said to occur, for example, between obligations, principles, duties, rights, loyalties, and so forth.

Let us examine different perceptions of conflicting moral claims. The nurse might perceive a conflict between adherence to two different principles, such as wishing to avoid the suffering a patient experiences as a result of hearing a bad prognosis, while at the same time respecting the patient's right to know. In this instance, the nurse might perceive a direct conflict between the principles of nonmaleficence (the wish to do no harm) and autonomy (assuring that the patient is self-governing). In another instance, the nurse might perceive a conflict of duties. This type of conflict can occur, for example, when nurse managers must make decisions regarding staffing patterns. The nurse manager will recognize a duty

Think About It

Facing Ethical Dilemmas

Put yourself in the position of the nurse in each of the examples noted in the previous discussion of ethical dilemmas.

- *How would the situation present a conflict for you?*
- *How do you think you would respond in each situation?*
- *Why would you respond in that manner?*
- *Think about a personal experience of a moral dilemma and describe why it was a dilemma for you.*

to the institution, but will also feel a duty to meet the needs of individual patients and nurses. When the needs of the institution conflict with the needs of individuals, this will often result in a conflict.

There are instances in which the nurse might feel conflicting loyalties. For example, in caring for a promiscuous patient with AIDS, the nurse might experience a conflict between being loyal to the patient and being loyal to society. In this instance, the nurse could experience a conflict between doing that which seems morally right and avoiding that which carries legal consequences. This situation can also be conceptualized as a conflict between the nurse's duty to maintain confidentiality and the duty to warn those at risk. All of these examples portray ethical dilemmas that nurses commonly experience. These moral problems offer conflicting moral claims, however conceptualized, and solutions that appear to be equally unfavorable.

Practical Dilemmas

One must be careful to differentiate between moral and **practical dilemmas**. Occasionally, situations present themselves in which moral claims compete with nonmoral claims. Nonmoral claims can often be identified as claims of self-interest (Beauchamp & Childress, 2001). Consider, for example, the nurse who must work overtime, caring for a gravely ill patient. The nurse might perceive a dilemma because she made a promise to take her children to the circus. Though the nurse might say that her duty to the children conflicts with her duty to care for the patient, it can be argued that the duties are not of equal moral weight. The duty to keep the promise to her children is a practical duty that is grounded in self-interest rather than having a moral claim. In decisions that involve practical dilemmas, moral claims have greater weight than nonmoral claims. Differentiating moral and practical dilemmas is an important facet of decision making.

Intervening Factors

Intervening factors are elements that appear in the situation in such a way as to interfere with, alter, or obstruct action. Intervening factors create a sense of mystery and add to the complexity of ethical problems. The skillful decision maker will anticipate and recognize intervening factors and attempt to gather as much data as possible. As more data is gathered, there is a greater likelihood that a rational decision will lead to a desirable outcome. In addition to the medical condition of the patient, the following section describes the anticipated intervening factors of uncertainty, context, stakeholders, power imbalance, extraneous variables, and urgency.

Uncertainty

Uncertainty refers to a lack of predictability because of insufficient evidence. Ethical decisions are more difficult because we can seldom accurately predict the outcome of a given act. Take, for example, a case in which an adult Jehovah's Witness sustains life-threatening injuries. She has decision-making capacity and refuses blood or blood products, but agrees to surgery. During the surgery, she hemorrhages profoundly. The hemorrhage is an unexpected, intervening variable. Because she is unconscious, the patient no longer has decision-making capacity. Her husband, who is not a Jehovah's Witness, demands that the physicians administer blood transfusions. The physicians and nurses respect the patient's autonomous decision; nevertheless, they are tempted to order the transfusion based upon the principle of beneficence. Of course, the decision would be easy if they knew that she would ultimately survive without the transfusion, but they cannot foresee the future. They can reduce uncertainty by gathering information about similar situations in the past. One of the goals of data gathering is to reduce uncertainty as much as possible.

Context

Context may present intervening factors. Context includes a person's unique life circumstances. Context describes the world in which the person lives—his or her culture, income, home, relationships, transportation, religion, and everything else. As you gather information about the context of a person's life, you discover the patient as a person. You learn about the patient's life and find out who the patient was before the illness. Each particular about the person is a piece of information that you may need to use when making a decision. Context is often the intervening factor that points toward one choice rather than another. For example, an elderly woman with dementia was discharged from a hospital and intentionally sent to Los Angeles's skid row wearing her hospital gown and slippers (DiMassa, 2006). The decision to discharge this woman was inappropriate and newsworthy because it ignored the context of her life.

Multiple Stakeholders

Stakeholders are persons with an interest in a given situation. As intervening factors, stakeholders can affect or be affected by a proposed action. The patient is always the major stakeholder, and full consideration should be given the patient's goals, desires, and intentions. Other stakeholders may include family members, close friends, and others. State laws may regulate who makes decisions in the event the patient does not have decision-making capacity. However, informal rules about stakeholders' input in ethical decision making are sometimes unclear. Occasionally, when making choices about an ethical problem, we are bewildered by multiple stakeholders with strong preferences. When this happens, key information may be obscured or distorted—especially if each stakeholder lobbies for his or her own interest. Consider this hypothetical example: An elderly woman lived for many years in the home of her daughter, who was kind and attentive. When the woman suffered a massive stroke, her son arrived and began arguing about what should be done. Before her illness, he rarely spoke to his mother, yet because he was the oldest sibling, he believed that he was the best person to make decisions for her. Since no one had medical power of attorney and there was no advance directive, the staff was unsure who should make decisions. They wondered if there were hidden motives that were affecting the decision-making process. The major stakeholder was, of course, the patient herself. But in this case, she could not speak for her own interests. The major challenge in cases like this is to create a safe forum that encourages people to discuss their interests candidly and search jointly for solutions.

Although we think in terms of patients' families, we might also find that health care professionals become stakeholders. This usually happens when a person with a strong bias seizes power. For example, a woman was pregnant with a seriously malformed fetus whose chances for survival were slim. Before the birth, the couple made the difficult decision to forego lifesaving treatments. Hospital policy required that a pediatrician attend the birth. Immediately after the child was born, the pediatrician carried the baby to the NICU and began resuscitation efforts. She ordered the nurses to continue resuscitation and limited the parents' access to the child. The baby survived for a short time (Nathaniel, 2003). Because of a strong religious bias, the physician became a stakeholder. This situation created tensions among the health care providers as well as between the physician and parents. Each person had strong beliefs about which option was right and which was wrong. Stakeholders in this case lacked a safe forum that would have allowed them to discuss their interests candidly and search jointly for solutions.

Power Imbalance

The preceding case is an example of power imbalance. The intervening factor of power imbalance, either real or perceived, affects the decision-making process by derailing honest and open discourse. A number of mechanisms are in place that maintain power imbalance within the health care institution. Even though nurses may sometimes be in the best position to know patients' wishes, physicians may have explicit power. Implicit social and institutional mechanisms may also disempower patients and nurses. Timid patients and their families may accept the advice of physicians. Afraid to make waves, nurses may feel constrained from expressing their opinions, even if they disagree (Nathaniel, 2006).

Physicians also feel the stress of power imbalance. Oberle and Hughes (2001) published results of a study that compared physicians' and nurses' perceptions of ethical problems. Nurses and doctors experienced problems around decision making, but their perspectives were different. Physicians bore the burden of having to make the decisions and write the orders, whereas the nurses' burden entailed living with the decisions made by someone else. Physicians questioned themselves, and nurses questioned physicians. Nurses expected physicians to make the "right" decision, even when right was unclear. This study exemplifies power imbalance that is stressful, even for those who have power.

Extraneous Variables

Intervening factors that influence decisions often consist of variables outside of the direct patient care setting. Decision makers must consider institutional policy, professional standards, third-party payers, and public policy when making ethical decisions. For example, even if you believe that euthanasia is the best choice for a terminally ill person, professional and institutional standards and the law all prohibit it. Sometimes the court will intervene, especially if there is disagreement on the course of action. Intervention of the court presents a strong intervening factor. For example, in the case of Baby K., the court favored the mother's request and ordered physicians and nurses to repeatedly resuscitate the anencephalic infant, even though all agreed that resuscitation was futile and there was no chance of recovery (Perkin, Young, Freier, Allen, & Orr, 1997).

Other Relevant Cases

Even though each situation may seem unique, there are few truly novel moral problems. Well-settled cases published in the legal and ethics literature can serve as intervening factors when they influence the decision-making process. Comparing the present situation with others in the past may help to clarify the situation and move toward a rational decision. For example, Terri Schiavo lay in a persistent vegetative state in 2005 as her husband and parents fought a highly publicized legal battle over whether or not to discontinue tube feedings. As you will read in Chapters 10 and 11, this case was very similar to the historical cases of Nancy Cruzan and Karen Ann Quinlan in which the courts supported the families' wishes to discontinue tube feedings. Although the media treated the Schiavo case as if it were the first of its kind, the Cruzan and Quinlan cases were among others that offered relevant information for the Schiavo case.

The salient difference between this case and the others was that Schiavo's family members were stakeholders with incompatible goals.

Urgency

Time itself may be an intervening factor. In certain urgent situations, you must make decisions before you have a chance to deliberate as much as you would like. This may occur when death is rapidly imminent. In these cases, failure to decide quickly is essentially the same as making a choice, since it directly affects the outcome. When you encounter an urgent situation, gather as many participants as possible and discuss known factors. Decisions are hard to make when pertinent data is unavailable and the future is uncertain. Most ethicists now agree that withdrawal of life support is no different than forgoing it in the first place. Therefore, you might decide to preserve life until such time that a more rational decision is possible. Recognize that the option you choose is the best one at that point in time.

ETHICAL DECISION MAKING

Four basic features constitute every type of decision. First, a problem must exist—otherwise a decision is unnecessary. Recall that a problem is a discrepancy between the current situation and a desired state. A clear statement of the problem is critical to finding a rational solution. A statement of the problem has two parts—the current situation and the desired state. When it is well articulated, the desired state becomes the goal of the decision-making process. Second, there must be at least two alternative solutions from which to choose. If no course of action will affect the outcome, there is no need to engage in decision making—the outcome is inevitable. Third, every action implies uncertainty. Uncertainties are elements that we can neither control nor predict absolutely. They are important because they affect the outcome. Uncertainties create angst among decision makers. Accurately anticipating, controlling, and predicting uncertainties assists with rational decision making. Fourth, every implemented decision, combined with the uncertainties, brings about an outcome. With decision making, our goal is to move from the current situation to a desired state. When the goal and outcomes are the same, people applaud the decision, even though uncertainties might have altered the outcome.

Making Decisions

As humans, we make decisions many times each day. Most decisions follow a similar pattern, whether they involve routine day-to-day problems or complex professional ones. Depending upon the situation, the decision-making process ranges from a subconscious one used for minor routine problems to a sophisticated one based upon scientific principles. The pattern for most types of decision making includes recognizing a problem, gathering data, comparing options, using some criteria for weighing the merits of each option, and making a choice. Evaluation of outcomes or circumstances surrounding the choice provides more data regarding the *rightness* of the choice. A simple example of this process is how you choose what clothes to wear each day. The data you gather includes such things as where you are going, what you will be doing, the weather, what is clean or handy, your mood, the colors you prefer, and the style of clothing you anticipate others will be wearing. You may narrow choices down to several options that would be acceptable or appropriate, and you compare these based on some criteria. The criteria may be what is least wrinkled, or feels most comfortable, or makes you look or feel more confident, or is more appropriate for weather conditions, or a combination of such considerations. Using the criteria, you narrow down options and make a choice. As you move through the day, you gather more data about the *rightness* of your decision. For example, are you comfortable? Do you feel dressed appropriately for the meeting? Are you warm enough? Does the color seem to make you stand out? Your evaluation of whether you made the right decision provides information about the strength or validity of the criteria you used to guide your decision, and whether to use these same criteria to guide similar decisions in the future.

Nursing Process and Ethical Decision Making

Knowledge of societal rules, ethical principles, and professional standards is as important to making ethical decisions as knowledge of principles related to physical, psychological, social, and human science is to other nursing judgments. But, the ability to make consistent ethical decisions requires a formal decision-making structure. When decision making follows an established procedure, the moral justification for an ethical decision can be as powerful as a scientific explanation for a medical decision. Ethical decision-making models are related to nursing care in the ethical realm in the same way that the *nursing process* is related to nursing care in the physical realm. If you understand the steps of the nursing process, the ethical decision making model will be clearer to you.

As nurses we commonly use the **nursing process** model for decision making. Utilizing logical thinking and intuitive knowing, the nursing process is a deliberate activity that provides a systematic method for nursing practice. The nursing process directs nursing practice, standardizes nursing care, and unifies nurses (Christensen & Kenney, 1995). Familiar to most nurses, the process generally includes the following interactive and sequential steps: problem identification based on assessment of subjective and objective data; development of a plan for care, guided by desired outcomes; implementation of interventions; evaluation of the outcomes; and revision of the plan over time. Criteria used in making nursing care decisions derive from areas such as knowledge of anatomy, physiology, psychology, pathophysiology, therapeutic communication, family dynamics, pharmacology, microbiology, nursing and other theories, and human energy fields; familiarity with standards of care and protocols; experience related to what has worked in similar situations; and intuitive knowing. The process is systematic and involves both logical thinking and intuitive knowing. As you will see, the ethical decision-making model is similar to the nursing process. It is a necessary tool that helps nurses make consistent decisions that are grounded in knowledge, yet sensitive to each individual case.

Approaching Ethical Decisions

We believe that nurses who are able to effectively engage in ethical decision making are less likely to experience moral distress and leave the bedside. Sadly, our research has shown that many nurses are unprepared to be equal participants in ethical decision making (Nathaniel, 2006). In an effort to make cogent and consistent moral judgments, you should familiarize yourself with the sociology and history of health care decision making and the basics of moral philosophy. You should make an effort to articulate and examine your core values and their relationship to nursing and institutional standards. In order to join decision-making groups, you should become fluent in the language of nursing and bioethics, and learn to appreciate the diverse moral perspectives of patients and colleagues. Jameton (1993) suggests that you take the perspective of the responsible actor, rather than the victim, dealing actively with morally troubling patient situations and working toward solutions to the larger problems.

Attributes of an Effective Ethical Decision Maker

In addition to the actions described previously, you can cultivate the following attributes that will prepare you to assume the decision-making role:

1. *Moral integrity.* Moral integrity binds all of a person's moral virtues into a coherent package—it creates a wholeness and stability of character that leads to trustworthiness. Beauchamp and Childress describe integrity as "soundness, reliability, wholeness, and integration of moral character" (2001, p. 35). It is a "coherent integration of aspects of the self—emotions, aspirations, knowledge and so on—so that each complements . . . the others" (p. 36). We believe that moral integrity

is integral to effective ethical decision making. The person with moral integrity does not hold stubbornly to one position, but rather encourages a climate of mutual respect and reasoned discourse. However, the person with moral integrity will not compromise beyond a certain point.

2. *Sensitivity, compassion, and caring.* Sensitive, compassionate, and caring nurses work intimately with patients—they hear what patients say and understand the meaning. They perceive the circumstances, attitudes, and feelings of others. They intimately know about suffering—from touch, sight, smell, and sound. Interests of patients become their own.

3. *Responsibility.* The nurse with responsibility has a sense of duty to the patient, an obligation to do whatever is necessary, within reason, to care for the patient or solve a problem. A nurse with responsibility, sensitivity, compassion, and caring will recognize moral problems, understand them from a human perspective, and accept a duty to work actively toward their solution. Responsibility also includes a duty to understand ethics in a way that informs consistent and fair application of ethics at the bedside.

4. *Empowerment.* Empowerment is the capacity of people to be active participants in matters that affect them. Empowerment suggests that a person has self-confidence that he or she can effect change. It includes courage and an exercise of power. Empowerment is an essential attribute for those making ethical decisions. It creates positive action flowing from sensitivity, compassion, caring, and responsibility.

5. *Patience and willingness to deliberate.* During a crisis, people struggle to understand the situation and their feelings. They work to clarify and articulate their views and relate them to a framework of values. The nurse must listen and be patient and able to live with vagueness, confusion, uncertainty, and paradox. The nurse should provide a safe environment and gently assist patients, families, and colleagues as they work through the ethical decision-making process.

Emotions and Ethical Decisions

Many approaches to ethical decision making describe a primarily cognitive process in which emotions are subordinated to reason. In a holistic view of people, however, both thinking and feeling are credible ways of knowing, each having a legitimate role in ethical decision making. Callahan (2000) suggests that heart and mind should not be viewed as antagonistic in the moral arena; rather, both reason and emotion should be active and in accord as we come to an ethical decision. Noting that emotions should influence reason while reason is monitoring emotions, she describes emotions as personal signals providing information regarding both inner processes and interactions with the environment.

It is important to appreciate not only what you *think* about what is right or wrong in a situation, but also what you *feel* in relation to the circumstances and decision to be made. If you feel discomfort, even though reason is pointing in a particular direction, then you should further explore both the arguments posed through reason and your reactions to them. Recognizing our health care culture's emphasis on technology and a tendency to devalue feelings and moral emotions, Callahan (2000) writes, "Numbness, apathy, isolated disassociations between thinking and feeling are also moral warning signals . . . the absence of emotional responses of empathy and sympathy become critical bioethical issues" (p. 29). The goal is to have head and heart in harmony as the decision is made.

In the same way that other people may approach an issue with differing moral reasoning, their emotional responses might be quite different from your own. In such situations you might see validity in the other's response and broaden your own view. On the other hand, you may recognize that the chasm between the two is too deep to bridge. Callahan suggests that such social conflicts and challenges present new ethical problems that may require dealing with the consequences of an ethical decision by repeating the decision-making process.

Think About It

The Role of Emotions in Decision Making

Consider your emotional response to the following situations and how it would affect your dealing with and caring for the people involved.

- *You work in a clinic primarily serving an indigent immigrant population, and you hear one of your coworkers comment that "it's a waste of time trying to do health education, because these people are all so stupid, and just a drain on the system."*

- *You just started working for a group of gynecologists, and you discover that the physician you are assigned to work with asks all of his young patients about their sexual fantasies.*

- *You are working in an emergency department at the local hospital, where a 2 year-old child dies as a result of injuries sustained while being "disciplined" by the mother's boyfriend. The child had previously been placed in foster care due to neglect, and had been returned to the mother's care only a week prior to this event.*

Ethical Decisions at the Bedside

Nurses at the bedside make decisions regarding issues of moral importance every day. In the next few pages, we introduce a formal decision-making model for you to use throughout your career. This model illustrates a process for using principles and theories to make those important, life-altering decisions. We acknowledge, however, that nurses make important—but less formal—decisions many times each day. These day-to-day decisions at the bedside require a consciousness of the moral nuances in each situation. Different from *ethics*, we use the term **ethic** to refer to a personal consciousness of the moral importance that guides personal action in particular situations. An ethic is derived from an individual's innate values. The term *ethic* can be combined with any morally important quality or virtue. For instance, nurses might be said to have an *ethic of care*, an *ethic of responsiveness*, an *ethic of attentiveness*, or an *ethic of respect*. As nurses seek to do that which is *good*, they call upon an innate consciousness of the moral value of day-to-day nursing actions. In a discussion of everyday ethics, Benner (1994) suggests that an *ethic of responsiveness* is central to the caring practice of nurses. On any given day, a nurse's ethic of responsiveness demonstrates respect for persons and a desire to do good for this particular patient on this particular day. The nurse with this quality responds with sensitivity to the concerns, needs, and preferences of each patient.

As we have suggested in the previous chapters, a nurse with a highly tuned consciousness of the moral importance of nursing actions engages with patients on a personal level and remains acutely vigilant to status changes. This nurse uses different ways of knowing to interpret all aspects of the patient and responds with sensitivity and caring (Benner, 1994). We mention everyday ethics at this point because we want to be clear that ethics and ethical decision making imbue every aspect of nursing. Ethical decisions are not limited to dramatic, life-altering issues. They surround us all the time. We ask you to seek to do good, recognize moral nuances, be conscious of the *ethic* that guides your comportment at the bedside, and employ the best qualities in yourself as you also attend to the ethical principles and theories that guide nursing practice. For those occasions when the larger dilemmas emerge, we offer a formal guide to ethical decision making in the following pages.

ETHICAL DECISION-MAKING MODEL

We approach ethical decision making with a problem-solving frame of reference and sensitivity to the human story. Similar to the nursing process, ethical problem solving includes a number of steps. On paper, these steps may seem linear; however, we believe they must remain non-linear. Ethical decision making is a process that overlays other dynamic biological, psychological, and social processes—layer upon layer. Physical conditions change, opinions change, knowledge evolves, and time passes. Nothing in the human sphere is static.

The nature of the ethical problem requires a decision-making process in which key facets are revisited from evolving perspectives, even as you move toward a decision or resolution. Other models for decision making describe step-by-step processes that are linear in nature, not reflecting the potential for an evolving perspective. The guidelines presented here provide a framework for entering a decision-making process that requires an ongoing evaluation and assimilation of information. This decision-making process is spiral in nature, with each step being revisited as often as is required and molded by the dynamics of changing facts, evolving beliefs, unexpected consequences, and participants who move in and out of the process. The following text describes a five-step process of ethical decision making.

Articulate the Problem

The first step in the decision-making process is to clearly articulate the problem. After you identify the problem, you will clarify the goal, since a problem consists of a discrepancy between the current situation and a desired state (goal). Ethical decision making begins when someone recognizes that there is a moral problem. If the problem is serious enough that it requires a decision, it is intolerable and should be relatively easy to identify. Once you name the current situation, there is a logical flow toward describing one or more desired states (goals). For example, if a terminally ill patient experiences intractable pain, one might describe the patient's current situation as "experiencing severe pain." It logically follows that the desired state (goal) would most likely be "being comfortable." In addition, clearly articulating the problem by identifying the current situation and the desired state will clear up confusion and streamline the decision-making process.

Identification of the problem serves other purposes, as well. You will notice that in the example above, the goal, "being comfortable," is a *state*, rather than a strategy. You must clearly identify the goal before you move toward strategies—step three of this model. Because strategies are often dramatic, establishing goals early will diminish conflict later in the process. In this case, the strategy might include increased analgesics, conscious sedation, or discontinuation of life support. When you clearly define the problem, you will be in a good position to judge whether the problem is an ethical dilemma or a practical dilemma. If you are a member of an ethics committee, you will likely eliminate all practical dilemmas at this point of the process.

Gather Data and Identify Conflicting Moral Claims

When an ethical problem occurs, gather information or facts in order to clarify the issues. Identification of the conflicting moral claims that constitute the ethical dilemma is the first part of the process. You should examine the situation for evidence of conflicting obligations, principles, duties, rights, loyalties, values, or beliefs. Additionally, data provides an understanding of the ethical components, principles of concern, and the various perceptions of issues and principles by those involved in the situation. You must pay attention to societal, religious, and cultural values and beliefs. Often, a situation you initially think constitutes an ethical dilemma will actually turn out to be a practical dilemma. This recognition allows the participants to appropriately weigh choices and expedite decision making.

Identify the key persons involved in the decision-making process and delineate each person's role. Determining the rights, duties, authority, context, and capabilities of decision makers is a critical component of the process (Curtin & Flaherty, 1982; Husted & Husted, 2001). The focal question is, "Whose decision is this to make?" Identification of the principal decision maker is sometimes all that is needed to facilitate the process. Recognition that one has the legitimate authority to make an important decision is an empowering event. Once the principal decision maker is identified, the roles of the other participants can be explicitly outlined. For example, nurses often feel the burden of difficult ethical decisions, even though the responsibility for the decision lies with the patient or the nearest relative. In these instances, the nurse serves as an advocate, a resource for information, a source of emotional support for those making the difficult decision, and a facilitator of the decision-making process.

Knowledge of moral development and ethical theory may provide a helpful framework for understanding participants and their perspectives and responses in the process. Assess how those involved fit into paradigms of moral development. It is valuable to recognize, for instance, whether the principal decision maker is at a developmental level in which choices reflect a desire to please others, and is thus susceptible to choosing an alternative solely on the basis of seeking approval. (See Chapter 5 for an in-depth discussion of moral development.)

It is also crucial to identify the participants' ethical perspectives. For example, if one of the major participants involved in discussions relative to discontinuing life support believes that it is always wrong to take a life (see discussion of deontology in Chapter 2), the process of negotiation with those who believe differently is likely to be frustrating. It would be more beneficial under those circumstances to begin the discussion by defining the point at which death actually occurs, thus finding common ground. When those involved present with diverse values, your role may be to facilitate their coming to a consensus around goals and understanding principles.

Explore Strategies

Having determined the desired outcomes, participants should identify possible alternative strategies. Various options begin to emerge through the assessment process. Participants must consider legal and other consequences. They must also determine which alternatives best meet the identified goals and fit their basic beliefs, lifestyles, and values. This process helps to narrow the list of acceptable alternatives. It is critical to eliminate all unacceptable alternatives and begin the process of listing, weighing, ranking, and prioritizing those that are found to be acceptable. Participants must make a choice among options with both head and heart, taking time to dwell on remaining alternatives and recognizing that there is rarely a good solution. Once the selection is made, the decision makers must be willing to act upon the choice.

Implement the Strategy

Taking action is a major goal of the process, but can be one of the most difficult parts of the process. It can stir numerous emotions laced with both certainty and doubt about the rightness of the decision. Participants must be empowered to make a difficult decision, setting aside less acceptable alternatives. Chapters 19 and 20 discuss empowerment in more depth. It is important to be attentive to the emotions involved at this point of the process.

Evaluate Outcomes of Action

After acting upon the decision, participants begin a process of response and evaluation. As in all decision making, reflective evaluation sheds light on the effectiveness and validity of the process. Evaluate the action in terms of the effects upon those involved. Ask, "Has the original ethical problem been resolved?" and "Have other problems emerged related to the action?" As the situation changes and new data emerge, participants must identify subsequent moral problems and adjust the course of action based upon both new information and responses to the previous decision.

Figure 7–1 is a guide for ethical decision making. Questions may need to be revisited several times and may emerge at various points as the process

Articulate the Problem

- What is the current undesirable situation?
- What is the desired state (goal)?

Gather Data

- What makes this situation an ethical dilemma? Are there conflicting obligations, principles, duties, rights, loyalties, values, or beliefs?
- What facts seem most important?
- What are the gaps in information?
- Who are the key participants?
- Who is legitimately empowered to make this decision?
- What are the issues of conflict and agreement among participants?
- Who is affected and how? What is most important to each?
- What emotions have an impact?
- What is the level of competence of the person most affected?
- What are the rights, duties, authority, context, and capabilities of participants?
- What are the moral perspectives and the level of moral development of the participants?
- What cultural factors are important?
- What potential strategies emerge from discussions?

Explore Strategies

- What are the risks and benefits of each strategy that emerged from the data-gathering process?
- How does each strategy fit the lifestyles and values of the people affected?
- What are the professional, institutional, and legal considerations of each strategy?
- What alternatives are unacceptable to one or all involved?
- How are alternative strategies weighed and prioritized?

Implement the Strategy

- Be empowered to implement a difficult decision.
- Give oneself permission to set aside less acceptable alternatives.
- Be attentive to the emotions involved in this process.

Evaluate Outcomes

- Has the ethical dilemma been resolved?
- Have other dilemmas emerged related to the action?
- How has the process affected those involved?
- Are further actions required?

FIGURE 7–1 Ethical Decision-Making Model

unfolds and new data are presented. For example, information about options may begin to emerge before all the parties involved are identified, and data regarding the ethical perspectives of the various parties may be clarified only at the point when options are being discussed. No matter how

Case Presentation

Facing a Difficult Choice

A couple in their mid-30s is pregnant with their second child after numerous unsuccessful attempts with artificial insemination. During a routine ultrasound at 28 weeks, the physician discovers that the fetus is anencephalic. The physician explains that anencephaly is a terrible condition for which there is no cure and no standard treatment. He informs them that the baby's prognosis is extremely poor and death will probably occur within a few hours to days after birth. He explains that major portions of the baby's brain, skull, and scalp will be missing. The baby will have no forebrain or cerebrum (the thinking and coordinating part of the brain). The baby will be disfigured and the brain tissue that remains may be exposed to view. The baby will probably be blind, deaf, unconscious, and unable to feel pain. The couple struggles with the choice to terminate the pregnancy at this time or to carry the child to term. They know that if they decide to carry the child to term, they will need to make future decisions about the level of aggressiveness of treatment such as resuscitation, life support, and artificial nutrition.

Think About It

Applying the Ethical Decision-Making Model to This Case

- *Articulate the Problem.* *The family must clarify the problem in terms of the present situation and the desired state. Of course, the couple would have liked to be pregnant with a normal child, but this is not a reasonable goal, so you encourage them to think about a rational goal that fits within the framework of their values. How can you assist the parents to sift through their emotions and articulate the problem? If you help them to write down their problem, how do you describe the problem in few words? If the mother says, "I don't want my baby to struggle to live when there is no hope," would this help you to clarify the problem? What is the present situation? Could you say that the present situation is a "terrible condition that leads to death"? What is the desired state? Do you think it might be, "no futile struggle"? Think of other problem statements that apply to the parents, rather than the baby.*

- *Gather Data.* *You will gather data about every facet of the case. You will discuss the biological implications of the disorder such as the potential treatments and the risks, harms, and benefits of possible*

(continued)

treatments. For example, the parents may ask if life-sustaining measures are painful to the child or if experimental treatments are an option. You will gather data on the context of the family's life. What are their religious and cultural beliefs? What is their living circumstance? You will also discuss the moral/ethical aspects of the case. For example, one moral conflict relates to the principle of nonmaleficence (the wish to do no harm). Terminating the pregnancy can be perceived as harmful to the baby, while carrying it to term may result in emotional or physical harm to the mother. Another conflict relates to the duty to preserve life, allowing the pregnancy, birth, and death of the baby to take its natural course, versus the duty to alleviate the suffering that carrying the pregnancy to term might impose on the mother. You will want to clarify the key participants and their relationship. Do they agree or disagree on the problem? What if the mother indicates that she will "go crazy" if she carries the pregnancy to term, and the father says "no one is going to kill my child"? What legal considerations would you need to review during the data-gathering phase?

- **Explore Strategies.** Once the parents are able to clarify the goal and identify possible strategies, how will you assist them to explore, weigh, and prioritize their strategies? In this situation, the parents might describe the desired outcome as prevention of unnecessary suffering for the mother and baby. Further exploration might reveal the sense that carrying the baby to term would create such anguish for the mother that her emotional health, even family integrity, would be threatened. In this instance, terminating the pregnancy would be more compassionate than prolonging the suffering of the mother and allowing the inevitable, yet slow, natural death of the baby. Abortion is one strategy. Think about other possible strategies in this case. Write a problem statement and list four different strategies. Which strategies are congruent with the goal statement? Among those that are congruent, which do you think will have a higher priority for this couple?

- **Implement the Strategy.** Whether deciding to terminate the pregnancy or prepare for the baby's birth, the parents move toward action. It is important at this point to attend to the parents' emotional response and ensure that they have other needed support. What if the parents feel that terminating the pregnancy is the better decision, but the local hospital has a religious affiliation that does not permit abortions? Imagine that they have no transportation to another hospital, a 2-hour drive away, where the procedure can be done. What is the present hospital's role? What is your role? How would you assist the parents? What are the ethical implications?

- **Evaluate Outcomes.** The parents resolved the dilemma of whether to terminate the pregnancy or carry it to term by choosing to proceed with termination. Reactions to the choice may emerge in the form of guilt, depression, acceptance, or always wondering how things might have been different if they had chosen the other path. If the parents have long-term reactions, such as deep guilt or depression, they may determine that, faced with the situation again, they would decide to carry the pregnancy to term. On the other hand, they may examine the emotional issues brought about by the decision to terminate and, in spite of the pain, they may recognize that they made the best decision at the time. What possible outcomes can you imagine for the nurses and physicians involved? What are the implications for nurses who oppose abortion because of personal beliefs?

much information the participants gather, they may make the decision with an awareness that they would like to have still more data, although having a long list of viable options may actually make it more difficult to come to a decision.

Moral Distress, Moral Outrage, and Moral Reckoning

Throughout this text, we see that moral problems in the workplace are inescapable. We examined moral uncertainty and moral dilemmas in the beginning of this chapter. Ethicist Andrew Jameton also described a third type of moral problem, *moral distress*. Nursing ethicists further clarified Jameton's types in the intervening years and discovered other complex processes, including *moral outrage* and *moral reckoning*, which are examined in the following section.

Moral Distress

Moral distress is a phenomenon first observed in nurses. As you recall, an ethical dilemma is a moral problem for which two or more choices carry equal weight, thus making decisions very difficult. In the early 1980s, Jameton (1984) asked a group of nurses to talk about the moral dilemmas they had faced during their careers. Jameton noticed that the nurses did not identify "dilemmas" according to the common definition, but they consistently described situations with compelling moral problems for which the nurses believed they knew the morally correct action, yet each felt constrained from following personal convictions (Jameton, 1993). Jameton concluded that nurses were compelled to tell these stories because of their profound suffering and their belief about the moral importance of the situations. Identifying this new category of moral problem, Jameton wrote, "**Moral distress** arises when one knows the right thing to do, but institutional constraints make it nearly impossible to pursue the right course of action" (Jameton, 1984, p. 6). Jameton (1993) later added that in cases of moral distress, nurses participated in the action that they have judged to be morally wrong. Based upon Jameton's work, Judith Wilkinson, a nurse, defined moral distress as "the psychological disequilibrium and negative feeling state experienced when a person makes a moral decision but does not follow through by performing the moral behavior indicated by that decision" (Wilkinson, 1987, p. 16). Further refining the definitions or offering examples for clarification, nearly every subsequent source relies on either Jameton's or Wilkinson's definitions of moral distress.

Moral distress occurs when a person is aware of a moral problem, acknowledges moral responsibility, and makes a moral judgment about the correct action, yet is constrained from the self-determined morally correct action. Different people vary in their moral judgment. Moral distress is not a response to a violation of what is unquestionably right, but rather violation of what the individual judges to be right. For example, nurses in the hurried atmosphere of a particular hospital's same-day surgery department report that managers expect them to have sedated patients sign consent forms, even though they know that the physicians have not fully explained the scheduled procedures. The nurses know that this does not respect patients' rights to informed consent, yet feel they believe themselves powerless to make the necessary changes. Jameton points out that in situations of this sort, it can be personally risky for staff to criticize a practice that helps the hospital make ends meet (Jameton, 1984).

Nurses' moral distress is more likely to occur in highly stressful situations or with vulnerable patients. Evidence-based studies over the years have shown that nurses who work in high stress areas such as critical care may end up with a greater proportion of moral distress (Cavaliere, Daly, Dowling, & Montgomery, 2010; Corley, 1995; Fenton, 1988; Forchuk, 1991; Gaeta & Price, 2010; Hefferman & Heilig, 1999; Kelly, 1998; Krishnasamy & Plant, 1998; Liaschenko, 1995; Millette, 1994; Perkin et al., 1997; Redman & Fry, 2000; Rushton, 2006; Solomon et al., 1993; Sundin-Huard & Fahy, 1999; Weissman, 2009). Moral distress has been documented in the following specific situations: prolonging the suffering of dying patients through the use of aggressive/heroic measures; performing unnecessary tests and treatments; lying to patients or failing to involve nurses, patients, or family in decisions; and incompetent or inadequate treatment by a physician.

The ethical climate in the facility may also contribute to moral distress. Most health care institutions are high-tech and fast paced and patients are older and sicker. Many nurses view themselves as powerless within rigid and highly structured health care systems (Corley, Elswick, Gorman, & Clor, 2001; Davies et al., 1996; Krishnasamy, 1999; Liaschenko, 1995; Perkin et al., 1997; Sundin-Huard & Fahy, 1999; Wilkinson, 1987). They perceive little support from nursing and hospital administration. Nurses may experience moral distress as a result of being socialized to follow orders, having experienced the futility of past actions, and having a fear of losing a job. Other organizational factors that contribute to nurses' moral distress include the quality of care, organizational ethics resources, nurses' satisfaction with the practice environment, and the law and/or lawsuits.

Relationships with physicians are the most frequently mentioned institutional constraints. Nurses experience moral distress as a result of physicians and nurses having different moral orientations, different decision-making perspectives, and adversarial physician-nurse relationships

(Corley, 1995; Davies et al., 1996; Liaschenko, 1995; Oberle & Hughes, 2001; Sundin-Huard & Fahy, 1999; Wilkinson, 1987). Specifically, nurses have voiced resentment when physicians are reluctant to address death and dying or when they ignore patients' wishes (Zuzelo, 2007).

Moral distress results in unfavorable outcomes for both nurses and patients. It can lead to physical and psychological problems, sometimes for many years. (Anderson, 1990; Davies et al., 1996; Fenton, 1988; Kelly, 1998; Krishnasamy, 1999; Perkin et al., 1997; Wilkinson, 1987). Among participants in one study, every respondent described some detrimental effect of moral distress (Elpern, Covert, & Kleinpell, 2005). Some nurses lose their capacity for caring, avoid patient contact, and fail to give good physical care because of moral distress (Austin, 2003; Corley, 1995; Hefferman & Heilig, 1999; Kelly, 1998; Millette, 1994; Redman & Fry, 2000; Wilkinson, 1987). Individuals may cope with moral distress in a variety of ways, including avoiding patient interaction, acting in secret, working fewer hours, leaving the unit in search of better conditions, or dropping out of nursing altogether (Austin, Kagan, Rankel, & Bergum, 2008; Kelly, 1998). Some nurses may have stopped listening to the call of their patients, having chosen to avoid engagement altogether (Austin, Bergum, & Goldberg, 2003).

Nurses experience psychosocial, physical, and emotional consequences of moral distress, including blaming others, excusing their own actions, self-criticism, self-blame (Kelly, 1998), anger, sarcasm, guilt, remorse (Fenton, 1988; Wilkinson, 1987), frustration, sadness, withdrawal, avoidance behavior, powerlessness, dispiritedness (Austin et al., 2003), burnout (Davies et al., 1996), betrayal of personal values, sense of insecurity, self-doubt, unease (Deady & McCarthy, 2010), low self-worth (Krishnasamy, 1999), and effects on spirituality (Elpern et al., 2005). Nurses may also choose to desensitize themselves by adapting or acquiescing to cultural pressures or by rationalizing, denying, or trivializing or distancing themselves from moral problems (Deady & McCarthy, 2010). In addition, evidence suggests that prolonged or repeated moral distress leads to loss of nurses' moral integrity (Kelly, 1998; Rushton, 1995; Wilkinson, 1987). Physical reactions to moral distress include weeping (Anderson, 1990; Fenton, 1988), sweating, palpitations, headaches, diarrhea, and sleep disturbances (Austin, 2003; Anderson, 1990; Wilkinson, 1987). Emotional reactions include anger, frustration, depression, shame, embarrassment, grief, sadness, and a sense of ineffectiveness (Austin et al., 2008).

Possibly heralding the nursing shortage, early studies indicated that up to 50 percent of nurses leave their units or nursing altogether because of morally troubling situations (Millette, 1994; Nathaniel, 2006;

Wilkinson, 1987). The nursing shortage is an indirect but strong threat that may perpetuate moral distress. Nurses report poor working conditions such as inadequate staffing, heavy workloads, increased use of overtime, and lack of sufficient support staff (General Accounting Office, 2001). As many as three-fourths of RNs believe the nursing shortage diminishes the quality of their work life and the quality of patient care. Nurses predict that the continuing nursing shortage will increase stress on nurses, lower patient care quality, and cause nurses to leave the profession (Buerhaus et al., 2005). Some research indicates that working in conditions with perceived unsafe staffing is the most distressing situation nurses face (Zuzelo, 2007). The situation creates a self-perpetuating downward spiral: the nursing shortage leads to moral distress, which causes more nurses to leave the workforce.

Researchers have been busy for the past 30 years examining the phenomenon of moral distress. Qualitative and quantitative research sheds light on the process and products of this troubling condition and suggests implications for practice. This is one facet of ethics that offers an opportunity for evidence-based practice.

Moral Outrage

Moral outrage occurs when someone else in the health care setting performs an act the nurse believes to be immoral (Wilkinson, 1987). In cases of moral outrage, nurses do not participate in the act, and therefore do not believe they are responsible for wrong, but perceive that they are powerless to prevent it. The nurse is more likely to be on the fringes of the moral situation rather than directly involved. For example, the charge nurse on a

ASK YOURSELF

Have You Experienced Moral Distress?

Moral distress occurs when moral problems seem to have clear solutions, yet institutional or other restraints prohibit morally correct action. This may occur in everyday life. For example, think about a used car salesperson who is encouraged to sell high-priced cars that are in poor condition. Think about a situation in which you or someone you know experienced moral distress.

- What were the circumstances?
- How did the person feel?
- How did the person resolve the distress?

medical/surgical floor on the evening shift is working at the desk when the nursing supervisor comes to the floor to use the telephone to call a hospital administrator. The charge nurse overhears the supervisor describing a situation in which a physician endangered a patient when he insisted on performing a surgical procedure in the hospital room. The surgeon was in a hurry and felt the patient would be safe, even though there were violations of patient privacy, informed consent, and safety. The charge nurse is uninvolved in the situation, but recognizes a grave moral problem.

Moral Reckoning

Moral distress and moral outrage are components of the larger process of **moral reckoning** that spans many nurses' careers (Nathaniel, 2006). Moral reckoning is a three-stage process that includes a critical juncture (Figure 7–2). After the initial novice period, the nurse begins professional life in a stage of ease in which there is comfort with rules and expectations. The nurse knows what is expected and has technical skill and a sense of at-homeness in the workplace. Internal and external values and expectations are congruent. Core values, professional norms, and institutional norms complement each other, or at least do not conflict. Unexpectedly, a situational bind with moral implications occurs in a particular patient care situation. The nurse's core beliefs come into irreconcilable conflict with social or institutional norms. This constitutes a critical juncture that forces the nurse out of the stage of ease and into the stage of resolution. At this point, the nurse attempts to resolve the conflict by choosing among conflicting values. Immediate and long-term resolution includes either giving up or making a stand. The nurse then moves into the stage of reflection, during which time he or she repeatedly examines past beliefs, values, and actions. At this point, the nurse tries to make sense of his or her experiences through remembering, telling the story, examining conflicts, and living with the consequences.

Stage of Ease

As illustrated in Figure 7–2, certain conditions are foundational to the **stage of ease**, the initial stage of moral reckoning. Conditions integral to the stage of ease include the properties of (a) *becoming*, which signifies core beliefs and values of the individual; (b) *professionalizing*, which relates to inculcation of the professional norms; (c) *institutionalizing*, which signifies the process of internalizing institutional social norms; and (d) *working*, the unique experience of the work of nursing. Conflicts between and among the conditions work together during a critical incident to produce a situational bind.

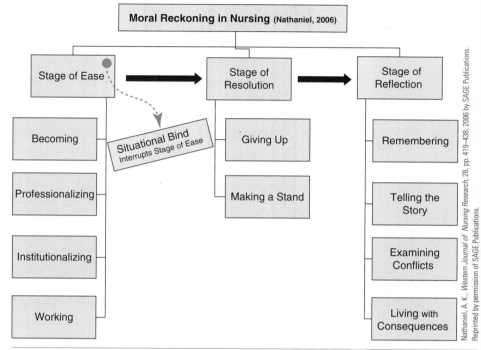

Nathaniel, A. K., *Western Journal of Nursing Research*, 28, pp. 419–438, 2006 by SAGE Publications. Reprinted by permission of SAGE Publications.

FIGURE 7–2   Moral Reckoning Model

Through the process of *becoming*, every person evolves a set of core beliefs and values, which are a product of lifelong learning about what is important and how to behave in society. Core beliefs evolve through experience, and from the modeling of parents, teachers, ministers, peers, and so forth.

In nursing school and in early practice, young nurses learn certain behavioral norms—they are *professionalized*. These professional norms are ideals about what a good nurse should be or do. For the most part, professional norms complement core beliefs. Nursing's moral norms include "the protection and enhancement of human dignity, the alleviation of vulnerability, the promotion of growth and health, and the enhancement of coping and comfort in the face of hardship" (Penticuff, 1997, p. 51). For some, professional norms might also include implicit rules such as the following: follow physicians' orders, complete assigned work with expert skill, and remain altruistic. Other implicit mores include "do not cry while on duty; be strong for the patient and for other nurses, do not let emotions interfere with the tasks to be done; [and] refrain from getting emotionally involved with your patients and their families" (Davies et al., 1996, p. 502).

When they become employed, nurses are *institutionalized*—they learn implicit and explicit institutional rules. Sometimes institutional norms are congruent with nurses' core beliefs and professional norms, and sometimes they are not. Explicit institutional norms include completing a job according to institutional standards and respecting lines of authority. Implicit institutional norms might include assuring that the business makes a profit, following orders, and handling crises without making waves.

The work of nursing is varied, challenging, and rewarding. Nurses' descriptions of the *work of nursing* include vivid sensual descriptions and heart-wrenching stories. The work of nursing requires technical skill and attendance to many facets of patients' lives. The work of nursing includes knowing the patients, witnessing their suffering, accepting the responsibility to care, desiring to do the work well, and knowing what to do. The conditions of *becoming, professionalizing, institutionalizing,* and *the work of nursing* are held in fragile balance as nurses enjoy the stage of ease.

During the stage of ease, core beliefs and values motivate nurses to uphold congruent professional and institutional norms. Nurses gain technical skills and feel rewarded. They know what their managers expect, and they feel a sense of confidence. During this stage, nurses have high standards and are proud of their abilities. The stage of ease may continue indefinitely, but for some, a morally troubling event will challenge the integration of core beliefs with professional and institutional norms. In those cases, nurses find themselves in *situational binds* that lead to changes in their professional lives.

Situational Binds

Sometimes, a morally troubling patient situation arises that places the nurse in a situational bind. The **situational bind** interrupts the stage of ease and causes turmoil when a nurse's core beliefs and other claims conflict. The turmoil may meet or exceed the traditional definitions of moral distress. Binds involve serious and complex conflicts involving professional relationships, divergent values, workplace demands, and other forces with moral overtones. Types of situational binds that occur most frequently include causing needless suffering by prolonging the life of dying patients or performing unnecessary tests and treatments, especially on terminal patients; lying to patients; incompetent or inadequate treatment by a physician; and coercing consent from poorly informed patients (Bassett, 1995; Corley, 1995; Nathaniel, 2003; Rodney, 1988; Wilkinson, 1987). When situational binds occur, nurses must make critical decisions—choosing one value or belief over another.

Often nurses' ability to follow through with their moral convictions is constrained. Wilkinson (1987) found that the external constraints nurses mentioned most often were physicians, the law or lawsuits, nursing administration, and hospital administration and policies. Nurses also experience internal constraints such as socialization to follow orders, self-doubt, and lack of courage (Nathaniel, 2006). Wilkinson (1987) and Anderson (1990) also found that nurses identified the constraints of futility of past actions and fear of job loss, particularly in non-responsive or defensive organizations.

Nurses often experience distress related to conflicting loyalties to patients, nursing peers, physicians, and institutions. In fact, loyalty may be a factor in determining the severity of nurses' distress. Conflict is strongest for nurses who take seriously their responsibilities, yet also have close bonds of allegiance and commitment to the profession, to colleagues, and to the organization (Anderson, 1990).

Sometimes professional or institutional expectations challenge core beliefs. For example, a nurse talked about a mentally competent patient who had a "no code" order. Because he experienced extreme discomfort when the nurses suctioned his nasotracheal tube, he refused the procedure. When he attempted to protect himself from the pain of suctioning, the nurse followed physicians' orders and tied his arms before suctioning him. In this case, the nurse was in a bind caused when actions prescribed by the profession and institution (suctioning excess respiratory secretions) conflicted with respecting the patient's wishes, which seemed to her to be the morally correct action (Nathaniel, 2003).

Nurses perceive themselves to be in binds when they recognize a problem, but cannot convince anyone about the problem or its solution. They may believe they are not part of the decision-making process. Some nurses feel that they do not have a voice as they struggle against authorities. For example, Andrews and Waterman (2005) described situations in which nurses recognized that patients' conditions were deteriorating, but encountered difficulty convincing physicians.

In some instances, nurses know the professional and institutional standards and are aware of their own core beliefs, yet are unable to uphold them because of workplace deficiencies. Workplace deficiencies might include chronic staff shortages and substandard equipment.

The Stage of Resolution

Nurses tell stories about how moral reckoning changes their lives. The move to set things right signifies the beginning of the stage of resolution. For many, this stage changes their professional futures. During this stage, nurses will either make a stand or give up. When confronted with a situational bind, some nurses decide to make a stand. Making a stand takes a variety forms—all of which include professional risk. They may refuse to follow physicians' orders, initiate negotiations, break the rules, whistle blow, and so forth. Sometimes nurses resolve a situational bind by giving up. In general, nurses give up because they recognize the futility of making a stand. They are unwilling to sacrifice themselves to no avail. They may also give up to protect themselves or to find a place where they can live with better integration of their beliefs and professional norms. Giving up includes participating with regret in an activity they consider to be morally wrong, leaving the unit or resigning, or leaving the profession altogether. Sometimes nurses seem to give up in the short term, but move toward preparing themselves for more advanced or autonomous roles or toward leadership positions—all of which prepare them to make a stand, on principle, in the future.

Stage of Reflection

Afterwards, nurses spend time thinking about their actions. The stage of reflection may last a lifetime and includes *remembering, telling the story, examining conflicts,* and *living with consequences.* These are interrelated and seem to occur in every instance of moral reckoning. Nurses retain vivid mental pictures. These memories evoke emotions many years later. As one nurse said, "I don't let go of it." Nurses invariably describe the sights, sounds, and smells. Even after 15 or 20 years, they are able to remember patients' faces, exact locations of the patients' beds, and sometimes a patient's position in bed. They remember particulars about patients such as their names, ages, and diagnoses (Nathaniel, 2006). Nurses also experience evoked emotion after many years, including feelings of guilt and self-blame, lingering sadness, anger, and anxiety.

Nurses continue the process of *moral reckoning* over time—telling and re-telling the story as they try to make sense of it. As they tell their stories, they examine conflicts in the situation. They examine their values and ask themselves questions about what actually happened, who was to blame, and how they can avoid similar situations in the future. As they think about the conflicts, some set limits or make decisions about future actions. Some identify new boundaries. Moral reckoning continues for a prolonged period. Nurses may move from one institution to another or from one specialty area to another. They may seek further education, many times intending to correct the type of moral wrongs they experienced in the past. Many leave the bedside.

Ways to Anticipate, Minimize, and Control Moral Reckoning

In order to anticipate and deal with moral problems in the workplace, you should internalize nursing codes of ethics and purposefully utilize nursing ethics in your practice. An effective form of ethics allows for consideration of the uniqueness and particularity of each patient and each situation, while acknowledging diverse moral perspectives. You should come to understand other professions' perspectives as different, yet complementary, understandings of reality. Nursing ethics should bind participants in shared symbolism, meaning, and purpose. It should recognize gender differences and discard gender and social bias. It should encompass the value of caring, which is integral to the profession of nursing, along with the value of curing, which is important to the profession of medicine. Nursing ethics should bring together men and women, physicians and nurses, patients and providers.

Case Presentation

Trying to Be Heard

Joanna is an experienced nurse. She has worked on the same medical-surgical unit for the past 15 years. During a Saturday night shift, Mrs. Kelly, an 82-year-old patient diagnosed with COPD, complains of abdominal pain. Joanna assesses Mrs. Kelly, who has been a patient on the unit many times in the past. The patient's vital signs are within normal limits and there is no significant change from past readings. However, Joanna still feels uneasy. Not only does Mrs. Kelly complain of pain, but also she looks sick to Joanna, who senses there is something seriously wrong. Joanna calls the medical resident, who tells her to call back if there are any changes in the vital signs. As the shift progresses, Joanna becomes more convinced that Mrs. Kelly is seriously ill. Although there are no changes in Mrs. Kelly's vital signs, she calls the resident a second time. The resident yells at Joanna and tells her to stop bothering him. After a couple of hours, Joanna decides to call her supervisor, who checks Mrs. Kelly and encourages Joanna to "get a grip." Joanna repeatedly checks on Mrs. Kelly, who remains awake throughout the night. The next morning, Joanna reports her assessment to the charge nurse and asks her make sure someone evaluates Mrs. Kelly's abdominal pain. The charge nurse responds, "Don't worry about her. If there is anything seriously wrong, she will let us know." When Joanna returns after 2 days off, she learns that Mrs. Kelly died on Sunday evening of a ruptured abdominal aortic aneurism. Joanna spends that evening crying at the nurses' station, barely able to take care of her patients.

Think About It

- *What is the ethical problem in this case?*
- *Were Joanna's actions sufficient?*
- *What were the institutional and professional constraints to action?*
- *How could Joanna have responded to the situation in a way that would result in a better outcome?*
- *Would you label Joanna's reaction as moral distress or moral reckoning? Why?*
- *How could Joanna prevent a similar situation in the future?*

With sufficient preparation, you should develop strategies to become more self-aware and to establish effective intra- and interprofessional relationships. You should closely examine implicit professional and institutional messages that inhibit meaningful dialogue and sustain conflict and power imbalance. You should learn strategies and language that prepare you to participate in ethical dialogue with other professionals and to deal with the realities of day-to-day practice.

To help anticipate sources of moral problems, you should uncover potential sources of conflict between core beliefs, professional traditions, and institutional expectations. You should prepare yourself to deal with situational binds related to asymmetrical power relationships, loyalty conflicts, and workplace deficiencies. If you are able deal with these problems in imagination, you may find better ways to avoid them or deal with them when they occur in the workplace. You might also prepare for the stage of resolution and its properties, giving up and making a stand. If you anticipate these ways to resolve moral conflicts, you may be better prepared to follow integrity-preserving courses of action when situations arise.

If you are an administrator, you should institute programs that encourage autonomy and collaboration in ethical decision making and implement strategies to support nurses who experience moral distress. As suggested in the recent literature, effective strategies include facilitating dialogue, encouraging nurses to be active participants in clinical and ethical decision making, developing support systems, providing opportunities for professional development, strengthening collaborative teamwork, and identifying and eliminating systematic patterns of dominance and subordination based on gender, race, and ethnicity (Donchin, 2001; Erlen, 2001; Hamric, 2000). Additionally, as suggested by Jameton (1992), you should budget nursing time for interpersonal care and facilitate dialogue in which nurses and physicians learn to understand and appreciate the other discipline's jobs and ethical perspectives.

SUMMARY

Ethical decision making requires knowledge and attention to many factors. Determining the existence of an ethical dilemma is the beginning step in the process that includes defining the problem, identifying desired objectives, listing and evaluating alternatives, choosing the best course of action based on one's knowledge and the current circumstances, and evaluating the outcomes of the action taken. One must consider both reason and emotion in making ethical decisions. Nurses are encouraged to utilize the decision-making process described in this chapter as a guide in dealing with dilemmas encountered in clinical settings. As with every other nursing skill, comfort and competency with ethical decision making comes with repeated practice.

CHAPTER HIGHLIGHTS

- Dilemmas exist when difficult problems have no satisfactory solutions or when all the solutions appear equally unfavorable.
- In decisions involving practical dilemmas, moral claims hold greater weight than nonmoral claims.
- Making thoughtful decisions in any arena follows a pattern that includes gathering data, comparing options based on particular criteria, making and acting on a choice, and evaluating outcomes or circumstances surrounding the choice.
- One's value system affects how one defines and deals with an ethical issue; thus, resolution of ethical dilemmas requires determining the ethical issue at hand and identifying the value systems of those involved.
- Both emotion and reason have legitimate roles in ethical decision making.
- Ethical decision making requires ongoing evaluation and assimilation of information, with revisiting of various steps in the process as often as required by the dynamics of changing facts, evolving beliefs, unexpected consequences, and participants moving in and out of the process.
- Familiarity with and practice in applying ethical decision making enables the nurse to develop competence and confidence with the process.

DISCUSSION QUESTIONS AND ACTIVITIES

1. Search an online database for full-text articles related to nurses' ethical decision making. How do other models compare to the one presented in this text?
2. Working in small groups, discuss ethical and practical dilemmas that you have experienced, then choose an example of each type of dilemma to illustrate for the class.
3. Describe a situation in which you or someone you know experienced moral distress, noting moral and nonmoral claims in the situation.
4. Talk with practicing nurses about their experiences of ethical dilemmas. Identify their approaches to dealing with such dilemmas, including their processes of ethical decision making.

5. Debate with classmates the role of reason and emotion in ethical decisions.

6. Use the ethical decision-making process to revisit an ethical dilemma that you have encountered in the past, or to guide you through a current dilemma. Examine your sense of comfort with each part of the process, noting areas of strength and areas needing more practice.

7. Discuss the interaction among moral development, moral perspective, and ethical decision making.

8. How would you approach an ethical dilemma in which the parties involved exhibit different moral perspectives?

9. How might legal considerations affect the process of making ethical decisions?

REFERENCES

Anderson, S. L. (1990). Patient advocacy and whistle-blowing in nursing: Help for the helpers. *Nursing Forum, 25*(3), 5–13.

Andrews, T., & Waterman, H. (2005). Visualizing deteriorating conditions. *Grounded Theory Review, 4*(2), 63–94.

Austin, W. J., Bergum, V., & Goldberg, L. (2003). Unable to answer the call of our patients: Mental health nurses' experience of moral distress. *Nursing Inquiry, 10*(3), 177–183.

Austin, W. J., Kagan, L., Rankel, M., & Bergum, V. (2008). The balancing act: Psychiatrists' experience of moral distress. *Medicine, Health Care, and Philosophy, 11*(1), 89–97.

Bassett, C. C. (1995). Critical care nurses: Ethical dilemmas a phenomenological perspective. *Care of the Critically Ill, 11*(4), 166, 168–169.

Beauchamp, T. L., & Childress, J. F. (2001). *Principles of biomedical ethics* (5th ed.). New York: Oxford University Press.

Benner, P. (1994). Discovering challenges to ethical theory in experience-based narratives of nurses' everyday ethical comportment. In J. F. Monagle & D. C. Thomasma (Eds.), *Health care ethics: Critical issues.* Gaithersburg, MD: Aspen Publishers.

Buerhaus, P. I., Donelan, K., Ulrich, B. T., Norman, L., Williams, M., & Dittus, R. (2005). Hospital RNs' and CNOs' perceptions of the impact of the nursing shortage on the quality of care. *Nursing Economic$, 23*(5), 214–221, 211.

Callahan, S. (2000). The role of emotions in ethical decision making. In J. H. Howell & W. F. Sale (Eds.), *Life choices: A Hastings Center introduction to bioethics* (2nd ed.). Washington, DC: Georgetown University Press.

Cavaliere, T. A., Daly, B., Dowling, D., & Montgomery, K. (2010). Moral distress in neonatal intensive care unit RNs. *Advances in Neonatal Care (Elsevier Science), 10*(3), 145–156.

Chinn, P. L. (2004). *Peace and power: Building communities for the future* (6th ed.). Boston: Jones & Bartlett.

Christensen, P. J., & Kenney, J. W. (1995). *Nursing process: Application of conceptual models* (4th ed.). St. Louis, MO: Mosby.

Corley, M. C. (1995). Moral distress of critical care nurses. *American Journal of Critical Care, 4*(4), 280–285.

Corley, M. C., Elswick, R. K., Gorman, M., & Clor, T. (2001). Development and evaluation of a moral distress scale. *Journal of Advanced Nursing, 33*(2), 250–256.

Curtin, L., & Flaherty, M. J. (1982). *Nursing ethics: Theories and pragmatics.* Bowie, MD: Brady.

Davies, B., Clarke, D., Connaughty, S., Cook, K., MacKenzie, B., McCormick, J., . . . Stutzer, C. (1996). Caring for dying children: Nurses' experiences. *Pediatric Nursing, 22*, 500–507.

Deady, R., & McCarthy, J. (2010). A study of the situations, features, and coping mechanisms experienced by Irish psychiatric nurses experiencing moral distress. *Perspectives in Psychiatric Care, 46*(3), 209–220.

DiMassa, C. M. (2006, March 23). Alleged skid row dumping is captured on videotape [Electronic Version]. *Los Angeles Times.* Retrieved July 25, 2006, from http://articles.latimes.com/2006/mar/23/local/me-dumping23

Donchin, A. (2001). Understanding autonomy relationally: Toward a reconfiguration of bioethical principles. *Journal of Medicine and Philosophy, 26*, 365–386.

Elpern, E. H., Covert, B., & Kleinpell, R. (2005). Moral distress of staff nurses in a medical intensive care unit. *American Journal of Critical Care, 14*(6), 523–530.

Erlen, J. A. (2001). Moral distress: A pervasive problem [Electronic version]. *Orthopaedic Nursing, 20*(2), 76–79.

Fenton, M. (1988). Moral distress in clinical practice: Implications for the nurse administrator. *Canadian Journal of Nursing Administration, 1*, 8–11.

Forchuk, C. (1991). Ethical problems encountered by mental health nurses. *Issues in Mental Health Nursing, 12*(4), 375–383.

Gaeta, S., & Price, K. J. (2010). End-of-life issues in critically ill cancer patients. *Critical Care Clinics, 26*(1), 219–227.

General Accounting Office. (2001). *Nursing workforce: Emerging nurse shortages due to multiple factors. Report to the Chairman, Subcommittee on Health, Committee on Ways and Means, House of Representatives* (GAO-01-944). Washington, DC.

Hamric, A. B. (2000). Moral distress in everyday ethics. *Nursing Outlook, 48,* 199–201.

Hefferman, P., & Heilig, S. (1999). Giving "moral distress" a voice: Ethical concerns among neonatal intensive care unit personnel. *Cambridge Quarterly of Healthcare Ethics, 8,* 173–178.

Husted, G. L., & Husted, J. H. (2001). *Ethical decision making in nursing* (3rd ed.). St. Louis, MO: Mosby.

Jameton, A. (1984). *Nursing practice: The ethical issues.* Englewood Cliffs, NJ: Prentice-Hall.

Jameton, A. (1992). Nursing ethics and the moral situation of the nurse. In E. Friedman (Ed.), *Choices and conflict* (pp. 101–109). Chicago: American Hospital Association.

Jameton, A. (1993). Dilemmas of moral distress: Moral responsibility and nursing practice. *Clinical Issues in Perinatal and Women's Health Nursing, 4,* 542–551.

Kelly, B. (1998). Preserving moral integrity: A follow-up study with new graduate nurses. *Journal of Advanced Nursing, 28,* 1134–1145.

Krishnasamy, M. (1999). Nursing, morality, and emotions: Phase I and Phase II clinical trials and patients with cancer. *Cancer Nursing, 22*(4), 251–259.

Krishnasamy, M., & Plant, H. (1998). Developing nursing research with people. *International Journal of Nursing Studies, 35*(1–2), 79–84.

Liaschenko, J. (1995). Artificial personhood: Nursing ethics in a medical world. *Nursing Ethics, 2*(3), 185–196.

Millette, B. E. (1994). Using Gilligan's framework to analyze nurses' stories of moral choices. *Western Journal of Nursing Research, 16*(6), 660–674.

Nathaniel, A. K. (2003). A grounded theory of moral reckoning in nursing Unpublished dissertation, West Virginia University, Morgantown.

Nathaniel, A. K. (2006). Moral reckoning in nursing. *Western Journal of Nursing Research, 28,* 419–438.

Oberle, K., & Hughes, D. (2001). Doctors' and nurses' perceptions of ethical problems in end-of-life decisions. *Journal of Advanced Nursing, 33*(6), 707–715.

Penticuff, J. H. (1997). Nursing perspectives in bioethics. In Kazumasa Hoshino (Ed.), *Japanese and Western bioethics* (pp. 49–60). The Netherlands: Khower Academic.

Perkin, R. M., Young, T., Freier, M. C., Allen, J., & Orr, R. D. (1997). Stress and distress in pediatric nurses: Lessons from Baby K. *American Journal of Critical Care, 6,* 225–232.

Redman, B., & Fry, S. T. (2000). Nurses' ethical conflicts: What is really known about them? *Nursing Ethics, 7*(4), 360–366.

Rodney, P. (1988). Moral distress in critical care nursing. *Canadian Critical Nursing Journal, 5*(2), 9–11.

Rushton, C. H. (1995). The Baby K case: Ethical challenges of preserving professional integrity. *Pediatric Nursing, 23*(1), 16–29.

Rushton, C. H. (2006). Defining and addressing moral distress: Tools for critical care nursing leaders. *AACN Advances in Critical Care, 17*(2), 161–168.

Solomon, M. Z., O'Donnell, L., Jennings, B., Guilfoy, V., Wolf, S. M., Nolan, K., . . . Donnelley, S. (1993). Decisions near the end of life: Professional views on life-sustaining treatments. *American Journal of Public Health, 83*(1), 14–23.

Sundin-Huard, D., & Fahy, K. (1999). Moral distress, advocacy and burnout: Theorizing the relationships. *International Journal of Nursing Practice, 5*(1), 8–13.

Weissman, D. E. (2009). Moral distress in palliative care. *Journal of Palliative Medicine, 12*(10), 865–866.

Wilkinson, J. M. (1987). Moral distress in nursing practice: Experience and effect. *Nursing Forum, 23*(1), 16–29.

Zuzelo, P. R. (2007). Exploring the moral distress of registered nurses. *Nursing Ethics, 14*(3), 344–359.

Part

III

PRINCIPLED BEHAVIOR
IN THE PROFESSIONAL DOMAIN

Part III examines various categories of issues that affect the profession of nursing and the everyday practice of individual nurses. Recognizing nursing as a profession, the chapters describe nurses' responsibilities related to ethical, legal, professional, and practice issues. These issues are examined in light of ethics and contemporary nursing. This part includes chapters discussing legal issues affecting nurses; professional issues such as autonomy, authority, and accountability; issues related to the relationship between nurses and the health care system; issues related to technology and self-determination; and scholarship issues.

Chapter

8

LEGAL ISSUES

We are caught in an inescapable network of mutuality, tied in a single garment of destiny. Whatever affects one directly, affects all indirectly.

(Martin Luther King, Jr., 1963/1996)

OBJECTIVES

After completing this chapter, the reader should be able to:

1. Recognize the difference between ethics and the law, and discuss the relationship of each to the other.
2. Describe sources of law.
3. Distinguish between constitutional law, statutory law, administrative law, and common law.
4. Describe the difference between public and private law.
5. Discuss instances in which nurses might be accused of breaches of public law.
6. Define *tort*, and distinguish between unintentional and intentional torts.
7. Discuss recent legal trends in health care.
8. Discuss methods that nurses can use to limit liability.
9. Describe the role of the expert nurse witness.

INTRODUCTION

Up to this point, the focus of this book has been upon values, morals, and ethics. You will recall from Chapter 2 that the prevailing cultural traditions influence individuals' moral values. Groups of people rely on these values, in turn, to help guide the formulation of formal and informal rules of action, usually referred to as ethics. Professional organizations, such as the American Nurses Association (ANA), the Canadian Nurses Association (CNA), and the International Council of Nurses (ICN), provide documents outlining a formal set of ethical guidelines. These guidelines offer some general rules that are intended for use as a tool to guide professional behavior but are not, in themselves, fully enforceable. Laws, on the other hand, consist of enforced rules under which a society is governed. Many laws either directly or indirectly affect the practice of nursing. Highly publicized issues such as termination of life support and "no code" status indicate a recent trend toward involving the legal system in issues that were previously thought to be ethical in nature. This chapter discusses the relationship between ethics and the law, general legal concepts, areas of potential liability for nurses, and recent legal trends. However, laws and statutes vary somewhat from state to state, so content in this chapter should be viewed as a general overview of basic concepts. The legal regulation of nursing is addressed in Chapter 6.

RELATIONSHIP BETWEEN ETHICS AND THE LAW

Law is the system of binding rules of action or conduct that governs the behavior of people in respect to relationships with others and with the government (Guido, 2010). Laws, meant to reflect the moral beliefs of a given population, are devised by groups of individuals serving in official capacities. Law has four basic functions in society: (1) to define relationships among members of society, and to declare which actions are and are not permitted; (2) to describe what constraints may be applied to maintain rules, and by whom they may be applied; (3) to furnish solutions to problems; and, (4) to redefine relationships between people and groups when circumstances of life change (Kozier & Erb, 1992).

The law establishes rules that define our rights and obligations, and sets penalties for people who violate them. Laws also describe how government will enforce the rules and penalties. In the United States and Canada, there are thousands of state, provincial, federal, and local laws. Among other functions, these laws ensure the safety of citizens, protect property, promote nondiscrimination, regulate the professions, provide for the distribution of public goods and services, and protect the economic and environmental interests of society.

How are ethics and laws related? Laws are intended to reflect popular belief about the "rightness or wrongness" of particular acts. Like ethics, laws are built upon a moral foundation. In most countries laws represent an attempt to codify ethics. Law can serve as the public's instrument for converting morality into clear-cut social guidelines, and for stipulating punishments for offenses (Beauchamp, 2001). One would expect that laws would be congruent with the prevailing moral values of a society; indeed, they usually are. For example, most people would agree that the murder of an innocent person is an immoral act. Laws that prohibit murder reflect this ethical standard. Murder of the innocent is both ethically and legally prohibited in every culture, though definitions of "innocence" vary from culture to culture. As society's needs and attitudes evolve, laws emerge to reflect these changes. Occasionally, however, governments create and enforce laws that many people believe to be unjust or immoral. In a democratic society, constitutional law provides mechanisms to change or abolish unjust or unpopular laws.

Some authors of nursing ethics texts take the view that professional ethical standards are congruent with the law—that is, that which is legal is also ethical, and vice versa. These authors imply that following a set of ethical guidelines, such as those provided by the ANA, the CNA, and the ICN, provides nurses with a legal safety net. This is usually, but not necessarily, true. Laws exist that can be considered (by some at least) to be unethical. Some illegal acts are considered by many to be ethical.

Think About It

Can legal actions and moral actions conflict?

The following examples may be considered illegal. Can you argue that they are morally permissible?

- *Breaking traffic laws to rush a severely ill child to the hospital*
- *Breaking and entering an isolated mountain cabin when you and your children are lost and suffering from cold and exposure*
- *Stealing a life preserver from someone else's boat to throw to a drowning person*
- *Injuring and restraining an armed person who broke into your family's home*

The following examples are legal. Can you argue that they are immoral or unethical?

- *Lying in social situations*
- *Habitually breaking promises and disappointing your children*

(continued)

- *Discriminating against someone because of race, gender, or age*
- *Telling a child she is ugly or fat*
- *Turning your back on elderly parents (Burkhardt, Nathaniel, & Walton, 2010)*

What are some reasons for the possible discrepancy between that which is legal and that which is ethical? First, there are differences between ethical points of view. Deontology and utilitarianism, for example, offer quite opposite answers to some basic ethical questions. While the utilitarian perspective would allow consideration of abortion or euthanasia, for example, to provide for the good of many, deontological views might require that life be protected regardless of circumstances. Thus, a law thought to be ethical by the utilitarian might be considered unethical by the deontologist. Second, human behavior and motivation are more complex than can be fairly reflected in law. Think back to Chapter 4. Individuals may consider the same act either right or wrong, depending to some extent on their stage of moral development. For example, acts of civil disobedience, such as those committed by Mahatma Gandhi and Martin Luther King, Jr., although unquestionably illegal, are generally considered to be motivated by high ethical standards. In his letter from the Birmingham Jail, Martin Luther King, Jr., wrote, "there are two types of laws: just and unjust. I would be the first to advocate obeying just laws. One has not only a legal but a moral responsibility to obey just laws. Conversely, one has a moral responsibility to disobey unjust laws" (1963/1996, p. 574). Third, the legal system judges action rather than motivation. For example, nurses following personal moral convictions or professional ethical codes can find themselves at odds with the policies or practices of their employer. In certain instances, the legal system may determine that an employer has the right to dismiss or discipline a nurse for laying aside institutional policy in favor of ethical considerations. Fourth, depending upon the political climate and other variables, laws change. Recent examples of laws that have changed include those related to expanded roles of nurses, abortion, fetal tissue use, organ transplantation, self-determination, confidentiality for AIDS patients, informed consent, and legal definitions of death. As defined in Chapter 4, integrity is fidelity in adherence to moral norms sustained over time. One should be able to predict that nurses with integrity will not alter their basic moral beliefs in response to changes in the law. Thus, there are several valid circumstances in which there may be a discrepancy between that which is legal and that which is considered ethical.

ASK YOURSELF

What Would You Do During a Disaster?

A recent example of the struggle of ethical versus legal received national attention during the Hurricane Katrina disaster. A New Orleans nurse described the appalling conditions she experienced in the wake of the hurricane. The hospital where she worked was the last one to remain open during the crisis. Conditions were horrific: there was no running water, no air conditioning, no food, no sanitation, and dwindling medical supplies. Temperatures exceeded 100 degrees, the staff snatched naps on stretchers, and people were "dying like flies." With the hospital filled to capacity, exhausted staff raided a hospital that was already evacuated for essential medicines such as insulin (Burnham, 2005).

- Stealing medications was illegal, yet it surely saved lives. Was stealing the medications justified in this circumstance?
- What are the determining factors?
- Apparently, many of the staff in this hospital remained to care for patients, even in the face of personal disaster and uncertainty. Television newscasts reported that some facilities were found to be without staff during the disaster. What are your thoughts about staying with patients versus fleeing danger to assure the safety of your own loved ones?

GENERAL LEGAL CONCEPTS

Nurses need to familiarize themselves with the law and legal system for several reasons. First, the law authorizes and regulates nursing practice. Nurse practice acts of the individual states describe both the activity of nurses and the boundaries of nursing. Chapter 6 discusses the legal regulation of nursing in greater depth. Second, knowledge of legal principles is a necessary component of ethical decision making. In order to make informed choices, nurses, physicians, patients, and families must be able to identify potential or real legal implications. Third, the legal system scrutinizes nursing actions and omissions. The profession is in a dynamic state of change: Advanced practice nurses expand the traditional boundaries; critical care nurses perform complex and vital tasks; staff nurses care for older and sicker patients; and many nurses practice in newly emerging settings. As we work in this demanding and quickly evolving health care environment, we must know about relevant laws, policies, and legal processes. This knowledge will help ensure that our actions are consistent with legal principles, and will help to protect us from liability.

Sources of Law

At least four different sources of law affect the practice of nursing: constitutional law, statutory (legislative) law, administrative law, and common law. Additionally, law can be divided into two main branches—private law and public law. Some laws are made by legislation, some by rule-making bodies, and some by judicial precedent. Adding to an already confusing mix, there is frequent overlap between the sources and branches of the law.

Constitutional Law

A constitution is a formal set of rules and principles that describe the powers of a government and the rights of the people. The principles laid out in a constitution, coupled with a description of how these principles are to be interpreted and carried out, form the basis of **constitutional law**. The Constitution of the United States is the preeminent source of U.S. law. Ensuring the legal rights and responsibilities of citizens and establishing the general organization of the federal government, constitutional law in the United States supersedes all other laws.

The Bill of Rights of the U.S. Constitution and subsequent amendments guarantee each citizen the rights, among others, of equal protection, due process, freedom of speech, and freedom of religion. Nursing actions must take into account these basic rights. Rights guaranteed in the Bill of Rights are consistent with the ethical principles of autonomy, confidentiality, respect for persons, and veracity. The same rights that apply to patients also apply to nurses. As participants in the health care system, we cannot be forced to forfeit any constitutionally guaranteed rights.

Statutory/Legislative Law

Formal laws (or statutes) that are written and enacted by federal, state, or local legislatures are known as **statutory** or **legislative laws**. Congress and the state legislatures pass thousands of laws each year; these are added to the hundreds of volumes of federal and state statutes already in force. Because many people think that every problem in society can be solved by passing a law, legislatures make more and more laws to satisfy the demands of society and special-interest groups. Changes in Medicare and Medicaid laws, statutory recognition of nurses in advanced practice (including prescriptive authority), and health care reform legislation are all examples of statutory or legislative law.

Administrative Law

Administrative law involves the operation of government agencies. National, state, and local governments set up administrative agencies to do the work of government. These agencies regulate such activities as education, public health, social welfare programs, and the professions. Administrative law consists mainly of the legal powers granted to administrative agencies by legislative bodies and the rules that the agencies make to carry out their powers. State boards of nursing are examples of this type of agency. These boards are granted the authority to execute the intent of state statutes by creating, implementing, and enforcing comprehensive and appropriate rules and regulations. As administrative bodies, the role of boards of nursing is to protect the public, rather than advocate for nurses. Rules promulgated by the individual states' boards of nursing carry the same weight as other law.

Common Law

The United States (except Louisiana), Canada (except Quebec), Great Britain, and other English-speaking countries have a **common law** system. Constituting the basis of the judicial system, this type of law is also known as **case law**. In the common law system, decisions are based upon earlier court rulings in similar cases. These are also known as **precedents**. In the common law tradition, case law strengthens and perpetuates itself when lower courts make decisions consistent with previous rulings of higher courts. The common law system is also self-correcting because higher courts revisit unfair or unworkable laws upon appeal. Over time, precedents take on the force of law.

Types of Law

Law can be divided into two different types: public and private. Recall that law is a system of enforceable principles and processes that governs the behavior of people in respect to relationships with others and with the government. In general, legal problems related to the relationship between people and the government are the domain of public law, and problems occurring as a result of relationships between people are the domain of private law.

Public Law

Public law defines a person's rights and obligations in relation to the government and describes the various divisions of government and their powers. One important branch of public law is **criminal law**. Criminal law deals with crimes—that is, actions considered harmful to society. Even though a crime might be committed against a particular person, the government considers the commission of a serious act, such as murder, to be harmful to all of society. In the United States, each state, as well as the federal government, has its own set of criminal laws. Nevertheless, the criminal laws of each state must protect the rights and freedoms guaranteed by the federal constitution. Crimes range in seriousness from public drunkenness to murder. Criminal law defines these offenses and sets the rules for the arrest, the appropriate procedures to ensure due process, and the punishment of offenders.

In the course of practice, nurses can be accused of a variety of criminal offenses. For example, nurses can be accused of directly injuring a patient, either intentionally or unintentionally. Nurses can also be accused of crimes related to their actual relationship with the government. These include such actions as falsifying narcotic records, failure to renew licenses, and fraudulent billing. Crimes are delineated according to seriousness as either felonies or misdemeanors.

Felonies are serious crimes that carry significant fines and jail sentences. Examples of felonies include first- and second-degree murder, arson, burglary, extortion, kidnapping, rape, and robbery. These crimes are punishable by jail terms. Nurses are rarely accused of felonies in the course of practice. However, this can occur. For example, it is possible that those participating in the unauthorized removal of life support from a terminally ill patient could be accused of first-degree murder, because of the intentional nature of the act that resulted in death. This could occur even though the act might be viewed as beneficent by a majority of people. A nurse who unintentionally causes the death of a patient by administering a medication to which a patient is allergic could be charged with second-degree murder (manslaughter).

Misdemeanors are less serious crimes, usually punishable by fines, short jail sentences, or both. Examples of misdemeanors include disturbing the peace, solicitation, assault, and battery (assault and battery are also considered intentional torts and can be decided by private or civil law). For example, a nurse who slaps a patient or gives an injection without consent can be accused of the misdemeanor of battery.

Think About It

Institutional Versus Individual Negligence

Occasionally, nurses find themselves in situations in which employer policies and practices are inconsistent with public law. In these instances, nurses and other staff members can be accused of crimes. In 1986, members of the staff of a nursing home in Louisiana were charged with cruelty, neglect, and

(continued)

mistreatment of the infirm. In the State of Louisiana v. Brenner *(1986), the staff was charged for the following reasons:*

1. *Failure to feed and care for the patients adequately*

2. *Failure to train the staff properly*

3. *Failure to provide adequate medical supplies*

4. *Failure to supply adequate staff*

5. *Failure to maintain a sanitary nursing home*

6. *Failure to maintain patients' records*

7. *Failure to see that the appropriate and necessary health services were performed.*

- *Ethics and the law are usually, but not always, consistent. Think about each of the seven accusations listed above in terms of breaches of ethical principles. What is the relationship between the accusations and ethical principles?*

- *Imagine that you live in a small community and are employed by a nursing home with similar problems. How do you think you would deal with the problems in a manner that is both legal and ethical? How do you think you would deal with the situation if you feel compelled to maintain your employment at the nursing home?*

- *Do you believe that individual nurses should be punished for actions that are clearly caused by institutional negligence? Substantiate your answer with ethical arguments.*

Private Law

Private law, sometimes called **civil law**, is different from public law in that it generally involves relationships between individuals, rather than between the state and individuals. Private law determines a person's legal rights and obligations in many kinds of activities that involve other people. These activities include everything from borrowing or lending money to buying a home or signing a job contract. More than a million civil suits are tried in the U.S. courts each year. There are six branches of private law: contract and commercial law, tort law, property law, inheritance law, family law, and corporation law. The branches of private law that are most applicable to nursing practice are contract law and tort law. When private laws are violated, individuals who are harmed (**plaintiffs**) bring lawsuits against violators (**defendants**). The government does not prosecute violations and a person cannot be sent to jail for violating private laws. In general, the penalties associated with violation of private laws are monetary. The courts grant monetary awards to the plaintiffs. Malpractice lawsuits are examples of private law.

Contract Law

Contract law deals with the rights and obligations of people who make contracts. A **contract** is a legally enforceable agreement between two or more people. Contracts may be either written or oral; however, in the presence of both a written and an oral contract, the written contract takes precedence. In health care, contracts may be either expressed or implied. Expressed contracts occur when the two parties agree explicitly to its terms, as in an employment contract. Implied contracts occur when there has been no discussion between the parties, but the law considers that a contract exists. The nurse-patient relationship is essentially an implied contract in which the nurse agrees to give competent care.

Tort Law

A **tort** is a wrong or injury that a person suffers because of someone else's action, either intentional or unintentional. The tortious action may cause bodily harm; invade another's privacy; damage a person's property, business, or reputation; or make unauthorized use of a person's property. The victim may sue the person or persons responsible. Tort law deals with the rights and obligations of the persons involved in such cases. Many torts are unintentional, such as damages that occur as a result of accidents. If a tort is deliberate and involves serious harm, it may also be treated as a crime. The purpose of tort law is to make the victim whole again, primarily through the award of monetary damages. Because it involves negligence and malpractice, tort law is the branch of law with which nurses are most familiar.

Unintentional torts. Unintentional torts occur when an act or omission causes unintended injury or harm to another person. Nurses are familiar with the unintentional torts of negligence and malpractice. You might hear these terms used interchangeably, but each has a technical meaning that is distinctly different from the other. As a nurse, you should understand the difference between negligence and malpractice and the relevance of each to safe and effective nursing care.

The term **negligence** is derived from the Latin term *negligentia* and literally means "not to pick up," thus to neglect. Negligence denotes failure to do something that a reasonable person would do in similar circumstances, or doing something careless that a reasonable and prudent person would avoid doing. Negligence refers to conduct that fails to use reasonable care.

As part of ensuring the safety of citizens, the law requires every person to be accountable for behaving in a reasonable way, particularly if the welfare of others is jeopardized. For example, there is certainly no law against throwing rocks into the air. However, within a crowd of people, this is not the act of a reasonable person. Although the person throwing rocks may enjoy the beauty of the arc or the distance of the throw and has no intention of harming others, a resultant injury would be the outcome of negligence. A nurse who pours liquid on the floor in a patient's room would be held to the same standard: That is, a reasonable person would recognize that wet floors often cause falls, and would immediately clean the floor and warn people who may be walking in the vicinity.

Negligence can also occur as a result of an omission. The nurse in the previous situation may have walked into the room and found that the patient had spilled water. Even though the nurse did not cause the spill, if he or she ignores it, the nurse will be responsible for the results. Acts of negligence in nursing can be judged upon the criteria of the knowledge and abilities expected of a reasonable and prudent nurse. Because the knowledge base of nursing is broad, technical, and specific to the profession, these criteria go far beyond those required of the ordinary person. **Malpractice** is a more specific legal term that refers to negligence committed by a person in a professional capacity, such as a physician, nurse, or lawyer. More stringent than simple negligence, malpractice is the form of negligence in which any professional misconduct, unreasonable lack of professional skill, or failure to adhere to the accepted standard of care causes injury to a patient or client. In one definition of malpractice, Creighton (1986) also includes lack of fidelity, evil practice, and illegal or immoral conduct. To be held liable for malpractice, the nurse must fail to act as other reasonable and prudent professional nurses who have the same knowledge and education would have acted under similar circumstances. There are six components of malpractice. The plaintiff (injured person) must prove each of the following elements to establish liability on the part of the defendant (the accused offender):

1. Duty owed to the patient

2. Breach of standard or care or failure to carry out duty

3. Foreseeability

4. Causality

5. Injury

6. Damages (Guido, 2010, p. 94)

The duty owed to the patient, often referred to as **duty of care**, is an overarching legal principle that calls for the nurse to act as an ordinary, prudent, reasonable nurse would act in similar circumstances. Duty of care is an obligation to adhere to a standard of reasonable care while performing acts that could foreseeably harm another person. For nurses, the duty of care is measured in terms of standards that define an acceptable level of care. In determining the extent of the duty to care, the court asks what a reasonable, prudent nurse with like experience and education would do under similar circumstances. This can be established by expert testimony, published standards, and common sense. In most cases, a duty of care does not exist in the absence of the nurse-patient relationship. When a nurse-patient relationship does exist, the duty of care requires that the nurse (1) possess the knowledge and skills required of a competent nurse engaged in the same specialty, and (2) exercise the care in the application of that knowledge and skill that is expected of a reasonably competent nurse in the same specialty, and (5) use nursing judgment in the exercise of that care (Louisville Law, n.d.). For example, when a patient is found to have a pneumothorax, a reasonable and prudent nurse would give immediate supportive care and notify a physician. At the same time, the duty to care would prohibit the nurse from attempting to insert a chest tube since the action is beyond the scope of practice, knowledge, and expertise of a registered nurse.

The second element of malpractice is **breach of duty** owed to the patient. When breach of duty is claimed, the patient must be able to establish that the nurse actually owed a duty to care—that is, that there was an implicit or explicit nurse-patient relationship. If such a duty is found to exist, the nurse may be found to be in breach of duty if his or her conduct falls short of the standard expected in similar circumstances. Standards of care are "yardsticks" by which the legal system measures the actions of a nurse in a malpractice suit. Standards include laws, rules, and regulations; statements of professional organizations; federal, state, and professional practice guidelines; educational content; and job descriptions, facility policies, procedures, bylaws, and so forth.

Foreseeability involves the concept that a person has the ability to reasonably anticipate that damage or injury may result from certain acts or omissions. The question may be asked, "Should the nurse have reasonably foreseen that his or her act could imperil or harm the patient?" Frequent legal cases concerning foreseeability include those involving medication errors and patient falls (Guido, 2010). For example, every nursing student learns about the actions and effects of insulin. So, a reasonable and prudent nurse could predict (or foresee) that administering a large dose of short-acting insulin to a patient who has been without food for 24 hours could cause life-threatening hypoglycemia. Standards of care provide insight into to the kind of specialized nursing knowledge that allows nurses to foresee potential benefits, harms, and risks of specific actions and omissions.

Causation refers to a causal relationship between an action and the resulting harm or injury. The court asks if the injury was directly caused by a breach of duty. To determine causation, the "but for" test is often used. For example, you might ask whether the NPO patient described previously would have developed life-threatening hypoglycemia, "but for" the short-acting insulin that the nurse administered. Causation presumes that injury was actually caused by the breach of duty.

As implied previously, in order for malpractice to occur, the breach of duty must have caused **injury**. The plaintiff must show that physical, financial, or emotional injury actually occurred as a direct or proximate result of the breach of duty. If a nurse commits an error or omission that does not result in injury, the case does not possess all the elements required to demonstrate liability. For example, a nurse may discover that she had inadvertently administered the wrong medication to a patient. Although the error is serious, if the patient is unharmed, the case does not meet the criteria for liability.

Remember, malpractice is almost always a "tort" offense—a civil, rather than criminal, matter. The purpose of tort law is to make the person whole again, primarily through the award of monetary awards to the plaintiff. These monetary awards are called **damages**. The purpose of awarding damages is not to punish the defendants, but to compensate the plaintiff and restore his or her previous financial position. Damages that are awarded might include financial losses and expenses incurred as a result of the injury; emotional damages, especially if there is apparent physical harm as well; and general damages inherent to the injury itself, including compensation for pain and suffering, permanent disability, and disfigurement. Punitive damages may be awarded if the court finds that there was malicious, willful, or wanton misconduct on the part of the nurse (Guido, 2010).

Aggregate data about nurses' malpractice suits in the United States are available to the public via the National Practitioner Data Bank (NPDB). Congress created the NPDB in 1986 to improve the quality of health care by encouraging state licensing boards, health care facilities, and professional societies to identify and discipline incompetent providers. The NPDB also restricts those who are found guilty of malpractice from moving from state to state without disclosing their prior records. Since 1997, registered nurses have been included in the data bank.

Slightly more than 1 percent of malpractice payment reports have been for registered nurses. The NPDB shows that non-specialized RNs have been responsible for the vast majority of these reports, with monitoring, treatment, and medication problems accounting for most awards. Nurse anesthetists, nurse midwives, and nurse practitioners account for the remainder of cases. As would be expected, awards against nurse anesthetists were anesthesia related and awards against nurse midwives were obstetrics related. Diagnosis- and treatment-related problems accounted for most of the awards against the nurse practitioners (U.S. Department of Health and Human Services [HHS], 2006).

Before the NPDB was established, data about malpractice awards was limited to research studies and anecdotal stories. Miller-Slade (1997) cites a study of malpractice claims against nurses that led to verdicts for the patients. Of 219 patient deaths, inadequate communication with the doctor led to 76; inadequate nursing assessment, 46; medication errors, 42; inadequate nursing intervention, 17; inadequate care, 21; unsafe environment, 7; improper use of equipment, 7; and inadequate infection control, 3. Another study found that the most common causes of malpractice lawsuits, in order of frequency, are medication and treatment errors; lack of observation and timely reporting about the patient; defective technology; infections caused by or made worse by poor nursing care; poor communication of important information; and failure to intervene to protect the patient from poor medical care (Physician Insurers Association of America, 1993).

O'Keefe (2000) suggests that nursing malpractice settlements can be viewed in terms of the nursing process, identified as a standard of care by the ANA and many state boards of nursing. Nurses can be accused of malpractice if they fail to assess, plan, implement, or evaluate the patient condition or response to treatment. Because the two actions are similar and the process is iterative, assessment and evaluation are considered together.

Assessment and evaluation are fundamental nursing duties. Because these basic nursing functions have a long history as standards of nursing care, failure to assess and evaluate may lead to malpractice judgments. O'Keefe (2000) identifies the following requirements in the duty to assess and evaluate:

1. The nurse must possess the knowledge and skill to properly assess and/or monitor a significant condition or change in the patient. There is a duty to know what the patient's condition should be, what it has been, and what it is now.

2. The nurse must actually carry out the assessment, monitoring, and evaluation.

3. The nurse must notify the physician if assessment, evaluation, or monitoring reveals a condition that should be reported. The nurse must report the patient's status and must thoroughly document the patient's condition and details of when and to whom the condition was reported.

4. The nurse must skillfully carry out appropriate nursing and medical interventions in an effort to correct the problem.

5. The nurse must continue to assess and monitor until the patient is stable. (p. 137)

The nursing standard of care is breached if any of these requirements are not met. *Ferris v. County of Kennebec* (1998) offers an example of a nurse's failure to assess so extreme as to be identified as "deliberate indifference." In the summer of 1996, a woman was arrested and placed in the county jail. When she was admitted, the woman told the jail officials that she was pregnant. Two days later she began having vaginal bleeding and pelvic pain. The woman complained to the nurse that she was having a miscarriage. The nurse took the woman's pulse, told her she was menstruating, instructed her to lie down, and refused to give her sanitary napkins. The woman was unable to continue to lie down because of her pain, but the nurse made no further attempt to assess her condition, telling her that she would be transferred to another cell if she continued to refuse to lie down and follow orders. Continuing to complain of severe pain, the woman was transferred to a smaller cell, and had no further contact with the nurse. A few hours later she had a miscarriage in her jail cell. After release, the woman filed a lawsuit. Finding in favor of the woman, the court determined that it was obvious that the woman was complaining of a serious condition that was ignored and untreated by the nurse. The nurse made no effort to assess or treat the woman beyond taking her pulse.

Because it is an integral part of the nursing process, a recognized standard of care, and a requirement of many federal program regulations, failure to plan may also result in accusations of malpractice. Though injury to the patient would directly result through the actions or omissions of the nurse, failure to record a plan of care stands as evidence that the nurse is negligent. In *Smith v. Juneau* (1997), nurses were found negligent for failing to develop a plan of care to protect an orthopedic patient's skin. There was no plan to reposition the patient or to assess the patient's skin under a traction sling. The court held that serious ulcers developed because the nurses failed to plan and implement care to protect the skin.

Nursing interventions include and exceed actions taken personally by the nurse (O'Keefe, 2000). Implementation is the embodiment of the ethical principle of beneficence. The nurse has a duty to do or promote good, to prevent harm, and to remove evil or harm. This includes such things as maintaining expertise in practice and reporting the dangerous practices of others. Medication errors are examples of failure to implement properly.

Accounting for thousands of deaths each year, medication errors are the most common type of adverse event, comprising nearly one-fifth of all reported adverse events (HHS, 2006). Research studies have shown that there may be as much as a 10 percent error rate for medication administration (Aspden, Wolcott, Bootman, & Cronenwett, 2011; Kohn, Corrigan, & Donaldson, 1999). Nurses can make errors of medication preparation and administration in many ways. The nurse can give the wrong medication, in the wrong dose, by the wrong route, at the wrong time, or to the wrong patient. Because of the frequency and likelihood of medication errors and the potentially serious consequences that can result, nurses need to be especially careful in administering medications. Nurses are responsible for safe and appropriate administration of medication, regardless of physician orders, workload, unusual circumstance, or institutional policy. The literature reveals many examples of medication errors. It is not unusual for damages to be awarded to victims or families when medication errors occur. In one case a nurse, in an attempt to assist on a busy pediatric unit, administered a lethal dose of digitalis to an infant. This nurse did not usually work with pediatric patients, and was unfamiliar with pediatric doses. Even though the nurse thought the dose ordered seemed high, she failed to check the literature, discuss the dose with a pharmacist, and question the physician. The parents in this case recovered substantial damages because the nurse's actions were determined to constitute malpractice (Creighton, 1986).

Think About It

Medication Errors

Medication errors constitute one of the most common areas for nursing liability.

- *What factors do you see that might influence rates of medication errors?*
- *How do you see technology either helping or hindering the medication error rate?*
- *What kinds of improvements could help prevent medication errors?*
- *Have you ever made a medication error? Did the error result in injury? Could you have foreseen the injury?*

Another area of frequent liability related to failure to implement nursing care is neglecting to remove foreign objects (Eskreis, 1998). Sponges and other small items can inadvertently be left in patients' body cavities after surgery. This can be a cause for serious postoperative complications. The nurse responsible for counting the sponges is often held liable for malpractice. In one malpractice lawsuit, two surgical nurses had to pay $4,000 apiece after a laparotomy sponge was left in a patient's abdomen. The nurses had reported a correct sponge count. Because the physician had ordered the nurses to remove metal rings from the sponges, he was also considered liable for the patient's injury (Creighton, 1986). In a similar case, a surgeon left a large surgical sponge in a patient's abdomen after a hysterectomy. The jury in the initial trial found that both the hospital and the physician were negligent, and further, that the nurses involved were agents of the hospital and not the physician. On appeal, the court found that it was a reasonable inference from the evidence that the sponge count done before surgery was performed negligently and that the procedure for counting sponges was below the standard of care (*Truhitte v. French Hospital*, 1982).

Since nursing care focuses on the psycho-social-spiritual realms as well as the physical, failure to implement care in these areas may result in nursing malpractice. Intentional infliction of emotional distress is an extreme example of this. There are certain contractual relationships, such as in the transmission and delivery of telegrams announcing the death of a close relative and services incident to a funeral and burial, that carry with them deeply emotional responses. Legal claims have been recognized that require a duty to exercise ordinary care to avoid causing emotional harm in such situations. Furrow, Greaney, Johnson, Jost, and Schwartz (2004) argue that this duty also applies to the delivery of medical and nursing services. They describe an interesting and complex case involving several instances in which nurses and other health care workers contributed to the emotional distress of Larry and Susan Oswald. In *Oswald v. LeGrand* (1990), the plaintiffs described a sequence of events that preceded the premature birth of their third child. Just prior to her 5-month checkup, Susan began experiencing bleeding and painful cramping. Her physician, Dr. Smith, ordered an ultrasound, subsequent to which Susan was examined by Dr. Smith's associate, Dr. LeGrand. Finding no explanation for the problems, Dr. LeGrand instructed Susan to go home and stay off her feet. Later the same day, Susan began bleeding heavily and was taken by ambulance to Mercy Health Center. The bleeding having spontaneously stopped, Dr. Smith discharged Susan with instructions to take it easy. The following day, with symptoms worsening, and fearing a miscarriage, Larry drove Susan to the Mercy emergency room. Another associate of Smith and LeGrand, Dr. Clark, examined Susan and advised her that there was nothing to be done and she should go home. Larry insisted that Susan be admitted, and Dr. Clark honored the request. Susan was transferred to the labor and delivery ward where her first contact was with a nurse who said, "What are you doing here? The doctor told you to stay home and rest." Later, another nurse told Susan that if she miscarried there would not be a baby but rather a "big blob of blood" (Furrow et al., 2004). Susan reported that she was scared. The next morning Susan overheard a loud argument outside her door, in which Dr. Clark was heard to yell, "I don't want to take that patient. She's not my patient and I am sick and tired of Dr. Smith dumping his case load on me" (Furrow et al., 2004, p. 166). Urged by Larry, Dr. Clark apologized and assured Susan that he would care for her until he left for vacation at noon that day, at which time Dr. LeGrand would take over. Susan began experiencing a great deal of pain at around 9:00 A.M., and Dr. Clark instructed the staff to schedule her for an ultrasound and amniocentesis. After viewing the ultrasound, Dr. Clark told the Oswalds that the situation was unusual and left without further explanation, one-half hour before his scheduled off-time. Susan was confused, distressed, in extreme pain, and still in the hallway outside the x-ray lab, when she began giving birth. Larry summoned two nurses, who delivered a one-pound baby girl. The nurses determined that the baby had no pulse or respiratory activity. They wrapped the baby in a towel, placed her on an instrument tray, and told the parents she was stillborn. After having called relatives to break the sad news, Larry touched the baby's hand and was startled when his grasp was returned. The nurses rushed the infant to the neonatal intensive care unit, where she died several hours later.

ASK YOURSELF

Emotional Harm

- In the Oswald case, do you think there was negligence on the part of any of the health care providers? If so, explain your thinking.

- If you believe there was negligence, do you think the premature birth or death of the infant was directly caused by the negligence?

- Larry and Susan contend that they have suffered severe emotional distress as a result of alleged breaches of professional conduct. Think about the several instances in which either the physicians or nurses may have contributed to the Oswalds' emotional distress.

- Do you feel there should be a duty to exercise ordinary care to avoid causing emotional harm? Was that duty breached in this instance?

- What are the ethical implications of the nurses' behavior?

Patient burns may also be considered a failure to implement nursing care. Burns can occur as a result of fires, baths, showers, hot water bottles, or heating pads. Patients who are comatose or have diminished sensitivity are especially prone to burns. In one case a 3-month-old infant suffered second- and third-degree burns on his buttocks after an operating room nurse placed him on a heating pad at the instruction of the anesthesiologist. The purpose of the heating pad was to help the child maintain body temperature during surgery. Though neither the nurses nor the surgeon noted anything unusual after surgery, arriving at home, the parents found the infant to have blisters draining bloody fluid. The child required subsequent skin grafting. Although admitting liability in this case, the defendants attempted to exclude from evidence the manufacturer's warning to avoid use of the heating pad on an infant, invalid, or sleeping or unconscious person. The manufacturers warned that burns could result from improper use (*Smelko v. Brinton*, 1987). In another case, a patient received a judgment against a hospital after he was seriously burned. The patient was paralyzed and had a speech impediment. He was left alone while smoking his pipe. The pipe fell from his mouth and set the bed on fire (Creighton, 1986, p. 145). Clearly a reasonable and prudent nurse would not leave a paralyzed person alone with a lit pipe in his mouth.

Errors have become so common and their expense has become so great that government and private organizations have begun to adopt initiatives to reduce errors and their costs alike. In 2002, the U.S. National Quality Forum (NQF) compiled a list of 28 Serious Reportable Events (SREs), which was updated in 2006. Because these events are the result of negligence and are considered preventable, they have come to be known as "never events"—that is, they should never happen. In addition to liability lawsuits, "never events" account for millions of dollars in insurance payouts. Below is the list of serious reportable "never" events:

- Surgical Events
  - Surgery performed on the wrong body part
  - Surgery performed on the wrong patient
  - Wrong surgical procedure performed on a patient
  - Unintended retention of a foreign object in a patient after surgery or other procedure
  - Intraoperative or immediately postoperative death of a previously healthy patient

- Product or Device Events
    - Patient death or serious disability associated with the use of contaminated drugs, devices, or biologics
    - Patient death or serious disability associated with the use or function of a device in patient care in which the device is used or functions other than as intended
    - Patient death or serious disability associated with intravascular air embolism that occurs while being cared for in a health care facility

- Patient Protection Events
    - Infant discharged to the wrong person
    - Patient death or serious disability associated with patient elopement (disappearance)
    - Patient suicide, or attempted suicide, resulting in serious disability while being cared for in a health care facility

- Care Management Events
    - Patient death or serious disability associated with a medication error (e.g., errors involving the wrong drug, wrong dose, wrong patient, wrong time, wrong rate, wrong preparation, or wrong route of administration)
    - Patient death or serious disability associated with a hemolytic reaction due to the administration of incompatible blood or blood products
    - Maternal death or serious disability associated with labor or delivery in a low-risk pregnancy while being cared for in a health care facility
    - Patient death or serious disability associated with hypoglycemia, the onset of which occurs while the patient is being cared for in a health care facility
    - Death or serious disability (kernicterus) associated with failure to identify and treat hyperbilirubinermia in neonates
    - Stage 3 or 4 pressure ulcers acquired after admission to a health care facility
    - Artificial insemination with the wrong donor sperm or wrong egg

■ Environmental Events

- Patient death or serious disability associated with an electric shock while being cared for in a health care facility

- Any incident in which a line designated for oxygen or other gas to be delivered to a patient contains the wrong gas or is contaminated by toxic substances

- Patient death or serious disability associated with a burn incurred from any source while being cared for in a health care facility

- Patient death or serious disability associated with a fall while being cared for in a health care facility

- Patient death or serious disability associated with the use of restraints or bedrails while being cared for in a health care facility

■ Criminal Events

- Any instance of care ordered by or provided by someone impersonating a physician, nurse, pharmacist, or other licensed health care provider

- Abduction of a patient of any age

- Sexual assault on a patient within or on the grounds of a health care facility

- Death or significant injury of a patient or staff member resulting from a physical assault (i.e., battery) that occurs within or on the grounds of a health care facility (NQF, 2008)

Since the NQF developed this list of serious reportable events in 2002, several states and other entities have enacted legislation or taken administrative action to require reporting of "never events" (NQF, 2006). In 2008, Medicare began denying payment for a number of these events, and Medicaid is following suit in some states.

Intentional torts. **Intentional torts** occur when someone intentionally injures another person or interferes with the person's property. The perpetrator intends to bring about a specific result or consequence. A tort must include three elements to be considered intentional: The act must be intended to interfere with the plaintiff or his or her property; there must be intent to bring about the consequences of the act; and the act must substantially cause the consequences (Figure 8–1). Examples of intentional torts include fraud, invasion of privacy, assault, battery, false imprisonment, slander, and libel. Damages awarded for intentional torts tend to be more generous than those awarded for unintentional negligence.

1. The defendant's act must be intended to interfere with the plaintiff or his or her property.
2. The defendant must intend to bring about the consequences of the act.
3. The act must substantially cause the consequences.
4. There is no legal requirement that the act causes damages or injury—proof of intention is sufficient.

FIGURE 8–1 Components of Intentional Torts

Fraud is a deliberate deception for the purpose of securing an unfair or unlawful gain. Although nurses are seldom accused of fraud, when this occurs it is usually prosecuted as a crime. Examples of potential areas of nurses' fraud include falsification of information on employment applications, untruthful billing procedures, false representation of a patient's physical condition in order to induce contracts for services, and falsification of patient records to cover up an error or avoid legal action. As is true with some other intentional torts, fraud can lead to both civil and criminal proceedings. Because of the deliberate nature and potential harm of fraudulent acts, court decisions tend to be harsh. Advanced Practice Registered Nurses' (APRN) third-party billing procedures are an area of potential fraud. Identified as one of the top priorities of the U.S. Department of Justice, fraudulent medical service billing can be intentional or unintentional. Complex billing procedures and inequality of reimbursement set the stage for errors in billing and "upcoding" for APRN visits. Complicated "incident to" codes and reimbursement levels for APRNs at a lower payment level than physicians lead some medical practices to try to find ways to bill for APRN services at the physician rate. "Incident to" is an awkward phrase that relates to a practice of billing services at the physician rate under stringent rules, even though the physician is not the person delivering care. Even though incident to billing is legal, this practice can lead to charges of fraud against both nurses and physicians when all regulations are followed. Each incident of fraud can result in up to 5 years of imprisonment, up to a $25,000 fine, and exclusion from Medicare and Medicaid reimbursement for at least 5 years (Mazzocco, 2000).

The **right to privacy** is the right to be left alone or to be free from unwanted publicity. Individuals have the right to withhold themselves and their lives from public scrutiny. The intentional tort of **invasion of privacy** occurs when a person's privacy is violated. There are four types of invasions of privacy related to patient care: (1) intrusion on the patient's physical and mental solitude or seclusion; (2) public disclosure of private facts; (3) publicity that places the patient in a false light in the public eye; and

(4) appropriation of the patient's name or likeness for the defendant's benefit or advantage (Fiesta, 1988). Many legal cases involve invasions of privacy. In *Berthiaume v. Pratt,* a dying patient being treated for cancer of the larynx was repeatedly photographed at the direction of his surgeon. On the day of his death the patient asked not to be photographed, but nevertheless the physician photographed him after lifting his head to place a pillow under it. A court decided that the physician be held liable for invasion of privacy (*Berthiaume v. Pratt,* 1976).

In another invasion of privacy case, Earl Spring, a senile 78-year-old man, resided in a nursing home where he was undergoing kidney dialysis. In an attempt to discontinue dialysis treatments, his legal guardians, his wife and son, were involved in a prolonged court battle. In opposition to the family's position, and without their consent, the nursing home staff permitted right-to-life advocates to interview the senile man. Interviews with the patient and four nurses were published. After winning a Superior Court ruling regarding discontinuing the dialysis, Mrs. Spring sued the nursing home and the four nurses for $80 million in damages. She claimed that her husband's right to privacy had been violated. Although the attorney for the nursing home maintained that the patient had become a "public figure," the jury found in favor of Mrs. Spring, awarding her $2.5 million.

The terms *assault* and *battery*, though usually used together, have different legal meanings. Both are intentional torts. **Assault** is defined as the unjustifiable, intentional attempt or threat to touch a person without consent that results in fear of immediately harmful or offensive contact. In order for assault to occur, touching does not need to actually occur. **Battery** is the unlawful, harmful, or unwarranted touching of another or the carrying out of threatened physical harm. Battery includes any intentional, nonconsented, angry, violent, or harmful touching of a person's body or clothes, or anything held by or attached to the person (such as a scarf or purse). Surgical procedures performed without informed consent are the most common example of battery occurring in the hospital setting. In the course of everyday activities, nurses have been accused of both assault and battery. For example, actionable assault occurs when a nurse threatens to give an injection to an unruly or noncompliant adult patient without consent. Battery is often thought of as such actions as slapping, shoving, or pinching, but the courts have upheld battery charges in actions that were much more subtle. Regardless of intent or outcome, touching without consent is considered battery. Even when the intention is beneficent and the outcome is positive, if the act is committed without permission, the nurse can be charged with battery.

Necessity and consent are two defenses that nurses can use when accused of battery in the course of administering care. **Necessity** refers to touching a person without consent in an emergency. It may be necessary to touch a person without consent to provide direct medical aid in an emergency or to protect self or others against a combative or violent person. In its most basic form, **consent** refers to approval or assent, particularly after thoughtful consideration. Consent may be explicitly expressed in verbal, nonverbal, or written form or it may be implied. Since most nursing acts do not require a formal consent process, consent is often considered to be implied. For example, if a nurse enters the room and asks, "May I change your dressing?" and the patient removes his blankets and positions himself for a dressing change, he can be considered to have given implied consent. For this reason, asking permission for even the simplest procedure is a good idea because it elicits implied consent and may constitute a good defense against a charge of battery. The informed consent process for invasive procedures is a common type of explicitly expressed consent.

The case of *Robertson v. Provident House* (1991) illustrates an example of battery involving nurses. Although having an order for an "as needed" indwelling catheter, a quadriplegic patient objected when nurses tried to insert one. He had experienced pain and complications with indwelling catheters in the past. The nurse reportedly told the patient to "shut up" and then proceeded to insert the catheter. The catheter was removed after repeated requests from the patient and family. Subsequently, ignoring the patient's objections, the nurse reinserted the catheter. Injury occurred when a nurse forcefully pulled the catheter out. The family eventually sued for damages and recovered $25,000. The Louisiana Supreme Court found that battery occurs when a nurse ignores the objections of the patient and performs an invasive procedure, such as the insertion of an indwelling catheter.

In another case, a practicing Christian Scientist who was committed to a mental hospital refused medications and other treatment. The patient was forced to take medication. The court awarded her compensation for both assault and battery since defense attorneys failed to prove that she was a danger to herself or others or that she was mentally ill or incompetent (Fiesta, 1988).

A patients' refusal to consent is more complex in some cases. An exception to the requirement of consent from competent adults may be made for prisoners. Some states permit nurses to obtain blood and other specimens without consent from persons under arrest if police request the tests as part of a criminal investigation. Institutions should provide nurses with very clear guidelines for cases such as this. Police can obtain a court order to get a blood sample if a patient refuses, but the nurse should not have to decide the issue without administrative support.

False imprisonment is defined as the unjustifiable restraint of a person within fixed boundaries, or an act intended to result in such confinement, without consent and without authority of law. False imprisonment can include physical restraint of the person, or acts intended to accomplish confinement, such as refusing the patient clothing or car keys. If false imprisonment is accompanied by forcible restraint or the threat of restraint, assault and battery may also be charged. However, each state has legal procedures granting authorization to detain, for a limited period of time, specific categories of persons who are disoriented, mentally ill, or substance abusers or who have contagious diseases. Generally, these persons can be held without consent while the hospital reports them to authorities and obtains commitment or custody orders (Trandel-Korenchuk, Rhodes, & Trandel-Korenchuk, 1997).

Nurses have been accused of false imprisonment for restraining patients, locking patients in rooms, and detaining patients for payment of bills. An example of false imprisonment is seen in the case of *Big Town Nursing Home, Inc. v. Newman* (1970), in which a 67-year-old man was kept against his will for nearly 2 months. Having been brought to the nursing home by his nephew, the man attempted to leave several times and was forcibly detained. The staff of the nursing home restrained him in a chair and denied him the use of a telephone and his clothing. The court found that the staff of the nursing home acted recklessly, willfully, and maliciously in unlawfully detaining him. In the case of *Blackman for Blackman v. Rifkin* (1988), the court held that some circumstances justify detainment. In this instance, the court upheld the hospital's duty to prevent further harm by detaining a highly intoxicated patient with a head injury, despite her insistence that she be allowed to leave. The court ruled that the hospital could assume that the patient would have consented to the treatment had she not been intoxicated.

Defamation occurs when one harms a person's reputation and good name; diminishes others' value or esteem; or arouses negative feelings toward the person in others by the communication of false, malicious, unprivileged, or harmful words. Only those remarks or statements that might arouse derogatory opinions about a person are considered defamation. Additionally, defamation only occurs when the words are communicated to a third person—that is, two persons directing remarks and epithets to each other are not liable for defamation. In most states there are two distinct forms of defamation, slander and libel. **Slander** occurs when one defames or damages the reputation of another by speaking unprivileged or false words. Slander can occur in nursing practice when nurses make cruel, false, or unsubstantiated claims against patients. By making value judgments or voicing the opinion that a patient is uncooperative, malingering, unintelligent, or drug-seeking, a nurse may be committing actionable slander. Nurses may also be accused of slander as a result of inappropriate defamatory remarks voiced against another professional. **Libel** consists of printed defamation by written words and images that injure a person's reputation or cause others to avoid, ridicule, or view the person with contempt. Nurses risk accusations of libel, for example, when writing information in patients' charts that can be damaging. Judgmental, critical, or speculative statements made in patients' charts such as, "The patient is drug-seeking," or "The patient is rude," can lead to charges of libel, particularly if the patient has reason to believe that the words adversely affect care given by others.

If the defamatory remarks have the potential of harming the business prospects of the person, proof of damage is not needed. An example of this can be seen in the case of *Schessler v. Keck* (1954). In this case, an unmarried female caterer had a false positive test for syphilis. Though the patient had never had the disease, a nurse seeing her catering at a party told the hostess that the woman was being treated for syphilis. This resulted in destroying the patient's business. The appeals court found that there was a valid basis for her claim of slander.

Nurses have also been the object of defamatory remarks. A physician accused his office nurse of having mixed up reports on a patient's chart and lying about it. He fired her the next day and called a meeting of his office employees. He told his staff that he could not work with anyone who was a liar, untrustworthy, and disloyal. A jury awarded the nurse $125,000 in damages (Creighton, 1986).

In certain instances, derogatory remarks may not constitute defamation. Two defenses to defamation include truth and privilege. In fact, there may be a legal or moral duty to pass on defamatory information in certain circumstances. For instance, a nurse has the duty to report suspected child abuse, a director of nursing services has a duty to report truthfully the character and qualifications of nurses to potential employers, and peer review groups are required to discuss privileged information for the purpose of improving services, disciplining providers, and so forth. Additionally, nurses are ethically obligated to report the illegal or incompetent practice of others. To avoid charges of defamation, prudent nurses will take care to observe appropriate channels of communication when making reports of this nature. In the absence of privileged communication, truth is a good defense for defamation.

CONTEMPORARY LEGAL TRENDS

The combination of an evolving health care delivery system, increased public awareness, and a vigorous legal system have led to changes in the delivery of care, exposure to potential sources of liability, and changing legal trends. The public has begun to subject both the individual provider and the health care system to intense legal scrutiny. The identification of "never events," litigation involving managed care organizations, increasing numbers of malpractice claims against nurses, and movement toward criminalization of negligence are four recent legal trends. Legal implications of confidentiality and telenursing are also mentioned here because of recent laws and the potential of both civil and criminal penalties for breaching patients' confidentiality.

Legal Trends Involving Managed Care Organizations

Promising efficiency and economy of health care delivery, managed care organizations (MCOs) began rapidly replacing traditional fee-for-service providers within the last three decades. MCOs are intended to reduce unnecessary health care costs and the intensive management of high-cost health care cases. As a result of policies that encouraged restrictions of expensive services, MCOs experienced significant financial corporate liability losses in the 1990s (Fiesta, 1996). Being both the insurer and the provider of care, MCOs have a vested interest in providing the most cost-efficient services. This can sometimes lead to diminution of the quality of care and liability. Managed care liability may be direct or indirect.

Direct liability occurs when negative patient outcomes result from the MCO's actions that are unduly influenced by cost-containment measures. Such actions may include improper denial of care, or financial incentives to providers that result in a denial (O'Keefe, 2000). Fiesta cites a case in Georgia in which a jury awarded $45 million to a family whose son had his hands amputated as a result of Kaiser Permanente's efforts to minimize health care costs. The malpractice occurred when the child's mother called the MCO's emergency line to report that her infant son was lethargic and had a temperature of 104 degrees. The nurse on duty first told the mother to place the child in a tepid bath and, after checking with a physician, instructed her to take the child to an approved Kaiser Permanente affiliate, even though there was a closer hospital. The child's heart stopped en route to the hospital and gangrene resulted from lack of circulation to his extremities. The family's lawyer argued that this was an example of what happens when cost-conscious managed care providers try to cut corners.

An MCO may be held indirectly liable because of its relationship with the physician or provider of care (O'Keefe, 2000). They choose the clinicians who provide care to members. Having a duty to investigate provider credentials and expertise and a duty to offer competent and qualified providers, MCOs take on potential liability under the corporate negligence doctrine (Fiesta, 1996). Courts have concluded that by limiting members' choices of providers to a select group, there is an unreasonable risk of harm if the clinicians are unqualified or incompetent. Managed care organizations must be careful that decisions regarding quality and availability of care are not negatively affected by financial considerations.

In the case of *Jones v. Chicago HMO* (2000), a managed care corporation was found liable in the care of a 3-month-old infant. The health maintenance organization (HMO) assigned Mrs. Jones's infant to a physician. The court later discovered that the physician was assigned as the primary care provider to as many as 6,000 other patients. On the day in question, the 3-month-old baby was constipated, crying, and felt very warm. An assistant to the physician told Jones that the doctor was not available and advised Jones to give the baby some castor oil. The physician returned Jones's call late that evening and repeated the advice. The next day, Jones took the baby to a hospital emergency room, where doctors diagnosed her with bacterial meningitis, secondary to bilateral otitis media. Because of the meningitis, the child is permanently disabled. A medical expert testified that when a 3-month-old infant is warm, irritable, and constipated, the standard of care requires a physician to schedule an immediate appointment to see the infant or to instruct the parent to obtain immediate medical care elsewhere. The court ruled that an HMO be held directly liable for failure to oversee the activities of network physicians whose patient load exceeded professionally acceptable norms and contributed to the physician's failure to timely treat an infant. Nine years after the incident, the child suffered regularly from seizures, was unable to feed herself, and weighed just 45 pounds.

Health maintenance organizations are sometimes accused of cutting corners in order to preserve profit. In 2006, a Los Angeles County jury found that the HMO, Kaiser Permanente, retaliated against one of its emergency room physicians after he raised concerns about the quality of care at a Kaiser hospital. The physician had complained about filthy treatment rooms, delays in care, and a shortage of supplies. The jury awarded the physician $200,000 for past economic losses. This case was the second to publicly spotlight the hospital's cost-saving practices. The first occurred in March 2006 when the hospital was accused of dumping an elderly patient on the streets of skid row, wearing a hospital gown and slippers (Omstein, 2006).

Some states allow "hold harmless" clauses that health providers sign with MCOs. Under these clauses, only providers, not MCOs, can be held liable for adverse outcomes, even if the treatment was guided by what the managed care company deemed medically necessary. Many states have passed laws prohibiting these hold harmless clauses.

Malpractice Claims Against Nurses

Although liability is a serious problem for nurses, only about 2 percent of all medical malpractice payments are for professional nurses' actions. Since the inception of the National Practitioner Data Bank, all types of professional nurses have been responsible for malpractice payments. Monitoring, treatment, and medication errors have been responsible for

Case Presentation

"Please Don't Let Me Die!"

In May 2006, a jury awarded $20 million to the family of Loren Richards, an 84-year-old Kentucky man. In addition to the nursing home corporation, two nurses were found culpable in Mr. Richard's death. In the final hours of his life, Richards screamed in pain as he pleaded for help, "I need a doctor. I need a nurse. . . . Please don't let me die" (Yetter, 2006). He died about 10 hours after he first complained of pain caused by an untreated bowel obstruction. Thirteen staff, three of whom were nurses, took care of 100 patients on that day. At one point, 10 of the 13 were on break, including all three nurses. That left three nursing assistants to care for everyone. The jury heard testimony that the nurses failed to monitor Richards' condition or respond to symptoms including pain and vomiting. The family alleged that there was an acute shortage of staff at the facility, owned by the nation's largest nursing home chain. Defendants' attorneys responded that the case was really about the family's greed (Kocher, 2006). In recent years, the nursing home corporation has been hit with wrongful-death lawsuits in five states.

Think About It

- If the nursing home was understaffed, why were the nurses found to be culpable?
- Why were the nurses judged responsible, rather than the nursing assistants?
- What standards of care did the nurses violate?
- What would you have done in that situation?

the majority of payments for RNs. Anesthesia-related problems are responsible for the greatest majority of malpractice payments against nurse anesthetists. Similarly, obstetrics-related problems were responsible for the majority of payments against nurse midwives. Diagnosis- and treatment-related problems were responsible for the majority of payments against nurse practitioners. It is predicted that as the health care system changes, nurses will be the target of a growing number of malpractice cases.

Criminalization of Nurses' Professional Negligence

Traditionally, nurses who make errors that cause harm to patients have been charged with the unintentional tort of professional negligence (malpractice). Either heard in civil court or settled out of court, charges of negligence against nurses have not resulted in criminal prosecution. It appears, however, that there may be a disturbing legal trend toward charging nurses with criminal negligence in particular cases. Until recently, the risk of criminal prosecution for nursing practice was nonexistent unless nursing action arose to the level of criminal intent, such as the case of euthanasia leading to murder charges. However, in 1997, three nurses were indicted by a Colorado grand jury for criminally negligent homicide in the death of a newborn. Public records show that one nurse was assigned to care for the baby. A second nurse offered to assist her colleague in caring for the baby. A third nurse was a nurse practitioner working in the hospital nursery. Because the baby was at risk for congenital syphilis, the physician ordered that the nurses give 150,000 units of intramuscular penicillin—which would have required five separate injections. In relation to other problems the same day, the baby was subjected to a lumbar puncture that required six painful attempts. To avoid inflicting further pain, Nurse Two asked the nurse practitioner if there was another route available for administration of the penicillin. Nurse Two and the nurse practitioner searched recognized pharmacology references and determined that IV administration would be acceptable. The nurse practitioner had the authority to change the route and directed Nurse Two to administer the medication intravenously rather than intramuscularly. Unrecognized by the nurses, the pharmacy erroneously delivered the medication prepared and ready to administer in a dose 10 times greater than was ordered—1.5 million units. As Nurse Two was administering the medication intravenously, the baby died. The Colorado Board of Nursing initiated disciplinary proceedings against Nurse Two and the nurse practitioner, but not against Nurse One. The grand jury indicted all three nurses on charges of criminally negligent homicide, but did not indict the pharmacist (C. A. Klein, personal communication, May 14, 1997). This case is an ominous reminder of the days of witch hunts, when bad outcomes of childbirth led to the execution of nurse midwives. It is a frightening example of the devastating and unpredictable consequences that can occur when a nurse makes a serious error. Although it happens rarely, several cases against nurses for criminal negligence or criminal prosecution of human error have been publicized in the last few years.

Confidentiality of Electronic Communications

This is the age of electronic communication. We use electronic media every day: wireless telephone, smartphone, fax, voice mail, pager, social media, Skype, satellite and microwave transmission, e-mail, and radio communication. We discuss patient care over telephones, send records via fax or e-mail, participate in video conferencing, and record protected patient data via smartphones. Because of the pervasive use of electronic media, we have a duty to be especially vigilant against invasions of privacy and confidentiality. Interception of electronic confidential material can occur in a variety of ways, either

ASK YOURSELF

Criminal Negligence Versus Malpractice

- What feelings are evoked as you consider the previous example?

- Should the courts take into consideration the fact that the nurses' error occurred because they wanted to avoid causing the baby unnecessary pain? Discuss your thinking.

- Can you think of other occupations in which the consequences of unintentional errors have greater legal implications? Discuss your answer with classmates.

- How should the profession respond to this frightening new legal threat?

unintentional or intentional. For example, unauthorized personnel may have access to electronic information on an institution's computer network, wireless and mobile telephone communications may be inadvertently intercepted, online communications pass through a number of nonsecure computers, and portable devices such as laptops and smartphones can be lost or stolen. Nurses' use of electronic communications raises a number of legal and ethical questions. What are the legal implications of electronic communications? What is our responsibility to maintain patient confidentiality? How does electronic communication affect the regulation of nursing practice?

Telenursing is the provision of nursing care utilizing any form of electronic media. In addition to confidentiality issues stipulated in codes of ethics and state nursing regulations, telenursing is regulated by other laws, such as the Uniform Health Care Information Act (UHCIA) and federal wiretap statutes. Any information transmitted over wire, cable, or like connection is subject to federal wiretap statutes. These statutes prohibit intercepting and recording of information and preclude its use in legal proceedings. Although there are no reported legal cases involving telenursing practice, in general case law supports the patient's right to confidentiality regardless of the type of media. The UHCIA identifies some legal implications of telenursing. These implications include identification of standards for disclosure, the nurse's potential for civil and criminal liability, and elements necessary for valid disclosure authorization from the patient (O'Keefe, 2000). In general, the nurse must follow the standard of reasonableness to protect the confidentiality of health care information. In other words, the nurse must reasonably believe that health care information is secure, or that authorization for its disclosure is authentic. The nurse may legally disclose health care information if there is valid authorization. Authorization must be written, dated, and signed by the patient; must specify the type or nature of information to be disclosed; and must identify the person to whom the health care information will be disclosed. Failure to use reasonable safeguards to secure the confidentiality of health information may result in criminal and/or civil liability. Criminal liability may include conviction of a misdemeanor, with a fine not exceeding $10,000 and/or imprisonment of no more than 1 year. Civil remedies include recovery of damages, particularly if the nurse is found to have obtained or disclosed information with malice or gross negligence (O'Keefe, 2000).

Different types of electronic media have different risks of unintentional disclosure. For example, wireless telephone communications are more likely to be intercepted than either land-based or cellular telephone communications, and non-encrypted e-mail is susceptible to interception. Nurses can be reasonably assured that institutional network communications systems provide privacy of information. Although many health care personnel have access to institutions' intranet computer network systems, employees are bound by a duty of confidentiality as required by the institution.

Telenursing also raises questions about the regulation of nursing practice. Many of these questions are yet to be fully addressed. What are the implications for nurses who staff telephone advice lines for hospital networks or managed care organizations with multistate networks? Can nurses offer advice to patients in states in which they are not licensed? If the purpose of a telecommunications system is to help to provide access to providers or specialists, what is the nurse's role in implementing orders from out-of-state physicians? The ANA (2006) developed a position statement on privacy and confidentiality, which focuses on use of electronic communication in nursing. The ICN and the National Council of State Boards of Nursing are studying the issue. We must recognize that we are at the cusp of a new era of health care information. We must be sensitive to the legal and ethical implications of telenursing, carefully safeguarding patients' rights to privacy and confidentiality.

RISK MANAGEMENT

Recognizing the litigious state of today's society, how can nurses limit the risk of lawsuits? Much of today's litigation occurs as a result of events over which nurses have little control. Unfortunate outcomes can result from institutional circumstances, errors or incompetence of other professionals, or unpredictable or intractable physical phenomena. Other litigation occurs as a result of thoughtless or negligent actions on the part of nurses or other professionals. Though it is impossible to completely eliminate the risk of litigation, attention to a number of critical factors may reduce the threat of malpractice suits. Critical factors include maintaining open communication with patients, conscientious practice, and autonomy (Figure 8–2).

I.   Maintain Good Communication
- Be courteous, show respect, and take time to listen attentively.
- Do not belittle patients or make value judgments.
- Involve patients in decision making.
- Assess patients' level of understanding.
- Explain in language that patients can understand.
- Clarify and verify telephone orders; whenever possible, avoid accepting telephone orders or giving advice over the telephone.

II. Maintain Expertise in Practice
- Keep up to date in both knowledge and skills.
- Do not attempt any task or give any medication that is unfamiliar.
- Practice within the professional and statutory scope of practice.
- Be familiar with and follow institutional and professional standards of care.
- Be attentive to patients' changing health status.
- Pay close attention to detail, avoiding distraction.
- Document objectively, thoroughly, and in a timely fashion.

III. Maintain Autonomy and Empowerment
- Challenge questionable physician orders.
- Seek attention for patients with changing health status.
- Challenge bureaucratic structures that threaten patient welfare.
- Avoid institutional settings that produce systematic and persistent threats to patient welfare.

FIGURE 8–2   Reducing the Risk of Malpractice Litigation

Maintaining Communication with Patients

On many occasions, nurses could have prevented malpractice lawsuits had they paid careful attention to interpersonal relationships and good communication techniques. Patients tend to become angry if they believe they are not being taken seriously, are not being listened to, are being belittled, or are denied involvement in the decision-making process. Regardless of the professional's knowledge or ability, angry patients are more likely to file lawsuits. One of the most important factors in reducing the risk of litigation is a genuine regard for others. This quality produces nurses who are courteous, honest, and caring. They maintain open lines of communication, spend the time that is required to show respect, have genuine interest and patience, and listen to understand. The value of untiring listening cannot be overemphasized. Anecdotal information reveals that a professional's lack of listening is a key element for patients who are inclined to file lawsuits. In addition to the psychosocial benefits, listening with a discerning ear can lead to clues of health status that might otherwise have gone undetected. Good communicators listen objectively, avoid making value judgments, and include patients in health care decisions.

Patients may also sue when there are negative outcomes resulting from a lack of understanding of self-care, treatment options, potential outcomes of treatments, side effects of drugs, and so forth. In addition to listening skills, good communication techniques include assessing patients' level of understanding and finding ways to help patients to understand important information. Nurses with a genuine regard for others are more likely to be aware of patients' level of understanding. They will teach and explain, being respectful, yet using language that patients understand. They will ensure that informed consent is truly informed. They will check and recheck patients' level of understanding and involve other family members when appropriate. Because lawsuits are frequent, and it is particularly difficult to assess patients' level of understanding, nurses need to be especially careful about giving advice or patient teaching over the telephone.

Maintaining Conscientious Practice

There are many factors related to conscientious practice. Expertise in practice is not only one hallmark of a professional but is also a legal and ethical imperative. There have been monumental advances in knowledge and technology in the past several years. With the advent of health insurance in the post–World War II era and malpractice litigation in recent years, standards of care have become very stringent. Society's expectations of nurses' knowledge and abilities are high. Consequently, nurses must strive to maintain up-to-date knowledge and technical skills. Lack of knowledge is no defense in a court of law. It is, in fact, tantamount to an admission of negligence. It is important that nurses know and uphold institutional, professional, and legal standards of practice and work within their scope of practice, never attempting to perform any task or administer any medication that is unfamiliar. Nurses' actions are examined in light of current information, professional or statutory scope of practice, and institutional and professional practice standards. Statements such as "Everyone does it that way," "That is what I learned in school 20 years ago," or "I did the best I could" will not protect a nurse from being found negligent.

Conscientious practice also includes close attention to detail. Nurses make serious errors when they become overly tired or distracted, are called away from tasks, are inattentive to patients' changing health status, or do not take the time to document thoroughly. Attention to detail will eliminate many errors that result in charges of negligence. Ethics and the law are closely related in regard to attention to detail. Recall from Chapter 2 that deontological ethics require that each person is seen as an end and not as a means only, and that one is compelled to fulfill one's duty to others, thus implying that nurses must focus clearly upon each patient and each task. Attention to detail will serve to improve patient outcomes and protect the nurse against lawsuits.

Maintaining Autonomy and Empowerment

As the examples in this chapter have illustrated, the courts demand that nurses practice autonomously. Time and again, court decisions indicate that society expects nurses to be courageous in questioning physicians' orders (particularly those given over the telephone), vigorous in seeking attention for patients with changing health status, and active in challenging bureaucratic structures that threaten patient welfare. The courts know that nurses have in-depth knowledge in areas such as pharmacology and pathophysiology, and expect nurses to protect patients from harm. Facing institutional situations that systematically present threats to patient safety and welfare, and being unable to bring about change, nurses may find they can protect themselves from liability only by leaving the situation.

Liability Insurance

Despite efforts to reduce the risk of liability, nurses are increasingly vulnerable to claims of malpractice. Regardless of nurses' level of expertise, patients can be injured. Even if a claim has no merit, the process of defense is time consuming, emotionally exhausting, and costly. Liability insurance is an important risk management strategy that protects assets and income and affords nurses peace of mind. Professional liability insurance provides for payment of lawyer fees and settlement or jury awards. It also provides nurses a mechanism of accountability in that they have the ability to pay should their actions cause injury. Nurses should never be without liability coverage.

Choosing a particular type of malpractice policy can be confusing and intimidating. How much coverage is appropriate? Are occurrence-based or claims-made policies better? Do nurses need individual policies if they have employer-sponsored coverage? Is it important that nurses be knowledgeable about their unique malpractice risks?

There are two basic types of insurance coverage. Occurrence-based policies provide broad coverage. These policies cover the nurse for claims arising from incidents that occur during the period of time that the policy is in effect. Occurrence-based policies protect the nurse when lawsuits are filed after the policy has expired, even if the policy was not renewed. In particular, nurses who work with children or infants run the risk of lawsuits being filed many years after an injury occurs. Claims-made policies provide coverage only in instances in which both the injury and the claim are made during the time in which the policy is in effect. This type of coverage is adequate if the nurse maintains continuous coverage and purchases a tail to provide uninterrupted extension for a period of time after the policy period. Occurrence-based policies are preferable for most nurses.

Another distinction is made between malpractice policies and professional liability policies. Generally speaking, *malpractice policies* offer coverage exclusively for claims of malpractice. Though specific coverage differs from policy to policy, *professional liability* insurance offers protection against various injuries that are not directly related to malpractice (Mitchell & Grippando, 1993).

Nurses also question whether they need individual coverage if their group or employer provides insurance. *Individual coverage* is purchased by the individual and offers the policy-holder 24-hour protection against liability claims for actions that fall within the scope of professional nursing practice, either paid or volunteer services (Guido, 2010). Individual coverage pays lawyer fees and monetary damages (in relation to limits of the specific policy) and offers the nurse some control over details of the defense strategy. Infrequently used by nurses, *group coverage* is purchased by professionals who have essentially the same job descriptions and covers only those activities performed during office hours. This is particularly attractive as a less expensive choice for nurse practitioners in group practice. *Employer-sponsored coverage* is purchased by the employing agency for the purpose of protecting business concerns. Coverage under employer-sponsored policies limits the protection to activities performed within the scope of employment. Though employers may claim that employer-sponsored coverage is adequate, it is actually the most limited type of liability insurance. In fact, if found negligent, nurses may be required to repay the employer a portion of the loss. Guido (2010) reports that nurses who rely solely on hospital policies have a greater chance of inadequate monetary protection and inadequate legal counsel.

NURSES AS EXPERT WITNESSES

The role of expert witness is relatively new to the nursing profession. Because of the complex and highly technical nature of nursing, attorneys require the assistance of knowledgeable and experienced expert witnesses. These witnesses may be hired by either the plaintiff or the defendant. Serving the legal system, expert witnesses are neither parties to the dispute nor patient advocates. Ideally, they remain honest and give objective opinions to the court.

Until very recently, most courts accepted physicians as expert witnesses in cases involving nurses. Historically, court rulings tended to reflect society's confusion about the relationship between nursing and medicine. There has been a slow evolution in the courts. In 1958, a California judge accepted a physician's testimony about nursing standards of care, saying,

"Surely a qualified doctor would know what was standard procedure of nurses to follow" (*Goff v. Doctor's Hospital,* 1958). More recently, a 1972 judicial opinion acknowledged that a physician might not be the best expert on nursing standards, but admitted physicians' testimony because, "all areas of medical expertise within the knowledge of nurses are also within the knowledge of medical doctors" (*Taylor v. Spencer Hospital,* 1972). A 2004 Illinois Supreme Court decision became a landmark case for nurses. In this case, the Supreme Court upheld a lower court ruling that the doctor who testified as an expert was not competent to give testimony as to the standard of care for nurses (*Sullivan v. Edward Hospital,* 2004).

Serving as an expert witness involves a complex and extensive process of examining evidence, reviewing pertinent nursing literature, giving depositions, and testifying in court. The expert witness is expected to be familiar with the following: all medical records of the patient during the time of the incident; pertinent written policies and procedures of the institution; the nursing care plan, including nursing assessment, diagnosis, plan, interventions, and evaluation; the state nurse practice act; the Joint Commission manual; applicable nursing standards; current professional literature outlining accepted practice at the time of the incident; and opinions from the state board of nursing (Dyke, 1989). The witness must describe the standards of care to the court, evaluate the nurse's actions against them, and discuss conclusions relative to the accusation of malpractice. Effectiveness of the expert witness is influenced by the breadth of experience, degree of preparation, depth of knowledge, and confident delivery.

The use of expert witnesses gives strength to the argument that nursing is a true profession. It supports the autonomy of nursing in that no other professional can appropriately judge the practice of nurses. Murphy (2004, 2005) believes that recent court decisions recognize nursing as a unique profession, different from medicine: Courts can no longer consider nursing a subcategory of medicine. Advertisements for educational courses and organizations for nurse expert witnesses are now common in nursing periodicals and websites. It is clear that the profession is taking seriously this newly acquired judicial recognition.

SUMMARY

As the enforceable system of principles and processes that govern the behavior of people, laws reflect moral and ethical tradition. Though there is sometimes disagreement regarding the rightness or wrongness of certain laws, the laws are generally consistent with popular beliefs.

Laws in the United States are constitutional, statutory, or administrative, and are divided into public and private realms. Public law deals with the relationship between persons and the government, and private law deals with the relationship between people. Nurses and other health care providers are more likely to be involved in liability cases related to tort law, a division of private law. Tort law includes unintentional torts, such as negligence and malpractice, and intentional torts, such as fraud, invasion of privacy, assault, battery, false imprisonment, and defamation.

Recent trends in health care delivery systems have both created new areas of liability and increased instances of traditional negligence. Managed care organizations, while assuming the roles of both insurer and provider of health care, are frequently charged with corporate negligence. Perhaps because of increased stressors in the workplace, nurses are experiencing an increasing number of malpractice claims related to the traditional kinds of errors.

With the increase in malpractice litigation, nurses are wise to take certain precautions to limit the risk of lawsuits. Critical factors include maintaining open lines of communication with patients through the use of good listening techniques, an accepting demeanor, and attention to patients' level of understanding; maintaining conscientious practice, including retaining expertise and ensuring attention to detail; maintaining autonomy through courageous and vigorous patient advocacy; and maintaining continuous professional liability insurance. When patients accuse nurses of malpractice, expert nurse witnesses can serve the court by describing standards of care, evaluating the nurse's action against standards, and discussing conclusions relative to the accusation of malpractice.

CHAPTER HIGHLIGHTS

- Ethics is the foundation of law; however, because laws are created by individuals and there are differences in beliefs among people, ethics and the law are not always congruent.

- Constitutional law is based upon the Constitution and supersedes all other law.

- Statutory law is created through the lawmaking process in state or federal legislatures; it is also called legislative law.

- Administrative law consists mainly of the legal powers granted to administrative agencies by the legislature, and the rules that the agencies make to carry out their powers.

- Common law, also known as case law, is a system of law based largely on previous court decisions.

- Public law defines a person's rights and obligations in relation to government, and describes the various divisions of government and their powers.

- Private law, also called civil law, determines a person's legal rights and obligations in many kinds of activities that involve other people.

- A tort is a wrong or injury that a person suffers because of someone else's action, either intentional (willful or intentional acts that violate another person's rights or property) or unintentional (an act or omission that causes unintended injury or harm to another person).

- Changes in health care financing and delivery have caused litigation related to corporate liability.

- Nurses can limit the risk of liability through maintaining open communication with patients, expertise in practice, attention to details, and autonomy.

- Supporting the autonomous nature of nursing, expert nurse witnesses serve the court through the process of examining evidence, applying nursing standards, reviewing pertinent nursing literature, and explaining conclusions.

DISCUSSION QUESTIONS AND ACTIVITIES

1. Search the Internet for references to recent court decisions. You may begin by visiting Google and searching for "recent malpractice cases." Find examples of recent court cases related to issues such as termination of life support, fetal tissue use, genetic engineering, and patient self-determination. Discuss your ethical beliefs related to the court decisions. What ethical principles are applicable?

2. Discuss with classmates opinions about the courts becoming involved in issues that have traditionally been considered ethical in nature.

3. Read the Bill of Rights of the U.S. Constitution found at http://www .usconstitution.net/const.pdf. How do the rights guaranteed in the Bill of Rights relate to patient care? How do they relate to nurses' employment?

4. Discuss recent examples of state or federal legislation that create changes in the health care delivery system or in the practice of nursing.

5. In the common law system, how do previous court decisions affect the outcome of current cases?

6. Discuss instances in which nurses can be charged with crimes of public law, even though acts were committed without malice in the process of giving nursing care.

7. Discuss specific examples of unintentional torts of which nurses have been accused.

8. How can you protect yourself from being accused of an unintentional tort?

9. In what instances can nurses be charged with intentional torts, even though they follow a professional code of ethics?

10. Discuss new areas of potential liability for nurses and the present health care delivery system.

11. Review the American Nurses Association ethics and human rights position statements page to examine official position statements at http://www.nursingworld.org/positionstatements.

12. Review the website for the NPDB at http://www.npdb-hipdb.hrsa.gov. Find the most recent annual report. Discuss the overall purpose of the data bank. Do you believe the data bank is achieving the intent of Congress? How do statistics differ among professions? Why are there vast differences in statistics from state to state? What type of nurse is most vulnerable to malpractice lawsuits?

REFERENCES

American Nurses Association. (2006). *Position statement: Privacy and confidentiality*. Retrieved June 21, 2011, from http://www.nursingworld.org/MainMenuCategories/Policy-Advocacy/Positions-and-Resolutions/ANAPositionStatements/Position-Statements-Alphabetically/PrivacyandConfidentiality.html

Aspden, P., Wolcott, J. A., Bootman, J. L., & Cronenwett, L. R. (Eds.). (2011). *Preventing medication errors*. Washington, DC: National Academies Press.

Beauchamp, T. L. (2001). *Philosophical ethics: An introduction to moral philosophy* (3rd ed.). Boston: McGraw-Hill.

Berthiaume v. Pratt, 365 A.2d 792, 795 (Me. 1976).

Big Town Nursing Home, Inc. v. Newman, 461 S.W.2d 195 (Tex. Civ. App. 1970).

Blackman for Blackman v. Rifkin, 759 P.2d 54 (Colo. App. 1988), *cert. denied* (1989).

Burkhardt, M. A., Nathaniel, A. K., & Walton, N. A. (2010). *Ethics and issues in contemporary nursing* (1st Canadian edition). Toronto, Ontario: Nelson Education, Ltd.

Burnham, H. (2005, September 14). New Orleans medical staff raid empty hospital for vital supplies. *Nursing Standard, 20*(1), 12.

Creighton, H. (1986). *Law every nurse should know* (5th ed.). Philadelphia: Saunders.

Dyke, R. M. (1989). The nurse expert witness: Professional implications. *Neonatal Network, 8*(3), 3–39.

Eskreis, T. R. (1998). Seven common legal pitfalls in nursing. *American Journal of Nursing, 98*(4), 34–44.

Ferris v. County of Kennebec, 44F. Supp. 2d 62—ME (1998).

Fiesta, J. (1988). *The law and liability: A guide for nurses* (2nd ed.). New York: John Wiley & Sons.

Fiesta, J. (1996). Legal update, 1995: Part 2. *Nursing Management, 27*(6), 24–25.

Furrow, B. R., Greaney, T. L., Johnson, S. H., Jost, T. S., & Schwartz, R. L. (2004). *Liability and quality issues in health care* (5th ed.). St. Paul, MN: West Group.

Goff v. Doctor's Hospital, 166 CalApp2d 314, 319 (1958).

Guido, G. W. (2010). *Legal & ethical issues in nursing* (5th ed.). Norwalk, CT: Appleton & Lange.

Jones v. Chicago HMO Ltd. of Illinois, 191 Ill.2d 278, 730 N.E.2d 1119 (Ill. 2000).

King, M. L., Jr. (1996). Letter from the Birmingham jail. In J. Feinberg (Ed.), *Reason and responsibility: Readings in some basic problems of philosophy* (9th ed., pp. 572–580). Belmont, CA: Wadsworth. (Reprinted from *Why we can't wait,* by M. King, Jr., 1963, New York: Harper & Row.)

Kocher, G. (2006, May 5). Man's estate to get $20 million. *Lexington Herald-Leader.* Retrieved on July 28, 2006, from http://www .wilkesmchugh.com/mans-estate-get-20-million.html

Kohn, L. T., Corrigan, J. M., & Donaldson, M. S. (Eds.). (1999). *To err is human: Building a safer health system.* Washington, DC: National Academies Press.

Kozier, B., & Erb, G. (1992). *Concepts and issues in nursing practice* (2nd ed.). Menlo Park, CA: Addison-Wesley.

Louisville Law. (n.d.). Elements of proof: Duty of care. *Kentucky Legal Resources on the Internet.* Retrieved from http://www.louisvillelaw .com/medical/malpractice/duty.htm

Mazzocco, W. J. (2000). "Mixed" billing raises questions. *Advance for Nurse Practitioners, 8*(10), 24–25.

Miller-Slade, D. (1997, May). Liability theories in nursing negligence cases. *Trial,* 52–57.

Mitchell, P., & Grippando, G. (1993). *Nursing perspectives and issues* (5th ed.). Clifton Park, NY: Delmar.

Murphy, E. K. (2004) OR nursing law. Judicial recognition of nursing as a unique profession. *AORN Journal, 80,* 924, 926–927.

Murphy, E. K. (2005) OR nursing law. The expert nurse witness. *AORN Journal, 82,* 853–856.

National Quality Forum. (2006). *Serious reportable adverse events in health care—2006 update: A consensus report.* Washington, DC: National Quality Forum.

National Quality Forum. (2008). Serious reportable adverse events: Transparency & accountability are critical to reducing medical errors. Retrieved June 20, 2011 from http://www.qualityforum.org/ Publications/2008/10/Serious_Reportable_Events.aspx

O'Keefe, M. E. (2000). *Nursing practice and the law: Avoiding malpractice and other legal risks.* Philadelphia: F. A. Davis.

Omstein, C. (2006, June 3). Kaiser is found liable in retaliation case. *Los Angeles Times.* Retrieved July 11, 2006, from http://articles.latimes .com/2006/jun/03/local/me-kaiser3

Oswald v. LeGrand, 453 N.W.2d 634 (Iowa 1990).

Physician Insurers Association of America. (1993). *Medication error study.* Rockville, MD: Author.

Robertson v. Provident House, 576 So. 2d 992 (La. 1991).

Schessler v. Keck, 271 P.2d 588 (Cal. Ct. App. 1954).

Smelko v. Brinton, 740 P.2d 591 (Kan. 1987).

Smith v. Juneau, 692 So. 2d 1365 (1997).

State of Louisiana v. Brenner, 486 So. 2d 101 (La. 1986).

Sullivan v. Edward Hospital, 806 NE2d 645 (Ill 2004).

Taylor v. Spencer Hospital, 292 A2d 449, 452 (Pa Super 1972).

Trandel-Korenchuk, D. M., Rhodes, A. M., & Trandel-Korenchuk, K. M. (1997). *Nursing and the law* (5th ed.). Sudbury, MA: Jones & Bartlett.

Truhitte v. French Hospital, 180 Cal. Rptr. 152 (Cal. Ct. App. 1982).

U.S. Department of Health and Human Services, Health Resources Service Administration. (2006). National practitioner data bank: 2006 Annual Report. Retrieved June 17, 2011, from http://www.docstoc .com/docs/44167324/National-Practitioner-Data-Bank-2006-Annual-Report.

Yetter, D. (2006, June 5). Law sought on nursing home staff levels: Ky. advocates say care suffers. *The Courier-Journal.* Retrieved on June 21, 2011, from http://blog.levinperconti.com/Law%20sought%20 on%20nursing%20home%20staff%20levels%20in%20Kentucky.htm

PROFESSIONAL RELATIONSHIP ISSUES

These virtues we acquire by first exercising them.... Whatever we learn to do, we learn by actually doing it.... By doing just acts we come to be just; by doing self-controlled acts, we come to be self-controlled; and by doing brave acts, we become brave.

(Aristotle, *trans.* **1925)**

OBJECTIVES

After completing this chapter, the reader should be able to:

1. Identify relationships and potential conflicts that nurses face in the professional realm.

2. Characterize the nature of various conflicts.

3. Examine beliefs about the relative strengths of various obligations.

4. Identify nurses' primary obligation.

5. Discuss issues related to nurses' relationships with other nurses, institutions, physicians, and subordinates.

6. Discuss issues related to racial discrimination, sexual harassment, and discrimination against persons with disabilities.

INTRODUCTION

Armed with knowledge about the physical, psychological, social, and spiritual realms of nursing care and proudly possessing a wide range of technical and professional skills, new nurses expectantly enter the workforce. Anticipating respect for our opinions and encouragement to focus our efforts on giving excellent care, we soon realize that our attention must be divided between giving patient care and dealing with problems among providers and within the institutional system. This dichotomy can present a confusing and frustrating challenge, forcing us to examine conflicting loyalties, question previously held values, make decisions based upon both practical and moral considerations, and test our skills of negotiation.

It is important that solutions to problems in the workplace consistently honor the uniqueness and value of each person and faithfully adhere to ethical principles. This process requires us to critically examine our personal values and determine an ethically sound method of conflict resolution, even before conflict arises. We must enter professional relationships with attentiveness and skill. This chapter provides the opportunity to examine critically selected problems related to nurses' relationships within the health care delivery system. We suggest that students further prepare themselves to deal with conflict by learning morally sound skills of negotiation and conflict management.

PROBLEM SOLVING IN THE PROFESSIONAL REALM

Nurses face practical and ethical dilemmas in everyday nursing practice. Though many moral problems involve patients, nurses can encounter as well troubling moral questions related to other facets of work. There are layers of meanings, expectations, and relationships in the workplace. Each person has unique values; each profession has certain values and expectations; each facility has explicit and implicit mandates; and each relationship has meaningful overtones of loyalty, power, and influence. These strata constitute a confusing, often contradictory arrangement. For example, you may believe you have a duty to your patient, yet the institutional budget may not provide the best equipment and staffing. You expect that others will respect your autonomy, yet feel that you are unheard. You may be friendly with a colleague, yet be concerned about his or her substance use. Professional relationship problems are often more troubling than problems directly involving patients and can affect patient well-being directly and indirectly. Therefore, workplace problems are important on a professional level and deserve serious exploration.

Problems in the workplace are frequent and troubling, so we must try to anticipate them and devise strategies to prevent or deal with them when they occur. Although there is no absolute formula with which to solve conflicts, the following general guidelines can be helpful:

1. Maintain attentiveness to personal and professional values.

2. Articulate and consistently follow a morally derived hierarchy of obligation.

3. Determine the nature of the problem.

4. Choose from alternative solutions thoughtfully.

The process above is congruent with the decision-making process described in Chapter 7. Much of the discussion in that chapter applies to workplace issues. The following section includes a brief discussion of these steps as they specifically relate to professional relationships and the workplace.

Maintain Attentiveness to Personal Values

Nurses who maintain integrity by confidently and consistently adhering to values strengthen professional relationships. Others perceive them as trustworthy. Attention to integrity is unrelated to self-interest and predicates action based upon coherent and integrated moral values. Integrity ultimately leads to trustworthiness and the respect of others. Beyond questions of loyalty or duty, nurses are compelled to maintain integrity as they seek to do the right thing. Often doing the right thing boils down to listening to one's conscience and paying attention to personal beliefs. Because the nursing profession expects nurses to accept personal responsibility, institutions should recognize and encourage ethical autonomy. This type of reciprocal respect enables nurses to act rationally, free from coercion or manipulation and in ways that are consistent with personally held values and principles.

In addition to enhancing professional relationships, nurses' integrity contributes to patient well-being. Gadow (1980) asserts that only nurses who act out of self-unity can truly assist patients in reaching decisions that express their complex totality as individuals. Integrity is required of us since the welfare of patients is our primary obligation.

Clarify Obligation

An **obligation** signifies being required to do something by virtue of a moral rule, a duty, or some other binding demand. **Loyalty** refers to faithfulness to a person, an ideal, or a duty. A loyal person is steadfast in his or her devotion. Unlike obligation, loyalty is a choice, not a requirement. Obligations and loyalty generally occur together, but may sometimes conflict.

Some obligations derive from a particular role or relationship. For example, parents have an obligation to feed and clothe their children. When you accept a position and a paycheck, you have an obligation to fulfill the requirements of your employer. You will likely also choose to be loyal to your children and employer. However, even nurses who possess a high level of integrity experience conflicting obligations or loyalties on occasion. There is, after all, a certain mix of obligations and loyalty owed to any of the following: the patient, the employer, peers and other coworkers, physicians, the broader society, family, and self. Before workplace problems arise, you should articulate and thereafter consistently follow a morally derived hierarchy of obligation and loyalty. Keep personal moral values and professional ethics in mind as you examine to whom you owe primary and secondary obligations. Recognize that these obligations may sometimes override certain loyalties, such as loyalty to a friend or coworker.

Obligation to Patients

As a part of professional nursing practice, nurses' first obligation is to patients. Because nurses are professionals, we have a moral obligation to maintain fidelity—that is, we must be faithful to the promises made to society, and thus give priority to meeting the needs of each patient. The codes of ethics from both the International Council of Nurses (ICN) and the American Nurses Association (ANA) are clear that the nurse's primary responsibility is to the patient. By following established professional codes of ethics and maintaining integrity and loyalty to patients, we also fulfill related obligations to the broader society, the profession, and ourselves.

Obligation to the Employer

Our secondary obligation is to the employer. By accepting and maintaining terms of employment and payment for services, we have both a legal and moral obligation to the institution. This obligation, however strong, does not suggest that we should jeopardize personal integrity or subordinate loyalty to the patient. To succeed in the age of technological advancement, competition, and litigation, institutions need the services of nurses who express the professional characteristics of autonomy, integrity, and ethically based practice. Conflicts arise when the institution's goals are focused more on profit margins than a moral responsibility and patient welfare. Conflict is inevitable when nurses, whose primary loyalty must be to the welfare of patients, are employed by institutions that eliminate important programs, employ poorly qualified staff or inadequate numbers of staff, and are otherwise ill-equipped to meet the needs of patients.

Case Presentation

When Economy Replaces Excellence

Community Hospital is a large metropolitan hospital that boasted the reputation of maintaining excellent nursing care services for many years. As a result of fierce competition and increasing financial strain, the hospital board of trustees decided to affiliate with a large hospital corporation. Television and radio advertisements describing the hospital corporation as having state-of-the-art equipment and services were far from reality. Immediately after the official affiliation was finalized, the hospital began dismissing nurses, cutting back supplies, eliminating unprofitable patient care services, and increasing patient charges. It was soon clear to nurses that patients would no longer receive the excellent nursing care that had been the hallmark of that hospital for many years. Nurses who remained on staff were faced with a changing environment that was no longer patient-centered, discouraged autonomous nursing practice, and led to ethical and practical dilemmas directly caused by an explicit focus on profit. Many felt trapped because of a shrinking job market and years of investment in the hospital retirement program. They also felt powerless to change impersonal policies that were created by faceless bureaucrats hundreds of miles away.

Think About It

How Do Nurses Respond to Bottom-Line Economics?

- *What kinds of dilemmas are likely to occur in this situation?*
- *Recognizing that a nurse's primary responsibility is to patients, how does the new hospital arrangement affect the nurse-patient relationship?*
- *Can nursing practice maintain a patient-centered, ethically sensitive focus in this type of setting?*
- *What alternative solutions to potential problems faced by nurses in this situation can you suggest?*

Determine the Nature of the Problem

When difficult situations arise, it is important that nurses clarify the nature of the problem. Is it a problem of a practical or ethical nature? Is it a problem of moral uncertainty, moral distress, moral dilemma, or moral outrage? It is important to know the answer to these questions because problems that seem immense on an emotional level are often truly unimportant. Ethical considerations should carry more weight than matters of self-interest—although, clearly, we owe some consideration to our own needs. For example, with changing patient demographics and increasing hospital bed vacancies, we are sometimes asked to "float" to unfamiliar settings. This practice redistributes the workload and offers the promise of improved nursing care. However, we frequently object to the prospect of being asked to float. Some nurses complain, "I've never worked there; I would be unsafe to practice in that setting!" They are tempted to refuse to float to unfamiliar settings. These nurses are faced with a moral dilemma. Recall that the nurse has obligations to both ensure the welfare of the patient and meet the needs of the institution. In either case—in assigning a nurse to float or in accepting the assignment—one must be guided by the principles of nonmaleficence and beneficence: The actions that the nurse is expected to perform must be relatively certain to do good and do no harm. In that regard, neither the nurse, nor the patient, nor the institution will benefit from requiring a nurse to perform beyond his or her ability. To do so would be unethical. On the other hand, to leave a patient unit critically understaffed would also be unethical. When faced with situations of this sort, we should look to our codes of ethics for help. Regarding this particular situation, for example, the ICN *Code of Ethics for Nurses* (2006) is very specific about the nurse's duty: "The nurse uses judgment regarding individual competence when accepting and delegating responsibility." Similarly, the ANA *Code of Ethics for Nurses* (2001) states, "As the scope of nursing practice changes, the nurse must exercise judgment in accepting responsibilities, seeking consultation, and assigning activities to others who carry out nursing care."

An ANA position statement clearly states that registered nurses have the "professional right to accept, reject or object in writing to any patient assignment that puts patients or themselves at serious risk of harm" (ANA, 2009). The Canadian Nurses Association (CNA) *Code of Ethics for Registered Nurses* (2008) also addresses this type of situation in a section on being accountable: "Nurses practise within the limits of their competence. When aspects of care are beyond their level of competence, they seek additional information or knowledge, seek help from their supervisor or a competent practitioner and/or request a different work assignment. In the meantime, nurses remain with the person receiving care until another nurse is available." It is clear that codes of ethics support nurses who recognize their own limitations.

Paradoxically, it could also be said that to refuse an assignment is unethical on a number of levels. We must not abandon patients in need of care. If there is no one else available to care for the patients, we are obligated to give care, but only the type of care for which we are prepared and competent. For example, nurses temporarily assigned to specialty units can be asked to give basic, supportive nursing care, but should not be asked to perform technical tasks for which they are unprepared. To do so is both ethically wrong and legally risky. In the same regard, we should not attempt tasks for which we are not prepared. To do so will compromise fidelity. We should not, however, refuse to accept float assignments simply because we fear the unknown, because familiarity is comfortable, or for other self-interested reasons.

Case Presentation

Facing a Dilemma in the Newborn Nursery

Angela is a registered nurse employed in the newborn nursery of a small hospital. She is working toward completing her bachelor's degree and has an important exam at 4:30 P.M. Though she is scheduled to leave work at 3:00 P.M., by 4:00 P.M. the nurse from the next shift has not yet arrived. There is an LPN who is capable of caring for the newborns, but hospital policy requires the presence of an RN in the unit at all times. The supervisor is unable to give her any assistance. All the babies are quiet; she expects the evening shift RN to arrive soon and feels the LPN can handle the nursery for a short time. Angela is torn between honoring her duty to patients versus leaving to take her exam.

Think About It

What Should the Nurse Do?

- *Is this a practical or an ethical dilemma? What factors make this either a practical or an ethical dilemma?*
- *Do you think Angela's duty to stay outweighs her obligation to take the exam?*
- *What is the harm that could occur if she leaves before the evening shift RN arrives?*
- *What is the harm that could occur if she stays and misses her exam?*

The situation in the Case Presentation above constitutes a practical dilemma. Moral and nonmoral claims are in conflict. Based upon the principles of beneficence, nonmaleficence, and fidelity, Angela has a moral obligation to the patients committed to her and to the institution. On the other hand, her obligation to attend class is a matter of self-interest and is not based upon moral principle. There is the potential for harm to the newborns if she leaves the unit inappropriately staffed. An emergency could arise for which the LPN is not prepared. Possibly the evening shift RN will not arrive at all. If Angela utilizes Kant's moral imperative—one should do only that which could become a rule for all people—a decision to leave the unit unattended by an RN would be untenable. By leaving, she would create a situation that should not become a rule for all nurses in all situations. A rule suggesting that all nurses should leave patients improperly attended would harm many patients in the future and as a result would harm society's faith in the profession of nursing. Based upon a comparison of moral versus practical considerations and the potential harm that could result if Angela left the unit improperly attended, it seems clear that she should not leave. This is not meant to imply that nurses should always subjugate personal needs to patient or institutional ones. Staying at work later than scheduled as a result of an occasional, unpredictable circumstance is one thing; being required to stay repeatedly is something entirely different.

Choose from Alternative Solutions Thoughtfully

Choose from alternative solutions thoughtfully and recognize that each person involved is an autonomous being, worthy of respect. Keep in mind your overriding goal and anticipate the potential for good and harm that each alternative might produce. Try also to foresee the long-term consequences, since some alternatives may seem attractive initially, yet may include undesirable long-term effects. Ideal solutions will diminish harm, engender good, preserve the integrity of each person involved, and maintain positive relationships.

NURSES' RELATIONSHIPS WITH INSTITUTIONS

We enter the workforce with very different perceptions than our employing institutions. Having learned that autonomy and accountability are valuable components of the nursing role, we believe we owe primary loyalty to patients. We also expect that our beliefs will be honored and that our opinions and knowledge will be respected. Hospitals and other health care facilities, on the other hand, tend to be sharply hierarchical and bureaucratic institutions that expect nurses' and other subordinates' primary loyalty to be toward the institution (Jameton, 1984). Moreover, institutions expect nurses' actions to be directed toward attaining the goals of the system—goals that focus strongly upon ensuring the well-being of the institution itself and sustaining patterns of power and control. Difficulties emerge when there is conflict between the goals of patient-centered nurses and the goals of the institution.

Problems arise, in part, because the institution's demands for loyalty are often inequitable. Though requiring employees to respond to certain requests, institutions rarely reciprocate with similar loyalty to nurses. For example, due to budget constraints, most institutions are fairly rigid about nurses' work hours. Nurses are expected to arrive ready to begin and complete work according to a set schedule. Nurses are sometimes directed to complete more work than can reasonably be done. Nurses, loyal to the institution and to the duty that they feel toward the patients in their care, are often willing to skip meals and breaks and complete work after "clocking out." In essence, these practices—though very stressful for nurses—are financially appealing to institutions (Jameton, 1984).

It becomes a real balancing act when nurses must consider personal commitments along with professional obligation and the ideal of compassionate service. The ANA *Code of Ethics for Nurses* (2001) supports the nurse's professional role, which may include working overtime and attending meetings at one's own expense, in order to improve patient care or to establish and maintain conditions of employment conducive to high-quality nursing care. However, habitual self-sacrificing, altruistic behavior on the part of nurses is self-defeating, and does not establish conditions of employment conducive to high-quality nursing care. It tends to support and perpetuate a flawed system: as long as nurses continue to work selflessly, the system (rather than the patient) benefits. Nurses willing to work for free devalue the work of all nurses and perpetuate the expectation that this type of one-sided self-sacrifice will continue. Of course, crisis situations can occur in any institution, but when nurses repeatedly accept workloads that are unreasonable, they become complicit in continuing the wrongs. On the surface, consistently working extra hours or assuming an unreasonable workload may appear to fulfill professional obligations and the ideal of compassionate service, yet ultimately it is harmful to nurses, the profession, and patients.

Case Presentation

When Patients Suffer from Lack of Nursing Care

Tim, an RN, works weekends on the skilled nursing unit of a small rural hospital. Recently purchased by a large corporation, the hospital was forced to dismiss nearly one-third of the staff of the skilled nursing unit. Lately, when Tim comes to work, he feels totally overwhelmed. Although he always considered himself efficient, Tim is distressed because he rarely has enough time to complete his work. He knows that many of the patients suffer because of lack of attention. Those who are bedfast are not turned on a regular schedule, they often wait for assistance with eating until their food is cold, and medications are rarely given on time. Suffering from expressive aphasia and hemiplegia secondary to a CVA, Mrs. Wallace was admitted to the skilled nursing unit after 2 weeks in the intensive care unit.

Mrs. Wallace has been on the skilled nursing unit for 3 weeks when her daughter, Nina, notices a large reddened area surrounding a small gray ulcer over her mother's coccyx. Concerned, Nina asks Tim what caused this problem. Even though Mrs. Wallace's nursing care plan calls for attention to activity including frequent turning and sitting in a chair twice daily, Tim suspects that this was not consistently done the previous week. He recognizes that the reddened area is the beginning of a large pressure ulcer, a problem that might have been prevented with proper attention to activity and good nutrition. Tim hesitates to tell Nina that the problem is a potentially serious one that might have been prevented by good nursing care measures. He believes she has a right to know but he is hesitant to implicate himself or the other nurses, and he is afraid that he will lose his job if he complains.

Think About It

How Do Nurses Make Decisions When Loyalties Conflict?

* *What are the ethical principles implicit in this situation?*

* *What are Tim's conflicting loyalties?*

* *The staff on the unit is efficient and hard working—skipping lunch and staying overtime to complete their work. Do you believe the staff is responsible for the apparently poor nursing care that Mrs. Wallace is getting?*

* *Do you believe Tim should tell Nina the truth about the pressure sore?*

* *Should Tim risk losing his job by whistle blowing?*

* *Is this an ethical or a practical dilemma?*

* *What harm can result from either option?*

* *What would you do?*

The previous Case Presentation is another example of a practical dilemma. The conflict that Tim is experiencing is between the principle of beneficence (the desire to do good for the patient) and a sense of loyalty to the institution or the other nurses with whom he works. There may also be an element of self-interest—Tim may not want to be implicated in the harm that the patients are experiencing as a result of the staff cutbacks. Tim's primary loyalty is owed to the patients—Mrs. Wallace, other patients suffering from the shortage of staff, and future patients who could be harmed by perpetuation of the problem. There are strong arguments that he should act to correct the situation. He may choose to take any number of actions: He can work through the administrative hierarchy to improve staffing; he can answer Nina's questions honestly; and, though his job will certainly be jeopardized, he can inform the media of the problems that were created by the drastic staffing shortages. In any case, if Tim fails to act to solve the problem, he will be complicit in its perpetuation and the subsequent harm to patients.

In some instances, nurses base the motivation for altruism on misguided beliefs about duty. Some believe that altruism is necessary to fulfill their duty to patients. Though many philosophers consider altruism and sacrifice a virtue, Ayn Rand (1996) suggested that altruism has a dehumanizing effect. Rand believed that those who are altruistic have a nightmare view of existence—believing that people are trapped in a malevolent universe. Rand viewed a persistent willingness to sacrifice as flowing from poor self-esteem and inappropriate priority-setting. Moreover, she believed that those with poor self-esteem have difficulty valuing others. Because genuine regard is partially a product of sympathy (imagining oneself in the situation of another), one must value oneself in order to value others. Additionally, nurses who repeatedly sacrifice for the good of an institutional system fail to assume the power to change the wrongs that are committed.

Another example related to institutions' inequitable demands for loyalty is seen in the customary practice of requiring nurses to complete incident reports. In an effort to prevent litigation, institutions discourage nurses from talking to patients about mistakes that have been made. They much prefer that nurses file incident reports. These documents, geared toward institutional goals, are filed and kept for use in the event the hospital needs a legal defense, in firing or disciplining workers, or in reorganizing services to prevent future incidents (Jameton, 1984). Thus, patient-centered goals based upon the principles of autonomy, fidelity, veracity, and respect for persons are subordinated to the institutional subgoals of employee control and risk management.

Nurses' loyalty to the institution is an important mode of control. Without loyalty, administrators cannot manage institutions. For this reason, supervisors and administrators sometimes react negatively when nurses support and cooperate with each other to make changes. The ensuing perception of nonsupportive supervisors is a contributing factor for job stress and dissatisfaction. In the end, this can be harmful to nurses and patients alike because it can interfere with nurses' expressions of loyalty to patients.

Nurses' Relationships with Other Nurses

Nurses work together in close proximity day in and day out. No other profession is so intimately connected with the essence of life. The knowledge gained from the intimate experiences of birth, illness, life, and death are both powerful and mysterious. Nurses are connected to each other and set apart from others—connected by common experience, language, and knowledge, and set apart through professional mystique. Nurses work together closely, identify with each other, and supervise or are supervised by other nurses. The practice of one affects that of others.

Loyalty among nurses is a natural product of long-term acquaintance and close working relationships. Some view loyalty among members as a distinguishing characteristic of a profession. Loyalty is a social, interpersonal phenomenon in which a person has devotion to another person. People who are loyal show sympathy and care toward those to whom they are loyal. Loyalty unites people together in their service. It is freely given, not coerced. Loyalty is actively practiced by words and deeds. People who are loyal keep promises and sacrifice personal interests to the relationship. They share common goals.

In most practical matters, loyalty is a productive virtue. It enhances unity, strength, and power. Facing bureaucratic, economic, and political forces, nurses' loyalty to each other and to the profession adds strength to the call for improved patient care, public welfare, nursing autonomy, and optimum employment conditions.

Though normally viewed as admirable, loyalty is seldom regarded as a virtue because it leads to the potential for misplaced loyalty, fanaticism, and blind injustice. While having the potential to strengthen the profession of nursing and improve the welfare of patients, loyalty among nurses can also be harmful. Misguided or fanatical loyalty can lead to a confused sense of obligation. Though nurses' primary obligation is to patients, those who are overly loyal to other nurses might act in ways that are harmful to patients' health status. For example, a nurse having blind loyalty to another might cover up the coworker's incompetent practice, illegal drug use, or other actions that have the potential to harm patients. For this reason, nurses must be careful to maintain objectivity in balancing loyalty to other nurses against the obligation owed to patients.

Case Presentation

Nurses' Loyalty to the Profession

A few years ago, politically active nurses in a small state lobbied for a bill mandating nurse representation on government bodies charged with considering health-related issues. Positions included membership on committees, task forces, advisory panels, and so forth. There was also a stipulation that required each public hospital to include one nurse on its governing board. As the largest group of health care professionals, nurses believed their knowledge and experience would be a welcome addition. Though there was strong and unified nursing support, the bill was fiercely opposed by both the state hospital association and individual hospitals. When public hearings were held, the politically active nurses found themselves testifying for the bill in opposition to commanding and articulate nurse administrators testifying against the bill. Representing individual hospitals, nurse administrators cited everything from nurses' lack of economic expertise to a gossipy tendency to spill industry secrets as reasons to oppose nurse members on hospital governing boards. The bill failed.

Think About It

Examining Differences in Loyalty

- *Can you think of moral justification for the diverse positions of nurses?*
- *To whom is each group of nurses loyal?*
- *How would you characterize each group's stance in relation to the professionalization of nursing?*
- *How would you account for the diverse positions of the nurses?*

Incivility among nurses in the workplace has received increasing attention over the past two decades. The phenomenon has been studied and extensively reported among nurses around the globe (Vessey, Demarco, & DiFazio, 2010). Most sources discuss incivility in terms of **lateral (or horizontal) violence**, or **bullying**. Lateral violence occurs when one directs hostile or aggressive behavior toward another member of the same group. In the work environment, lateral violence is directed toward nurses who are otherwise equals. By contrast, bullying occurs when the aggressor has a position of power or authority over the victim. The Task Force on the Prevention of Workplace Bullying (2001) defines bullying as "offensive abusive, intimidating, malicious or insulting behavior, or abuse of power conducted by an individual or group against others, which makes the recipient feel upset, threatened, humiliated or vulnerable, which undermines their self-confidence and which may cause them to suffer stress. Bullying is behavior which is generally persistent, systematic and ongoing." Bullying, lateral violence, and incivility in general are prevalent in the workplace as well as in schools of nursing.

The exact prevalence is not known, but recent studies have estimated that up to three-quarters of nurses have experienced incivility in the workplace. Often directed toward new, inexperienced nurses and nursing students, incivility warrants attention because of its prevalence in the nursing workplace and its potential to lead to serious consequences.

The description of aggressive and bullying behavior is far too familiar. The 10 most frequent forms of incivility are nonverbal innuendo, verbal affront, undermining activities, withholding information, sabotage, infighting, scapegoating, backstabbing, failure to respect privacy, and broken confidences (Griffin, 2004). Incivility includes a long list of antagonistic behaviors, including gossip, putdowns, blaming, bullying, lack of respect, undue criticism, scapegoating, undermining, impatience, passive aggression, angry outbursts, condescending language, competitiveness, rudeness, humiliating comments, and refusal to answer questions. These offensive behaviors lead to a number of negative outcomes.

The consequences of incivility are immense, including physical and psychological effects on victims, decreased productivity, decreased patient safety, and loss of nurses from the workforce. Nurses who have experienced incivility in the workplace complain of symptoms such as headaches, gastrointestinal problems, sleep disturbances, fatigue, increased blood pressure, anorexia, loss of libido, fear, depression, sadness, anxiety, nervousness, mistrust, suicide ideation, and suicide (Vessey et al., 2010). However, the effects of incivility extend beyond individual nurses.

Incivility disrupts the critical components of nursing work, including communication, the exchange of crucial health information, and collaborative decision making. Creating a barrier to effective communication, incivility is associated with increased medical errors and poorer patient outcomes (Vessey et al., 2010). Nurses who experience incivility have poor morale, decreased productivity, increased errors, and significantly lower levels of job satisfaction. Many leave the workforce within the first 6 months. Jones (2008) calculated that the cost to replace even one newly graduated nurse is an estimated $88,000 per nurse.

What is the solution to the pervasive problem of incivility in nursing? In 2008, the ANA approved a position statement on lateral violence and bullying in the workplace, proposing that nursing leaders should have a zero tolerance (Center for American Nurses, 2008). Leaders should be encouraged to recognize the signs of lateral violence and bullying in the workplace, and institute education programs and devise strategies to reduce incivility. Since significant bullying is perpetrated by nursing leaders, heightened awareness of the problem through education and training is essential. Organizations should eliminate behaviors such as finger-pointing and view mistakes as opportunities for learning and improvement. After all, nurses share a common goal.

NURSES' RELATIONSHIPS WITH PHYSICIANS

The nurse-physician relationship is an important factor in the quality of patient care. Ideally, the work of nurses and physicians should be complementary and synergistic. Because both professions hold claim to the primary goal of patient health, one would expect a sense of collegiality and collaboration between them. When this type of relationship exists, it is rewarding and productive. When there is conflict between nurses and physicians, the relationship is stressful and damaging to nurses, physicians, and patients alike. Because nurses and physicians work in close proximity, conflict that occurs between them is a strong contributor to nurses' lack of job satisfaction.

Nurse-physician relationships have generally reflected the prevailing gender roles in society. These roles were well defined for centuries. The traditional nurse was expected to obey the physician, much as the wife was expected to obey her husband. Physicians demanded obedience, and nurses hesitated to disagree with physicians, even if there was good reason to do so.

Given the bureaucratic nature of most health care institutions, particularly hospitals, today's relationship between physicians and nurses is complex and peculiar. Generally, nurses are employees of the institutions, while physicians are independent practitioners who have the privilege of institutional practice. Physicians, who are not employees of the institutions, have no formal chain-of-command relationship with the nurses who care for their patients. This tradition of self-employed physicians having power over a large group of nurses who are employees of the institution defies explanation. Though they issue orders to nurses directly, physicians are not employed by, subordinate to, or even responsible to the institutional administration. These bizarre lines of authority are confusing, and have the potential to severely limit the autonomous decision-making role of the nurse. Because most nurses are employees with either expressed or implied contracts with institutions, they have an obligation to perform the tasks required by the institutions. One of the major tasks that most institutions require of nurses is the implementation of physicians' orders. When nurses question or disagree with physicians, they may feel distressed, believing they are being disloyal to both the physician and the institution.

Another contributor to conflict in the nurse-physician relationship is the rapid advent of advanced practice nursing. With an expanded knowledge base and a scope of practice that includes many functions that were once limited to physicians, advanced practice nurses can contribute to tensions with physicians. The outdated tradition of the nurse who blindly obeys the physician conflicts with the concept of the autonomous nurse who thinks independently.

What actions should be taken by the nurse who questions or disagrees with an order or an action of a physician? The nurse must remember that the primary obligation is owed to the patient, not the physician. Nurses are autonomous practitioners. They have the knowledge and experience and the legal and ethical responsibility to make independent judgments, even when carrying out physicians' orders. If medical care constitutes incompetent, unethical, or illegal practice, the nurse is clearly obligated to disobey orders (ANA, 2001). When deciding what course to take in situations in which nurses disagree with physicians' orders, nurses can apply the test of urgency. Low-urgency problems are minor and may be solved at a leisurely pace. Very urgent problems require quick solutions and immediate actions. With low-urgency problems there is little risk of serious harm, or there is significant time available to examine all aspects of the situation. High-urgency situations consist of emergencies in which life-saving actions must be carried out at once. Nurses may have time to discuss and negotiate satisfactory solutions to problems at the low-urgency end of the spectrum, but problems at the high-urgency end of the spectrum require immediate, sometimes drastic action.

Case Presentation

Making a Decision in an Urgent Situation

Marta is night shift charge nurse in the emergency department. She has advanced certification and 25 years of experience. Marta works well with the other members of the emergency room staff, and is comfortable and efficient in situations of extreme urgency. The emergency department is usually staffed by board-certified emergency physicians. Because one of the regular physicians recently moved to another state, there has been a series of physicians with various degrees of preparation and ability moonlighting in the department, particularly on the night shift. During an unusually busy shift, an ambulance arrives with a middle-aged man having severe chest pain and dyspnea. His condition quickly deteriorates, and after a few minutes he experiences cardiac and respiratory arrest. The physician on duty, Dr. Andrews, is a family practice physician moonlighting after his regular shift at a local community health center. Marta perceives Dr. Andrews as nervous and hesitant. During the first phase of the "code," Dr. Andrews seems uncertain of every detail. As the nurse in charge, Marta begins instituting a seldom-used protocol that was developed for use in the event that the nurses are faced with a cardiac arrest when no physician is present. All the nurses are trained in intubation techniques, but hospital policy prohibits them from performing that particular procedure. Marta suggests to Dr. Andrews that he intubate the patient. After several clumsy attempts, Dr. Andrews angrily orders Marta to call an anesthesiologist at home to come and intubate the patient. Marta realizes that the patient's chances of survival are best if he is intubated quickly. She asks the unit clerk to call the anesthesiologist. Over his angry objections, Marta removes the laryngoscope and endotracheal tube from Dr. Andrews's trembling hands and proceeds to intubate the patient quickly and successfully. The patient responds to resuscitation attempts and is discharged 5 days later.

Think About It

Was Marta's Decision Correct?

- *What is your immediate response to the situation in which Marta finds herself?*
- *Where would you place this situation on the "spectrum of urgency"?*
- *What are the arguments in favor of Marta's actions?*
- *What are the arguments in favor of Marta's following Dr. Andrews's orders?*
- *Do you consider Marta's actions to be based upon ethical principle?*
- *Did Marta place herself at risk of reprisal or legal action?*
- *What would you have done?*

Nurses are charged with making thoughtful, fair, and knowledgeable decisions in relation to physicians' orders, while also being careful to consider the overall harm that can result from any given action. Recognizing that the physician's goal, like that of the nurse, is the welfare of the patient, nurses must be mature and objective when questioning orders. Nurses have an ethical obligation to protect the patient from medical incompetence. Nevertheless, they must be careful, keeping in mind the overall harm that can result from the practice of constantly and inappropriately questioning insignificant aspects of physicians' orders.

Nurses' Relationships with Subordinates

Most nurses are leaders. They may be informal leaders of a small number of assistive personnel or they may be leaders of large organizations. The actions of a leader send value messages. The quality of a nurse's leadership is reflected in the quality of the work of subordinates. Good leaders are those who inspire, motivate, and pay attention to individuals. They inspire others to work toward a common goal. Poor leaders may be abusive bullies who degrade, ridicule, and otherwise terrorize; or they may be passive and ineffective to the point that problems become so serious that they demand attention. Because nurses work toward the goal of caring for patients, the quality of nurses' leadership carries moral weight.

Nurses must be sensitive to those who work beside them. Each person is a moral agent and must be recognized as worthy of dignity and respect. As the coordinator of patient care, the professional nurse is accountable for the quality of nursing care rendered to patients. This accountability includes supervision, delegation of nursing care functions, and disciplining of other health care providers. The inherent practical, moral, and legal implications of these functions are facets of the role of the professional nurse that must be undertaken with sensitivity and respect.

The structure of health care delivery in some institutional settings makes the professional nurse responsible for delegating a number of nursing functions to subordinate staff members. The nurse has a moral obligation to ensure that each patient receives excellent nursing care, to respect the value of each individual, and to make sure the situation is conducive to high-quality nursing care (ANA, 2001). The following is an excerpt from the ANA *Code of Ethics for Nurses* regarding the nurse and delegation of nursing activities:

> Since the nurse is accountable for the quality of nursing care given to patients, nurses are accountable for the assignment of

nursing responsibilities to other nurses and the delegation of nursing care activities to other health care workers. The nurse must
make reasonable efforts to assess individual competency when
assigning selected components of nursing care to other health
care workers. This assessment involves evaluating the knowledge,
skills, and expertise of the individual to whom the care is assigned,
the complexity of the assigned tasks, and the health status of the
patients. The nurse is also responsible for monitoring the activities of these individuals and evaluating the quality of the care
provided. (2001, p. 9)

As the coordinator of patient care, the nurse is accountable for all nursing
care that patients receive, whether from the nurse or subordinates.

In addition to delegation, the supervisory role of professional nurses
occasionally includes disciplining subordinates. Disciplining is a difficult
task that must be done with insight, respect, compassion, and logic. The
nurse must be keenly aware of the effect of disciplinary action upon others
and must focus on the intended goal. The traditional methods of discipline,
such as punishment and chastisement, are damaging to the spirit and coun-
terproductive in practice.

Nurse managers' method of disciplining may set the tone for the entire nursing unit. Discussing poor leadership, Dilley says, "Nurse managers
from hell can be easily identified. They use coercion—as in, 'do as I say or
you'll find yourself on the night shift.' They belittle their employees in front
of patients or other staff. They communicate by memo rather than face-to-
face. They change policies without input from others. They are rude and
thoughtless" (2000, p. 9).

A good nurse manager may also set the tone of the unit through the
style of discipline. Quoting the great teacher Maria Montessori, Leah
Curtin writes, "'Our aim is to discipline for activity, for work, for good; not
for immobility, not for passivity, not for obedience'" (1996, p. 51). Curtin
suggests that the most meaningful method is self-discipline, which corrects
the problem, strengthens the character of the worker, and improves performance. She defines self-discipline as a process by which the rules are
internalized and become a part of the individual's personality. This process
is possible only if the person knows the rules, understands their purpose,
and agrees that they deserve compliance. To achieve this result, the nurse
must model the expected standard daily and have few rules—all of which
are applied consistently, change infrequently, and apply to all personnel
equally. The nurse has a moral obligation, to both patients and personnel,
to uphold rules that protect the health or safety of patients, other employees, the institution, and oneself as leader.

Discrimination and Harassment

Claims of discrimination or harassment in the workplace are becoming more frequent. In fact, millions of Americans have experienced employment discrimination. Recent literature points to evidence of continuing discrimination in nursing related to gender, age, race, disability, and sexual orientation. A 2005 Gallup poll found that 15 percent of all workers perceived that they had been subjected to discrimination (U.S. Equal Employment Opportunity Commission [EEOC], 2005). In 2011, the EEOC recorded record highs in discrimination charges (EEOC, 2012).

Discrimination is ethically prohibited. Because this prohibition entails treating others fairly and equitably, the ethical principle of justice is key to discussions of discrimination. Discrimination is professionally prohibited. In a 2010 position statement, the ANA outlines the role of the nurse in upholding human rights and preventing discrimination (ANA, 2010). Discrimination is also legally prohibited. The Bill of Rights of the U.S. Constitution, the Civil Rights Act of 1964, the Americans with Disabilities Act of 1990 (ADA), and the Civil Rights Act of 1991 provide legal protection against discrimination in the workplace.

Racial Discrimination

The Civil Rights Act of 1964 made it unlawful for an employer to fail or refuse to hire or to discharge any individual, or to otherwise discriminate against any individual, because of the person's race, color, religion, sex, or national origin. Unlawful acts include discrimination in terms of compensation or payment, conditions of employment, or privileges of employment. Considered one of America's strongest civil rights laws, the Civil Rights Act of 1964 primarily protects the rights of African Americans and other minorities. Attempting to correct a long tradition of racial discrimination, this act ensures that minorities receive fair and equal treatment from government, other persons, and private groups, including schools and employers. The act is enforced by the EEOC. It also specifically forbids discrimination by any program that receives money from the federal government.

The Civil Rights Act of 1964 enjoins employers to provide equal employment opportunities to individuals from the initial recruitment or application process through termination of employment. When considering claims of discriminatory practices, the legal system looks at two discriminatory outcomes: disparate treatment and disparate impact. *Disparate treatment* occurs when an individual is treated differently by a superior or by organizational policy. For example, if a supervisor passes over all Hispanic nurses who apply for promotion, regardless of their qualifications or abilities, disparate treatment exists. *Disparate impact* occurs when employers consistently apply policies that appear to be fair to all employees but actually adversely affect one group. For example, 346 men received a $5 million settlement in a disparate impact claim. The men were denied medical and dental insurance coverage for their children because of a former requirement that children of employees and pensioners live with them full time (EEOC, 2001). Denial of coverage for these men was considered disparate impact, because certain social and ethnic groups are less likely to have intact families living together in one home.

Because stereotypes are slow to change, it can be very difficult for non-majority group members to enter and succeed in any occupational group. Though the landmark civil rights legislation was passed decades ago, there is some indication that discrimination continues to exist in the health care system. Swart, Wendt, and Slonaker (1996) studied a group of nurses who had filed discrimination claims. Among nurses reporting discrimination, 47 percent based their claims on race discrimination.

In a study of nurses in California, Seago and Spetz (2005) reported that more than four times more African Americans and Asians reported feeling isolated in the workplace than Caucasians. Over 40 percent of African Americans and slightly fewer Asians believed they were denied promotions for which they were qualified. Most felt that favoritism and race were the primary factors. Only 29 percent of Caucasians reported being denied promotions for which they were qualified. Paradoxically, Caucasians were the least likely to believe they had the opportunity to advance in the workplace. Nearly all African American and Filipino nurses believed they had a good relationship with supervisors (over twice as many as Caucasians) and minority nurses were generally satisfied, while Caucasians were very dissatisfied.

Another source of race discrimination may be a lack of recruitment and retention of minority nursing students. Although African Americans, for example, constitute 12 percent of the U.S. population, only 4 percent of nursing students are African American (U.S. Census Bureau, 2010; Minority Nurse, 2011). There are a number of barriers to recruitment of minority nursing students, including a lack of full scholarships, scarcity of minority groups in certain geographic areas, lack of effective minority recruitment strategies, a negative attitude from administrators, and a lack of minority role models.

Both the ICN *Code of Ethics for Nurses* (2006) and the ANA *Code of Ethics for Nurses* (2001) identify racial discrimination as an ethical issue. Racism is prohibited by both. The ANA is active in identifying and eradicating racism in the profession. According to the ANA's position statement on discrimination and racism in health care, "ANA abhors the recent rise in racism and discriminatory behavior in this country. . . ." and ". . . is committed to addressing the need for racial and ethnic diversity among nurses" (1998).

Discrimination Against Persons with Disabilities

The ADA was signed into law on July 26, 1990. Seen by some as the most significant piece of legislation since the Civil Rights Act of 1964, this act provides comprehensive protection to Americans with disabilities. Challenged to combine the legal concepts of disability and equality, the aim of Congress in drafting this legislation was to ensure equality for the disabled without creating "undue" hardships on employers (Guido, 2010). The ADA considers one to have a covered *disability* if there is record of physical or mental disability that causes an impairment substantially limiting one or more of the major life enjoyments of the person, and if the person actually has such an impairment. *Major life enjoyments* include activities that the average person can perform with little or no difficulty, such as caring for oneself, performing manual tasks, walking, seeing, hearing, speaking, learning, and working. A *physical impairment* includes any physiologic disorder or condition, cosmetic disfigurement, or anatomical loss affecting any body system. A *mental impairment* includes any mental or psychological disorder, such as mental retardation, organic brain syndrome, emotional or mental illness, and learning disabilities. Mental or psychological conditions that result from such conditions as diabetes, cancer, AIDS, alcoholism, and drug abuse qualify under this definition (Guido, 2010).

Related to the Civil Rights Act of 1964, the ADA has several provisions. The act ensures that people with disabilities are not excluded from job opportunities or adversely affected in other aspects of employment unless they are unqualified or unable to perform the job. This protection extends to application, salary, promotion, discharge, transfer, and all other aspects of work. The ADA prohibits the practice of requiring medical examinations before employment except for drug testing, which may be performed. Medical examinations may be done only after a job offer has been extended. Employers may question individuals about their educational qualifications, experience, and their ability to perform the job safely with or without accommodation. To avoid the suggestion of discrimination, the prospective employer may not ask questions about disabilities, past medical problems, or previous workers' compensation claims. Upon request from employees with disabilities, employers must make necessary physical accommodations to the workplace, such as wheelchair accessibility, telephone systems for the hearing impaired, and so forth, but may be exempted from hiring persons with disabilities if the necessary accommodations cause *undue hardship* because they are extremely expensive or difficult to implement. The employer must have investigated the required accommodations and offer data proving the hardship. Undue hardship is based on cost, number of employees, and type of business (Guido, 2010).

The ADA does not require employers to hire individuals with disabilities. It demands, however, that employers base employment decisions solely upon job qualifications and ability, without regard to physical or mental disabilities. It also protects employers from financial ruin in the case of undue hardship related to making workplace accommodations for persons with disabilities.

SEXUAL HARASSMENT AND DISCRIMINATION

Sexual harassment is a widespread problem. As many as 76 percent of nurses and nursing students have been affected by sexual harassment (Bronner, Peretz, & Ehrenfeld, 2003). Sexual discrimination and harassment is not new in nursing. In the nineteenth century certain occupations were redefined as feminine. Nursing and teaching, for example, became accepted as feminine lines of work, and women in these occupational groups were seen and treated as "ladies." Florence Nightingale struggled with this identity: "In effect, she violated the gender norms of the day and threatened male power. Very much aware of her threat to the men, she continually emphasized that she was doing only what a proper lady should do—extending the role by accepting what society said women were especially qualified to do" (Bullough, 1990, p. 6). While allowing women to function as nurses, this attitude sustained the social order. Defined today as sexual harassment, there was an effort to sustain male power by treating women as sexual objects and inferiors.

Sexual harassment is a form of sex discrimination that violates the Civil Rights Act of 1964. The EEOC defines sexual harassment as "Unwelcome sexual advances, requests for sexual favors, and other verbal or physical conduct of a sexual nature constitute sexual harassment when this conduct explicitly or implicitly affects an individual's employment, unreasonably interferes with an individual's work performance, or creates an intimidating, hostile, or offensive work environment" (EEOC, 2006). Recognizing sexual harassment as a significant problem, federal and state courts have struggled with the issue for the past several decades. In October of 1991, the problem was brought to the attention of the public with the Senate confirmation hearings of Supreme Court nominee Clarence Thomas. A direct result of these hearings, the Civil Rights Act of 1991 was signed into law on November 21, 1991. This act defines sexual harassment and identifies two categories of the offense—quid pro quo sexual harassment and hostile work environment sexual harassment.

When submission to or rejection of the sexual conduct of an individual is used as a basis for employment decisions, *quid pro quo sexual harassment* is said to occur. There are four requirements to prove quid pro quo sexual harassment. The employee must show first that there was unwelcome harassment in the form of sexual advances or requests for sexual favors; second, that the harassment was based on sex; and third, that submission to the unwelcome sexual advances was required for receiving job benefits or that refusal to submit to the advances resulted in job detriment. Fourth, the individual who claims to be a victim of sexual harassment must be a member of a group that is lower on the chain of command than the person making the unwelcome advances. In quid pro quo harassment suits, employers are liable for the conduct of supervisory personnel (Guido, 2010).

Hostile work environment sexual harassment occurs when the employee is subjected to sexual innuendos, remarks, and physical acts that are so offensive as to create an abusive work environment. The two factors that must be shown in claims of hostile work environment are that the harassment unreasonably interfered with work and that the harassment would affect a reasonable person's work. The employer is only liable in such an instance when it can be shown that there was knowledge of the harassment. In hostile work environment sexual harassment cases, it is not necessary that the conduct be directed toward the individual who files the complaint, merely that the employee's psychological well-being was affected because the conduct was observed or known. This can occur, for example, with the unwanted posting of pornographic pictures or cartoons, sexually explicit comments or jokes, or sexual propositions. It is not necessary to prove that terms of employment are attached to this type of sexual harassment (Guido, 2010).

Although the majority of sexual harassment claims are filed by women, men can also be the object of real or perceived sexual harassment or discrimination. In one study, male student nurses reported effects of gender on their nursing school experiences such as few or no male nurses in clinical settings, no male faculty, and the exclusive use of women in textbooks as evidence of gender issues (Smith, 2006). In addition to the same type of sexual discrimination experienced by women, there are potential areas for sexual discrimination targeted specifically against men. These might involve such behaviors as stereotyping all male nurses as being gay, or assigning an inequitable portion of tough patients to men because of perceived physical stamina or strength.

Sexual harassment entails emotional costs such as anger, humiliation, and fear, and direct costs such as counseling and lawyer's fees. To avoid these costs, nurses must be sensitive in recognizing and protecting themselves and their colleagues from sexual harassment. Madison and Minichiello report on a study of nurses that identifies cues for recognizing harassment as follows:

- Invasion of space: Someone corners you or enters your personal space.

- Confirmation: Another person or colleague recognizes and confirms your suspicions of harassment.

- Lack of respect: Past or present behavior of the harasser is perceived to be disrespectful.

- Deliberate nature of behavior: Harassment is intentional, planned, and orchestrated.

- Perceived power of control: Circumstances put the harasser out of the control of the harassed organizationally, hierarchically, and physically.

- Overly friendly behavior: Behavior is considered too friendly, or falsely friendly.

- Sexualized workplace innuendos, explicit jokes, or pictures are common. (2000, p. 407)

Prevention of sexual harassment in the workplace is difficult. Sexual harassment is difficult to identify and difficult to prove, and many nurses are afraid to report incidents, fearing reprisal. Monarch (2000) suggests some guidelines for sexual harassment policies. A good policy should provide a clear description of prohibited conduct; assure employees who file complaints that they will be protected from retaliation; assure confidentiality to the greatest extent possible; identify reporting and investigative procedures that are free of chain-of-command entanglements; guarantee prompt investigations; assure immediate and appropriate action when sexual harassment is found to have occurred; pledge thorough investigation; identify sanctions; and offer counseling to the person complaining of sexual harassment.

SUMMARY

In the professional realm, nurses are faced with the dichotomy of striving to meet their primary obligation to patients while dealing with problems among providers and within the institutional system. Nurses must be prepared to examine personal beliefs, prioritize obligations, and devise morally sound solutions to problems. Solutions must reflect an overall respect for persons and recognize the moral agency of individuals. Nurses are guided in this endeavor by personal values and beliefs and by professional codes of ethics.

CHAPTER HIGHLIGHTS

- As a moral agent, each person has the duty to pursue solutions to moral problems.
- Solutions to practical and ethical problems in the professional realm must be sensitive to personal values and beliefs.
- Nurses must be able to identify and prioritize conflicting obligations.
- It is important for nurses to determine the nature of conflicts in the professional realm.

- Problem resolution requires thoughtful consideration and weighing of alternative solutions.
- In solving problems, nurses must recognize that each person is an autonomous being, worthy of respect.
- Nurses must seek solutions to moral problems related to conflicting role expectations in the institutional setting.
- Nurses must seek solutions to moral and practical problems related to relationships among nurses, physicians, and subordinates.
- Discrimination is prohibited by the ethical principle of justice, because it entails claims related to fair and equitable treatment of persons.

DISCUSSION QUESTIONS AND ACTIVITIES

1. Explore the EEOC website at http://www.eeoc.gov. Identify three recent court cases involving discrimination or harassment. Report the court decisions to the class.

2. Explore the ANA website at http://nursingworld.org. Read two position statements on discrimination or harassment. How do these position statements fit with your experience in the health care system?

3. Describe potential problems in the professional realm that fall into each of the following categories:
   - Conflicts of obligation
   - Conflicts of principle
   - Practical dilemmas
   - Conflicts of loyalty

4. Discuss with your classmates situations that could reasonably occur in the work setting that would constitute an appeal to conscience.

5. Review the nursing codes of ethics. List statements that apply to problems related to nurses' relationships with other professionals. Discuss the practical application of each of these statements.

6. Interview nurses who have been in practice for 1 year or less. Ask them to compare their expectations of the work environment with the reality that they faced upon graduation.

7. Discuss the conflict that results as shrinking institutional budgets require cutbacks in nursing staff.

8. List the positive and negative aspects of loyalty. Do you feel loyalty is a virtue?

9. Describe experiences that you've seen or heard about in which nurses experienced bullying or lateral violence.

10. Describe the ideal professional relationship between nurses and physicians.

11. Role-play a situation in which a nurse is sensitive and respectful in disciplining a subordinate—focusing on the goal of improving performance rather than punishing.

12. Discuss racial discrimination, discrimination against persons with disabilities, and sexual harassment in terms of ethical principles and legal mandates.

13. Visit websites for impaired nurses. Discuss sensitive, yet effective ways to approach an impaired nurse with these resources. Which resources would be most helpful to the nurse who is impaired?

REFERENCES

American Nurses Association. (1998). *Position statements: Discrimination and racism in health care.* Washington, DC: Author. Retrieved from http://www.nursingworld.org/MainMenuCategories/Policy-Advocacy/Positions-and-Resolutions/ANAPositionStatements/Position-Statements-Alphabetically/Copy-of-prtetdisrac14448.html

American Nurses Association. (2001). *Code of ethics for nurses.* Washington, DC: Author. Retrieved from http://www.nursingworld.org/MainMenuCategories/EthicsStandards/CodeofEthicsforNurses/Code-of-Ethics.pdf

American Nurses Association. (2009). *Patient safety: Rights of registered nurses when considering a patient assignment.* Washington, DC: Author. Retrieved from http://www.nursingworld.org/MainMenuCategories/Policy-Advocacy/Positions-and-Resolutions/ANAPositionStatements/Position-Statements-Alphabetically/Patient-Safety-Rights-of-Registered-Nurses-When-Considering-a-Patient-Assignment.html

American Nurses Association. (2010). The nurse's role in ethics and human rights: Protecting and promoting individual worth, dignity, and human rights in practice settings. Retrieved from http://www.nursingworld.org/MainMenuCategories/Policy-Advocacy/Positions-and-Resolutions/ANAPositionStatements/Position-Statements-Alphabetically/Nursess-Role-in-Ethics-and-Human-Rights.pdf

Americans with Disabilities Act of 1990, Pub. L. No. 101–336, § 2, 104 Stat. 328 (1991).

Bronner, G., Peretz, C., & Ehrenfeld, M. (2003). Experience before and throughout the nursing career: Sexual harassment of nurses and nursing students. *Journal of Advanced Nursing, 42*(6), 637–644.

Bullough, V. (1990). Nightingale, nursing and harassment. *Image: Journal of Nursing Scholarship, 22,* 4–7.

Canadian Nurses Association. (2008). Code of ethics for registered nurses. Retrieved from http://www2.cna-aiic.ca/CNA/documents/pdf/publications/Code_of_Ethics_2008_e.pdf

Center for American Nurses. (2008). Lateral violence and bullying in the workplace. Retrieved from http://www.can.affiniscape.com/associations/9102/files/Position%20StatementLateral%20Violence%20and%20Bullying.pdf

Civil Rights Act of 1964, 41 U.S.C.A. § 2000e *et seq.*

Civil Rights Act of 1991, P.L. 102–166, 105 Stat. 1071 (1991).

Curtin, L. (1996). Ethics, discipline and discharge. *Nursing Management, 27*(3), 51–52.

Dilley, K. B. (2000). Out from under their thumbs. *American Journal of Nursing, 100*(5), 9.

Gadow, S. (1980). Existential advocacy: Philosophical foundation of nursing. In S. F. Spicker & S. Gadow (Eds.), *Nursing: Images and ideals, opening dialogue with the humanities* (pp. 90–91). New York: Springer.

Griffin, M. (2004). Teaching cognitive rehearsal as a shield for lateral violence: an intervention for newly licensed nurses. *Journal of Continuing Education in Nursing, 35*(6), 257–263.

Guido, G. W. (2010). *Legal & ethical issues in nursing* (5th ed.). Norwalk, CT: Appleton & Lange.

International Council of Nurses. (2006). The ICN code of ethics for nurses. Retrieved from http://www.icn.ch/icncode.pdf

Jameton, A. (1984). *Nursing practice: The ethical issues.* Englewood Cliffs, NJ: Prentice-Hall.

Jones, C. B. (2008). Revisiting nurse turnover costs: Adjusting for inflation. *Journal of Nursing Administration, 38*(1), 11–18.

Madison, J., & Minichiello, V. (2000). Recognizing and labeling sex-based and sexual harassment in the health care workplace. *Journal of Nursing Scholarship, 32*(4), 405–410.

Minority Nurse. (2011). Minority nursing statistics. Retrieved from http://www.minoritynurse.com/minority-nursing-statistics

Monarch, K. (2000). Protect yourself from sexual harassment. *American Journal of Nursing, 100*(5), 75.

Rand, A. (1996). The ethics of emergencies. In J. Feinberg (Ed.), *Reason and responsibility: Readings in some basic problems of philosophy* (9th ed., pp. 541–545). Belmont, CA: Wadsworth.

Seago, J. A., & Spetz, J. (2005). *Advancement of minorities in nursing: A study by the discrimination research center.* San Francisco: University of California, San Francisco.

Smith, J. (2006). Exploring the challenges for non-traditional male students transitioning into a nursing program. *Journal of Nursing Education, 45*(7), 263–269.

Swart, J., Wendt, A., & Slonaker, W. (1996). Employment discrimination experiences of registered nurses. *Journal of Nursing Administration, 26,* 37–43.

Task Force on the Prevention of Workplace Bullying. (2001). *Report of the task force on the prevention of workplace bullying: Dignity at work—the challenge of workplace bullying.* Dublin Health and Safety Authority. Retrieved from http://www.djei.ie/publications/employment/2005/bullyingtaskforce.pdf

U.S. Census Bureau. (2010). The Black population: 2010. Retrieved from http://www.census.gov/prod/cen2010/briefs/c2010br-06.pdf

U.S. Equal Employment Opportunity Commission. (2001). EEOC, private plaintiffs and American Cast Iron Pipe Company settle lawsuit. Retrieved from http://www.eeoc.gov/press/1-4-01.html

U.S. Equal Employment Opportunity Commission. (2005). New Gallup poll on employment discrimination shows progress, problems 40 years after founding of EEOC. Retrieved from http://www.eeoc.gov/eeoc/newsroom/release/12-8-05.cfm

U.S. Equal Employment Opportunity Commission. (2006). Sexual harassment. Retrieved July 18, 2006, from http://www.eeoc.gov/types/sexual_harassment.html

U.S. Equal Employment Opportunity Commission. (2012). Private sector bias charges hit all-time high. Retrieved from http://www.eeoc.gov/eeoc/newsroom/release/1-24-12a.cfm

Vessey, J. A., Demarco, R., & DiFazio, R. (2010). Bullying, harassment, and horizontal violence in the nursing workforce: The state of the science. *Annual Review of Nursing Research, 28,* 133–157.

Chapter 10

PRACTICE ISSUES RELATED TO TECHNOLOGY

There is an appointed time for everything, and a time for every affair under the heavens.

(Ecclesiastes 3:1)

OBJECTIVES

After completing this chapter, the reader should be able to:

1. Discuss the impact of technology on nursing and health care.

2. Apply beneficence and nonmaleficence to decisions about technology.

3. Discuss issues and dilemmas related to current technology and to life-sustaining interventions.

4. Relate the concept of medical futility to health care decisions.

5. Relate economics to decisions regarding health technology.

6. Discuss considerations in decisions about cardiopulmonary resuscitation and artificial sources of nutrition for patients.

7. Describe legal issues associated with health care technology.

8. Discuss issues and dilemmas associated with technologies affecting reproduction, genetics, and organ transplantation.

9. Identify issues and dilemmas associated with research into controversial technologies.

10. Describe nursing considerations for patient care in the midst of technology.

INTRODUCTION

Nursing care is inextricably intertwined with ever-expanding advances of scientific knowledge and technology. Few would deny the benefits of medical advances, often referred to in terms such as wonders or miracles. However, the many benefits brought to the health care arena by technology are often accompanied by serious dilemmas for both practitioners and patients. Technology brings to the fore many questions related to issues of living and dying as well as the changing definitions of both that are brought on by scientific advances. Dilemmas include availability of technologies, what patient situations warrant the use of available technologies, and who decides when to initiate and when to withdraw particular interventions. Additionally, nurses must be concerned about the amount of nursing energy and attention that technology requires. As much as we say that nursing focuses on holistic caring for the patient, nurses are faced with increasing demands to focus attention to technology rather than on their patients.

This chapter focuses on common issues related to technology encountered in today's health care settings. Issues of technology, patient self-determination, and economics are intertwined. Nurses who are directly involved in dilemmas, as well as those who are more on the periphery, must be aware of considerations regarding the effect of technology on patient care. These considerations include values, attitudes, communication, and attention to the humanistic caring role. The term *technology* includes the vast range of scientific advances that affect health and health care. Changing technologies bring with them the challenge of dealing with new issues, and nurses need to be prepared to face this challenge.

BENEFITS AND CHALLENGES OF TECHNOLOGY

Scientific advances in the past 100 years have been phenomenal. They include medications, surgical techniques, machines and equipment, diagnostic procedures, specialized treatments, expanded understanding of the causes of and progression of disease, gene diagnosis and therapy, and greater insight into what is required for people to stay healthy. New interventions have saved lives, improved quality of life, alleviated suffering, and significantly decreased the incidence of some diseases. Before the advent of many modern health-related technologies, people experienced illness and death as an inevitable part of the cycle of their lives. Although death was not necessarily welcomed, it was expected as the natural outcome when the body could no longer ward off the effects of certain diseases or injuries. If someone was born with, or developed, a deformity, it may have been seen as a curse, but was also considered part of who the person was. Life began when the infant started breathing, and life ended when the heart and breathing stopped.

Current technology makes it possible to restart arrested hearts, use machines to breathe for people, correct deformities, assist the body in dealing with disease through use of medications and other interventions, eliminate diseased parts through surgery, and even to replace malfunctioning or diseased vital organs. The ability to prolong life, or at least to extend the functioning of the physical being, has prompted the necessity of dealing with some very important issues. One dilemma relates to questions of quality of life, and whether physical existence is synonymous with living. Another issue relates to whether the availability of certain technologies means they should always be used. Many issues relate to decisions about how and for whom technologies will be used.

Quality of Life

The ability to keep people alive and physically functioning through use of technology has led to much reflection and discussion about what constitutes life and living. Some people believe that biological life must be preserved, regardless of the effect on the person whose body is being kept alive. A frequently asked question is whether a person is truly alive in situations where there is merely physiological functioning, without awareness of oneself or others. Many suggest that living implies a quality that goes beyond physical existence. **Quality of life**, a subjective appraisal of factors that make life worth living and contribute to a positive experience of living, means different things to different people. It is difficult to find a clear and concise definition of quality of life, because of the multidisciplinary usage and variable cultural understandings of the concept. Definitions of quality of life vary from global understandings of the concept, such as satisfaction with life, to focused definitions used for research—for example, health or functional ability (Plummer & Molzahn, 2009). Discussions of quality of life encompass physical, emotional, spiritual, and social considerations. Ideas incorporated in understandings of the concept include fulfillment; satisfaction/dissatisfaction; meaning and purpose; conditions of life; happiness/unhappiness; experiences of life; and factors such as comfort, functional status, socioeconomic status, independence, and conditions in one's environment.

Evaluating dimensions of the concept presents challenges in defining quality of life (Clark, 2004). For instance, when assessing personal quality of life, which does a person rank as more important: happiness or functional status, such as the ability to get around and care for oneself? Nurses need to understand patient perspectives of what constitutes quality in their lives in order to incorporate these factors into goal setting and care planning.

Quality of life is a personal perspective that is determined by each individual. Recognizing this, we should not judge the quality of another's life based on our own values. If judgments are made about a person's worth and quality of life based on factors such as contributions to society, age, mental capacity, or ability to function, then discrimination against those who are judged to have a lesser quality of life may easily follow. Perceptions of quality of life often change with age and life experiences. For example, persons with debilitating health concerns may rate the quality of their lives quite positively, although others might feel that they could never live with such limitations. When patients and families are confronted with technological options, nurses need to help them clarify their perceptions regarding quality of life, and discuss not only how life might be extended, but also how quality of life may be affected by various options.

Principles of Beneficence and Nonmaleficence

When dealing with issues of technology, the principles of **beneficence** and **nonmaleficence** may be in conflict. A particular technology, which may be implemented with the intention of *doing good* (beneficence), may result in much suffering for the patient. Inducing such suffering is counter to the maxim of *do no harm* (nonmaleficence). In some circumstances this is accepted as part of the treatment process, such as pain associated with surgery or side effects of chemotherapy. We are willing to endure the discomfort because there is an expectation of recovery, that we will ultimately be or feel healthier. In circumstances in which there is little or no expectation of recovery or improved functioning, the essential question is whether the harm imposed by technology outweighs the good intended by its use. Suffering associated with technology may include physical, spiritual, and emotional elements for both patient and family. Making decisions regarding use of technology may cause pain, and there is suffering in living with the unknown results of these ongoing decisions. Relief of suffering, a goal of healing from its earliest days, needs to be addressed in all patient encounters.

CURRENT TECHNOLOGY: ISSUES AND DILEMMAS

Current technologies related to organ and tissue transplantation, genetic engineering, reproduction, and sustaining life have profound potential for affecting our lives and health in positive ways. Their use also presents dilemmas for patients, families, professionals, and society. Nurses generally do not make the decisions regarding implementing or withdrawing particular technologies (except perhaps in situations such as initiating cardiopulmonary resuscitation following specific protocols), yet we are involved as the caregivers of those receiving interventions and in many levels of patient care that involve technology. One of nursing's primary responsibilities is to help patients and families deal with the purposes, benefits, and limitations of the specific technologies. This section focuses primarily on the issue of withdrawing or withholding treatment as a prime example of a dilemma related to technology. Other issues related to technology are discussed briefly, and the reader is encouraged to further explore particular areas as the need or interest arises.

Treating Patients: When to Intervene and to What End

One of the most controversial bioethical topics of recent years relates to withholding or withdrawing life-sustaining treatments when they are deemed to have poor outcomes or offer no benefit. Decisions about withholding or withdrawing medical treatment are generally made by physicians in consultation with patients and family members. Approaches to dealing with these decisions reflect varying attitudes and concerns and may be confusing for all involved. A brief look at history sheds light on current attitudes regarding dealing with contemporary medical treatment. Questions related to the ethical limitations of medical care date back to the time of Hippocrates, when physicians were taught that the goal of medicine was to relieve suffering and reduce the effects of disease by lending support to natural processes. When the body was overpowered by disease, there was a concern that using medical interventions might merely prolong the suffering. The limitations of medicine were recognized and it was considered ethical to withhold treatments that held little potential for healing.

The scientific era that began emerging in the seventeenth century fostered a change in this ethical stance. Rather than revering and working with natural processes, conquering and dominating nature became the goal of science. In the nineteenth century, as medicine began to align more with science, and as biologic causes for diseases were discovered, the goal of medicine became the conquest of disease by exercising power over nature. Within this narrow focus of curing disease, ethical issues often relate to aggressive medical treatments, and issues of personal quality of life and dimensions of suffering are often unrecognized and neglected. With their attention to healing and caring, nurses play an important role in calling attention to concerns that go beyond the narrow focus of curing.

Issues of Life, Death, and Dying

Ethical dilemmas faced in health care settings often relate to issues of, and attitudes toward, living and dying. Important questions that are deliberated by those involved include "When does life begin?" "When does life end?"

"How can we be sure that someone has died?" and "Who decides?" Technology has stretched the boundaries and clouded the waters surrounding life's beginning and ending. Perspectives range from the belief that life begins at conception to the view that it begins when an infant can survive outside the womb. Technology makes this discussion even more complex and raises questions such as "What happens when conception cannot occur 'naturally' and artificial processes are employed either in vivo or in vitro?" and "Is the laboratory embryo a life?"

Today, many low-birth-weight infants and those with certain birth defects, who would not have survived in prior eras, survive with the support of machines, medications, and surgical procedures. In the process, however, some babies are kept alive only to die after months of expensive treatment. Others survive to face chronic health problems, with their associated financial, emotional, and physical strains on families and the health care system. There is no definitive way to predict which infants will have problems as they grow and develop. Dilemmas arise regarding how much effort to invest in "saving" a few infants who have a high probability of living only a short time or with significant health problems.

ASK YOURSELF

When Does Life Begin?

- What are your beliefs about when life begins? What shaped these beliefs?

- Consider that you are a member of a special task force called together by your hospital to establish guidelines for allocating dwindling funds for support of low-birth-weight infants in the neonatal intensive care unit. What criteria would you use to determine which of the infants who cannot survive without technology at birth will receive such interventions?

- If an infant will die without technology and the technology is withdrawn, do you consider that a natural or unnatural end of life? Why?

In our society, death has become an unnatural event, frequently associated with hospitals and other institutions, surrounded by tubes, machinery, and heroic efforts. Determining when life ends has become a critical issue related to use of technology, prompting the involvement of courts in decision making. The general attitude, especially among health care providers, is that death is the enemy to be overcome or kept at bay for as long as possible, regardless of the age or health condition of the person. Thus death is often viewed as a failure on the part of the health provider. It is understandable, therefore, that many health care providers have difficulty dealing with death as a possible outcome for patients, and thus find it a difficult topic to discuss. Another reason that the topic of death may be avoided is that discussing death requires us to face issues of meaning in life as well as anxieties and fears regarding our own mortality. However, lack of discussion of death as a possible outcome may lead families and patients to have unreasonable expectations and false hopes of what the system can offer. Demands for inappropriate interventions, or accusations that not enough was done, may arise from such situations. Patients and families need support in recognizing and honoring their own responses, beliefs, and fears regarding death. By facing our own issues about death, we are better able to facilitate this process with patients.

In many cultures, death is viewed as part of our life cycle that comes in its own time. Health care focused on curing is provided when there is reasonable hope of benefit, but people recognize when it is time for care to mean letting go and facilitating the transition through the dying process. In such cultures, dying often occurs at home, surrounded by family and friends.

ASK YOURSELF

What Are Your Views of Death and Dying?

What many people fear most regarding death is suffering and dying alone.

- How does technology contribute to this concern or attitude?

- What has your experience been related to death, what has shaped your attitudes regarding death, and what are your fears related to death?

- How can nurses minimize or deal with the effects of technology on patients in the dying process?

- How can nurses support patients and families in recognizing and honoring their own responses and beliefs regarding death?

- If machines and medication are keeping a body functioning, even if the person is apparently unaware, is that person still alive? Discuss your response.

- Do you think that brain wave activity in the midst of severe deterioration of major systems constitutes living? Discuss your response.

Personal attitudes prompt different expectations and scenarios when we are faced with decisions about heroic efforts and life-sustaining technologies. We must be aware of our own attitudes concerning living and dying, as well as the beliefs and expectations of patients, families, and other health care providers. Such awareness alerts us to situations in which there are differing attitudes among the parties involved, and provides an opportunity for opening lines of communication before a serious dilemma arises. Consider, for example, the patient who tells the nurse that he feels that his body is just giving up in spite of all the medications and treatments he is receiving, and he would like to go home to die peacefully, yet the physician is considering another surgery that is helpful about 30 percent of the time. In such a situation it would be important for the nurse to explore this area further with the patient, and either communicate his wishes to the physician or facilitate the patient's talking with the physician about his wishes.

Case Presentation

A Child with Leukemia

Lucia, a 12-year-old child with leukemia, has relapsed in spite of routine chemotherapeutic interventions. This child has suffered the side effects of the treatment, including nausea, hair loss, and frequent hospitalizations with infections, and is deteriorating physically. She says she feels as if she is being tortured with all the needles, spinal taps, and bone marrow samples; that she has no friends; and that this kind of life is not worth living. A bone marrow transplant (the only hope for a cure at this point) would mean subjecting her to intensive chemotherapy, total body irradiation, and weeks in isolation following the transplant. The family is told that there is a 40 percent chance that the transplant will be effective. The procedure is very expensive, and the family has already had to obtain a second mortgage for their home because their insurance has not covered many of the expenses to date.

Think About It

Factors Influencing Choices Regarding Medical Technology

- *What factors do you think need to be considered in making the decision about having the bone marrow transplant?*
- *How do percentages of risk and benefit affect your decision making?*
- *In this situation, do you think a 40 percent chance of success is enough to go ahead with the transplant? What if it were 60 percent? What about 20 percent?*
- *How can you help patients and families use statistical information in thinking about their decisions? What other factors would you help them to consider?*
- *Who should be involved in making this decision?*

Dying is more than a medical occurrence; it is a spiritual process touching the individual, family, and community. Although medical interventions can assist and support those in the dying process, current technologies can prolong suffering by prolonging the dying process, and can separate people from their families by actual physical barriers and institutionalization. Relieving suffering and supporting a dignified death are important elements of the nursing role. Addressing patient needs may require nurses to make decisions to go against institutional policy regarding such things as visitors and visiting hours, in order to ensure that the patient is not alone, or to risk confrontations with physicians over pain management or other aspects of care.

Medical Futility

Ethical and legal arguments for initiating or discontinuing life-sustaining treatments are based primarily on the relative benefits and burdens for the patient. Most ethical and legal discussions regarding life-sustaining treatments make little if any distinction between not implementing a life-sustaining treatment and discontinuing one that has been initiated. Withholding or removing life-sustaining treatments in situations in which the burden or harm has been determined to outweigh the benefits is, in essence, allowing the person to die as a result of the natural progression of the illness process. This is different from **euthanasia**, which is causing the painless death of a person in order to end or prevent suffering. Ethicists argue that it is the deterioration of the patient's condition that causes death, not the removal of the technology that is artificially supporting life.

In deliberations regarding withholding, initiating, or withdrawing life-sustaining interventions, **medical futility** related to the patient's situation is a major consideration. Medical futility refers to situations in which interventions are judged to have very little or no medical benefit, or in which the chance for success is low. Futility is often discussed in relation to cardio-pulmonary resuscitation (CPR), but it relates as well to interventions that preserve patients who are in persistent vegetative states or dependent on the technology of tertiary care settings. One difficulty associated with medical futility is that there is no set definition of the concept, only suggested parameters that vary greatly in guiding health care providers. Literature on futility discusses both quantitative definitions of futility that would justify unilateral decisions by physicians to withhold or withdraw interventions and qualitative, value-laden definitions such as situations in which interventions do not lead to acceptable quality of life for the patient (Clark, 2007; Day, 2009; Jacobs & Taylor, 2005; Lo, 2009). Quantitative definitions of futility include interventions that have no pathophysiologic rationale, have already failed in the patient, or will not achieve the goal of care, and situations where maximal treatment is failing. Objective data and the clinical expertise of the physician are the basis of determining futility in these situations. Medical ethicists generally agree that physicians have no ethical duty to provide interventions that are futile in the quantitative sense, and may well have an ethical obligation not to provide them even if they are requested (Lo, 2009).

Qualitative definitions of futility include situations that prompt variable interpretations and thus are more confusing—for example, situations in which the likelihood of success is very small, no worthwhile goals of care can be achieved, patient quality of life is unacceptable, and the prospective benefit is not worth the resources required. In these situations, the meaning of futility must consider perceptions of the patient and family and judgments of the health care team. In the absence of clear external guidelines, these less-clear situations require more skillful nursing care, as the persons involved draw on their own understandings and resources shaped by personal beliefs and cultural values.

ASK YOURSELF

What Constitutes Medical Futility?

- What do you think about these definitions of futility? Where would you envision potential problems or dilemmas based on these definitions?

- Would you consider an expensive treatment that works 20 percent of the time to be futile? What if it only works 5 percent of the time? Explain.

- Should medical futility be an issue when treatments are not expensive? Explain.

- Do you think a decision about futile treatment should be different with children and younger adults than with the elderly? Discuss your response.

- How would you see a patient's inability to pay for treatment affecting decisions about futility?

Because personal values come into play, health care providers, patients, and families may have differing views of what is a benefit or burden. The difficulty in defining and developing clear guidelines for medical futility has prompted health practitioners to focus more on the process of working with the patient and family to explain fully the medical circumstances, and to negotiate care that is in the best interest of the patient. For example, a patient or family may find hope and be willing to consider a treatment that has a 5 percent likelihood of success, while the health care providers see this as a futile effort. When considering quality of life, the perspective of the patient and family is essential in any determination of futility. Deciding when it is not worth continuing life-sustaining treatment is another circumstance in which the views of the parties involved may differ. Consider, for example, a 72-year-old quadriplegic patient on a ventilator at home who has been deteriorating and having frequent infections. She had to be resuscitated when recently hospitalized for severe respiratory infection. The physician discussed the situation with the patient and the family and suggested a **do not resuscitate (DNR) order**, which is a written directive placed in the patient's medical chart indicating that cardiopulmonary resuscitation is to be avoided. (See further discussion of DNR orders later in this chapter.) Even though the patient and most family members indicated agreement, the daughter who is the caregiver says she wants every effort made to keep her mother alive, saying that God will take her mother when He is ready. In another situation, health care providers might view continuing treatments that prolong a patient's life a few more days to be causing unnecessary suffering, while for the patient and family this is important "saying goodbye" time.

Case Presentation

Mr. Mason and His Son

Mr. Mason is a 78-year-old retired, widowed ironworker. He has been estranged from his adult son, an only child, for many years. He was recently diagnosed with advanced lung cancer. He recognized that he needed to make some plans for his immediate future, so he contacted his son and allowed him power of attorney. Mr. Mason is admitted to your unit in severe pain. He is somewhat confused, and you are unable to elicit information from him about his wishes regarding life-sustaining measures. You carefully begin discussing this difficult subject with his son, as it is your hospital's policy that everyone admitted to your oncology unit be informed about advance directives. Following are three possible twists this case could take, each of which is based on a real-life situation.

Ending 1. Mr. Mason's son begins to sob uncontrollably, saying, "I was never a very good son. I left home when I was barely 19 and didn't even write or call for many years. I am just getting to know my dad, and now this happens. I want as much time with him as possible. He told me a few days ago that he was ready to die and didn't want to be kept alive on machines. But it is so unfair to me. I want him alive and more time with him. Please, do everything you can to keep him alive. I need some more time with him. I need for him to forgive me."

Ending 2. Mr. Mason's son seems impatient, continually looking at his watch as you talk to him. Finally, seeming exasperated, he says, "Look, he's going to die anyway, right? Two things: First, I'm a busy man, and the quicker we get this over with the better; second, I have an appointment in 20 minutes with a real estate agent, and later with Dad's stockbroker. I'd really like to start arranging to sell his house and cash in some of his stocks. My son starts college in 2 months, and we could use the money. I suppose you think this is cruel, but realistically, would Dad rather we spend the money he worked so hard for on keeping him alive, when he's bound to die anyway, or on his grandson's education? It's pretty clear to me. I say, just let Dad go; that would be the best for everyone concerned."

Ending 3. The son quickly acknowledges that he understands the question. Without hesitation he says, "Do all you can to keep him alive. The tyrant was mean to me all of my life. I hate him. I want him to suffer as long as possible."

Think About It

Family Reactions to Medically Futile Situations

- *What is your response to the son's statement in each of these scenarios? Include both your thinking response and your feeling response.*
- *How would your feelings lead you to advise one option over another?*
- *How do you think the nurse should react to each response?*
- *What values and dilemmas are evident in each scenario?*
- *Identify your personal and professional values related to each scenario.*
- *Who should make the decision? Do you feel conflicting loyalties?*
- *How would you respond to the son's decision?*

Economics and Medical Futility

The cost of health care, particularly in relation to technology, has brought economic factors into discussions of futility. Some suggest that the principle of justice indicates that if a particular intervention is judged to be of limited or no benefit for one person, it should be discontinued so it is available for another patient who can make better use of the scarce resource. Political and economic developments in medicine, particularly prospective payment systems, have prompted physicians and hospitals to look more closely at futile treatments. Under prospective payment systems, physicians and institutions lose money if patients are maintained on particular treatments beyond a predetermined length of time. Because reimbursement for medical care requires justification that the care is medically indicated, the physician's responsibility to limit excessive treatments has become a kind of social mandate (Baily, 2011). Many argue that it is ethical and justifiable for physicians to limit access to treatments that are expensive while offering limited benefits, and that, given limited health care resources, such decisions are socially responsible. Such an argument is consistent with utilitarian ethics, a perspective often used by government agencies when deciding about distribution of goods and services. While economic issues do impact health care decisions, and some raise concerns that medical futility may be a subtle form of rationing, the important focus is not the cost of the therapy, but whether the benefits outweigh the disadvantages for the patient. Whatever the decision regarding the therapy, nursing must focus on high-quality care for and communication with the patient and family.

ASK YOURSELF

How Are Economics and Decisions About Medical Futility Related?

- Under what circumstances do you feel physicians or institutions should be able to limit a patient's access to expensive treatments?
- How do you think economics affects decisions about medical futility?
- How might patient care be affected by these decisions?
- What are the potential legal ramifications of such decisions?

Do Not Resuscitate Orders

In decisions regarding cardiopulmonary resuscitation (CPR), nurses have an active role in initiating or withholding life-sustaining treatment. Considering whether to initiate CPR with a patient requires attention to professional, ethical, legal, and institutional considerations. Principles utilized to justify decisions regarding resuscitation include autonomy, self-determination, nonmaleficence, and respect for persons.

The general practice regarding CPR is that it must be initiated unless: (1) it would clearly be futile to do so, or (2) the practitioner has specific instructions not to do so. The legal definition of do not resuscitate (DNR) is not to initiate CPR in the event of a cardiac or pulmonary arrest. As noted previously, DNR orders are written directives placed in a patient's medical record indicating that the use of cardiopulmonary resuscitation is to be avoided. DNR orders should be documented immediately in a patient's health care record, noting the reason the order was written, who gave consent and who was involved in the discussion, whether the patient was competent to give consent or who was authorized to do so, and the time frame for the DNR order (American Nurses Association [ANA], 2003). In situations of medical futility, decisions to withhold or stop CPR are appropriately made by physicians in consultation with patients and families and need not be offered as an option for patients (Bishop, Brothers, Perry, & Ahmad, 2010; Hayes, 2004;

Lo, 2009). Some suggest that nurses are as well qualified as physicians to write DNR orders. Because nurses are the professionals who are in close and continuous contact with patients, they are perhaps better able to help patients and families articulate their views regarding end-of-life care and concerns (ANA, 2003). DNR decisions require open communication among the patient or surrogate, the family, and the health care team. This communication needs to include explicit discussion of the efficacy and desirability of CPR, balanced with the potential harm and suffering it may cause the patient. People often overestimate the effectiveness of CPR, and do not understand that CPR is not always medically indicated. Many people derive their concept of CPR from what they see in the media. Diem, Lantos, and Tulsky (1996) conducted an interesting study that indicated that rates of survival after CPR in television dramas were much higher than the most optimistic survival rates in the medical literature. In order to make informed decisions regarding CPR, patients and families need to understand the patient's clinical condition and prognosis. People rarely appreciate that CPR is a harsh and traumatic procedure, and that patients with multiple, severe, chronic health problems who receive CPR rarely survive to be discharged (Cadogan, 2010; Feen, 2010).

The relevance of considering the patient's or family's values in justifying DNR orders may vary, depending on the rationale given for the decision (ANA, 2003; Cadogan, 2010; Feen, 2010; Hayes, 2004; Hickman et al., 2009). In situations in which CPR would be medically ineffective, patient autonomy and consent are considered less relevant. However, when the rationale for the decision is based on the patient's quality of life, either after or before CPR, determination of whether the benefit of continued life outweighs the risk of harmful consequences, such as debility or suffering, must flow from the values of the patient or the patient's surrogate. Competent patients have the right to refuse CPR and may request DNR orders after they have been informed of the risks and benefits involved. Good communication is the most critical factor in assuring that any DNR decision is acceptable to all parties involved.

DNR orders apply only to resuscitation. The fact that CPR might be considered futile does not necessarily imply that other life-sustaining interventions are futile or that other treatments will not be used. Health care providers often fail to make this distinction, thus causing confusion for patients as well. Many institutions require more specific instructions regarding what is and is not to be done for a patient. These interventions might include treatment of physiological abnormalities such as fever or cardiac arrhythmias, nutrition, or use of mechanical ventilation and CPR. Plans for and parameters of DNR orders need to be discussed with all members of the health care team so that the goal of care is clear. The presence of DNR orders requires nurses to become even more focused on providing supportive and comfort interventions, and to ensure that there is no reduction in the level of care for the patient and family. A DNR order means only that, in the event of cardiac or respiratory arrest, there are to be no attempts to resuscitate. Presuming no arrest occurs, the patient may recover from the problem necessitating hospitalization and return home.

Many years ago Scofield suggested that decisions to not resuscitate ask us "individually and collectively, to arrive at a consensus on how to integrate death and decisions about it into the legitimating values of our moral universe. Deciding what kind of life we want involves deciding what kind of death we can face" (1995, p. 184). He noted that death, which was once considered fate, is now often a matter of a choice that we do not want to

Case Presentation

Mistaken Resuscitation

Jacob has had a chronic lung condition for the past 10 of his 32 years. The condition causes some restrictions on his life, but he has kept up with a regular job and is very involved in his church. He is currently hospitalized with a severe respiratory infection. Although his condition did not seem to be that serious, when he was admitted he made sure that there was a DNR order in his chart, noting that he has a firm religious conviction that the Creator, and not the doctor, is to decide when it is time for him to die. Because of a staff shortage, Lashanda, a registered nurse who usually works on another unit, has been assigned to Jacob's unit. Although she has been working on the other side of the unit, she is presently covering the whole unit while other staff are at lunch. As she answers a call light from Jacob's roommate, she notices that Jacob is not breathing and has no pulse. Since she is unfamiliar with Jacob's DNR request, she immediately calls a "code" and initiates CPR, figuring that there would be no question that this would be the appropriate action for someone this age. Although Jacob is successfully resuscitated with no serious sequelae, he is intensely angry, saying that this was interference in the Creator's plan.

Think About It

Decisions Regarding Resuscitation

- *What do you think about Jacob's request for a DNR order? What ethical principles are involved in his choice?*

- *What do you think about Lashanda's response in the situation? Do you think she acted appropriately under the circumstances?*

- *How do you think you might respond in a similar situation? What principles would guide your actions?*

- *Describe potential legal ramifications in this situation.*

- *What guidelines would your state's laws regarding DNR status offer to Lashanda? Would they support her actions?*

have to make. His comments are still relevant today because those involved in DNR decisions face this dilemma.

Nursing Considerations Related to DNR Orders

Although it is generally considered the domain of the physician to write a DNR order, nurses need to be aware of parameters surrounding such orders. In some states, persons with serious medical conditions keep a special medical order form documenting end-of-life wishes posted in a prominent place at home (or in the chart if the person is in a long-term care facility). This form specifies end-of-life wishes (including DNR orders), is readily available to emergency personnel, and travels with the person to the hospital or other treatment facility. A copy of the form used in one state (Physician Orders for Scope of Treatment, or POST form) is available at http://wvethics.org/POST-Forms. Other forms of "portable" DNR orders include wallet cards, bracelets, and necklaces. Nurses need to know which patients under their care have DNR orders, and these orders need to be documented clearly in a patient's chart, and perhaps at the bedside, and reviewed periodically as the patient's condition changes. Nurses are often the bridge between patient and physician. If a patient or appropriate surrogate indicates to the nurse the desire not to be resuscitated and there is no order in the chart, the nurse should document the request in the patient's chart and bring this to the immediate attention of the physician. The nurse may wish to explore the request with the patient or surrogate, and may need to facilitate discussion of the issue between patient and physician. Orders should specify which interventions are to be withheld, and considerations regarding circumstances in which they are to be withheld. All persons involved in the care of the patient need to know about the orders. Since attitudes affect one's approach to others, nurses need to reflect on their own attitudes toward decisions regarding withholding of interventions, both in general and in particular patient situations.

Artificial Sources of Nutrition and Hydration

Maintaining nutrition is a natural life-sustaining measure and a common part of the nursing role. Once a person has difficulty with functions associated with nutrition, such as chewing or swallowing, or is not conscious enough to participate in these activities, decisions about artificial sources of nutrition and hydration must be made. Ethical dilemmas arise concerning whether to classify such interventions as feeding or as medical treatments, or as ordinary or extraordinary measures. ANA's (2011) policy on *Forgoing Nutrition and Hydration* stresses the importance of determining whether food and fluid are more beneficial or harmful to a patient, noting that artificially-provided nutrition and hydration may not be ethically justified.

Utilizing artificial sources of nutrition may present dilemmas in situations involving persons in persistent vegetative states or end-stage dying processes for whom this intervention is maintaining physical life. We know that withholding food will eventually lead to starvation and death and, under most circumstances, is not considered an ethical action. However, it is considered appropriate to withhold or discontinue life-sustaining medical interventions when they are not benefiting the patient or are contrary to the patient's wishes. There are fewer complexities surrounding decisions to withhold artificial sources of nutrition than there are regarding decisions to withdraw medical interventions.

As with any such decision, we must consider the wishes of the patient or surrogate. Quality of life is an important factor, and if interventions contribute more to, rather than relieve, a patient's suffering, the principle of nonmaleficence may sway one toward a decision of not implementing or of discontinuing such therapies. Evidence suggests that tube feeding does not improve outcomes and may have substantial risks in some patients, particularly those with dementia or multisystem illness (ANA, 2011; Geppert, Andrews, & Druyan, 2010; Williams, 2006). Additionally, there is little evidence to suggest that either using or withdrawing hydration alleviates discomfort at the end of life (ANA, 2011). Health care providers need to ensure that patients and families understand the benefits and burdens of artificial nutrition and hydration so that they can make informed decisions. Once artificial measures have been implemented, it is often psychologically more difficult to decide on their removal. With any technological intervention we must consider whether its use is prolonging living or prolonging dying. When competent patients refuse food or fluid, respect for persons directs nurses to honor this refusal. Nursing's role of providing high-quality care with attention to providing comfort and promoting a patient's dignity is especially important when a decision has been made to forgo artificial nutrition or hydration. Nurses need to help family and other caretakers understand that people who are dying often have a decline in appetite, and that the care of keeping the person comfortable does not need to include efforts to maintain nutrition. It is often helpful to involve family in providing comfort measures such as offering ice chips or using mouth swabs to keep the mouth moist.

Legal Issues Related to Technology

As noted in Chapter 8, what is considered an ethical decision by some may not be upheld as a legal action. In the area of health care technology, the courts have intervened in some decisions related to withholding or withdrawing life-sustaining treatments when there has been disagreement among the involved parties. Legal precedents regarding issues such as what constitutes clear evidence of a person's wishes related to these treatments and what is considered standard practice have been set in the process. Examples of two such cases are presented here. When one looks at dilemmas faced by families, health care providers, institutions, and the legal system in situations such as these, the importance of having advance directives becomes evident. **Advance directives** are instructions indicating one's wishes regarding health care interventions or designating someone to act as a surrogate in making such decisions in the event that one loses decision-making capacity. These directives are discussed in Chapter 11.

When issues arise related to technology or other aspects of care that may have an ethical component, it is appropriate for nurses to initiate an ethics consult with the institution's ethics committee. An ethics committee is generally made up of representatives from various disciplines such as nursing, medicine, social work, and chaplains. The role of the ethics committee is to gather information about the issue from all involved (including patient, family, key health care providers, and other key persons involved in the situation); to arrange for a patient care conference, if appropriate; to develop recommendations related to resolving the issue and communicate these to the patient and health care team; to work with those involved as needed to come to some resolution of the issue; and to follow up on the outcome of the issue.

Case Presentation

Karen Quinlan

The well-known case of Karen Quinlan (Devettere, 1995; Pence, 1995) is the story of a 21-year-old woman who, in 1975, was found to have suffered cardiopulmonary arrest at home alone after having been drinking at a local bar. After the ambulance crew restored heartbeat through CPR, she was admitted to the local hospital and placed on a ventilator. Within a few days she was transferred to a larger hospital where she was kept alive with the assistance of a respirator and feeding tube. Over months she lost weight, developed contractures, and was given no hope of regaining awareness. After much deliberation, the family asked that the respirator be discontinued, but the hospital indicated that it could not grant the request unless the father was named as her guardian. When the father asked the court to appoint him guardian with authority to make decisions to discontinue extraordinary interventions, the court appointed him guardian of her property, but not of her person, and appointed a **guardian *ad litem*** to represent Karen. The guardian *ad litem* felt responsible for preserving Karen's life, and opposed removing the respirator. The physician's lawyer argued that removing a respirator from a living person was not standard medical procedure, and the judge sided with this view. When the family appealed the ruling to the New Jersey Supreme Court, the decision of the lower court was reversed and the father was appointed as her guardian. When the father requested that the respirator be removed, the physicians initiated a process of weaning her from it, resulting in her being able to breathe without the machine. Totally unconscious with severe contractures, she was transferred to a nursing home, where she died 10 years later.

Case Presentation

Nancy Cruzan

In another well-known case, Nancy Cruzan (Angell, 1990; Annas, 1990; Pence, 1995) was found un-conscious and not breathing after her car went into a ditch in the winter of 1983. Although emergency personnel restored her breathing, she never regained consciousness. After a year of being sustained through the use of a gastrostomy tube for artificial nutrition, it was determined that she was in a persistent vegetative state. When her parents, acting as her guardians, asked that the artificial feeding be discontin-ued because she had indicated previously that she would not want to be kept alive in this condition, the physicians and hospital refused. When the case went to court, the evidence supporting discontinuing the feeding was based primarily on a statement she had made to a roommate that she would not want to live if she were a vegetable. The judge ruled that the medical nutrition could be removed, but that decision was appealed to the Missouri State Supreme Court by a guardian *ad litem.* The Missouri supreme court reversed the previous decision, claiming that there was no clear and convincing evidence that this would be her wish; that she was not terminally ill or suffering; and that there was no reason to act contrary to the state's interest in preserving life, regardless of how minimal that life had become. An appeal to the U.S. Supreme Court upheld the decision that medical nutrition could not be withdrawn because of the lack of clear and convincing evidence. In 1990, almost 8 years after her accident, Nancy's parents appealed again to the local court with the evidence of three of her friends who stated that she had told them that she would not want to live in a vegetative state. At that time, the physician agreed that it was no longer in her best interests to be medically nourished, and the judge agreed that there was now clear and convinc-ing evidence indicating that it was in her best interests to terminate artificial nutrition.

Think About It

When the Courts Intervene

- *Reflect on these two cases (and the case of Terri Shiavo, presented in Chapter 11). Which position do you support, that of the family or that of the guardian* ad litem?
- *Which court decisions do you think are more valid? Defend your position.*
- *Describe the ethical dilemmas and principles involved in these situations.*
- *If one of your family members was in a similar situation, how do you think you would respond? Would you expect solidarity or disagreement with this position from other members of your family?*
- *Consider that you are a nurse caring for Karen or Nancy at various stages in her situation. How would you respond to the various parties involved as decisions about her care are being discussed?*
- *What do you think about the role of the legal system in decisions regarding use of technology?*

The reader is encouraged to review the information about ethics committees and consultation found at http://www.wvnec.org/Ethics-Committee-Tools.

Palliative Care

Two primary obligations that we have to people who are dying are comfort and company (Rushton, Spencer, & Johanson, 2004). When life-sustaining interventions are no longer of benefit or are not desired by the patient, the focus of care becomes palliative, that is, directed toward comfort and support. **Palliative care** is comprehensive, interdisciplinary, and total care, focusing primarily on comfort and support of patients and families who face illness that is chronic or not responsive to curative treatment (ANA, 2010; Arraf, Cox, & Oberle, 2004; Rushton et al., 2004). Palliative care focuses on the best quality of life for patient and family through meticulous control of pain and other symptoms, a personalized plan to optimize quality of life as defined by patient and family, and spiritual and psychosocial care. Palliative care requires delivery of coordinated and continuous services in home, hospice, skilled nursing facilities, or hospital, and includes support in bereavement. Members of the palliative care team include nurses, physicians, spiritual support persons, pharmacists, social services, mental health services, and pain services.

The backbone of palliative care is good nursing care that continues to support the dignity and self-respect of patient and family. In addition to providing care to the patient and the family, nurses often coordinate palliative care teams. When families are in disagreement about when it is time to stop other interventions and focus on palliative care, the nurse's ability to communicate effectively with and facilitate communication among those involved is crucial. Families often need time to see what we see regarding the patient's condition and expected outcomes of various interventions. We have to be willing to take as much time as necessary and as often as needed to explain and negotiate care decisions. Palliative care conferences may take different forms. An example of an approach outlined by a palliative care nurse follows (Robin Shirley, personal communication, January 18, 2001).

Palliative Care Conference

- Have a holistic view of the patient, including present health status, prognosis, significant relationships, living situation, family dynamics, decision-making capacity, advance directives or surrogate, and spiritual support.

- If the patient does not have decision-making capacity and there is no surrogate, seek to have a surrogate named.

- Prior to scheduling the conference, inform the surrogate that the purpose of the meeting is to determine the best way to provide quality end-of-life care to the patient and family, and stress the need for all family and significant persons, including spiritual support persons, to participate. The conference is set at a time when most people can be there. Primary nurse, physician, and other involved health care team members are included.

- In opening the meeting, the palliative care nurse describes the process that will be followed in order to allow everyone an opportunity to speak and ask questions, and to arrive at a consensus regarding what is truly best for the patient.

- The meeting is opened by introducing everyone present and their role or relationship with the patient. In order to prevent disorder that can occur with the high emotions of the circumstances, those present are then asked one by one to name things that the patient enjoyed in life. This process also helps the physician and other care providers to step back from the clinical picture and see the patient as a person with individual values and meaning. Next, the physician is asked to discuss current status and prognosis, allowing an opportunity for the family to ask any questions. The primary nurse is then asked to discuss daily care and interactions with the patient, and to respond to any questions. Through this process the family is often able to acknowledge that their loved one will not return to the state they once enjoyed, which leads to the beginning of acceptance and consideration of what is truly best for the patient at this time.

- Everyone in turn is then asked what they know or believe to be the desires of their loved one regarding end-of-life care. This includes the values of the patient, and what family members consider to be in the best interest. This process often prompts tears and reminiscing. Spiritual support persons may comment about the patient's spiritual values and considerations, or intervene as needed to support those participating.

- Throughout this process the palliative care nurse periodically restates what the general consensus of the group seems to be. This helps to clarify what is being said, and provides those not in agreement an opportunity to bring up concerns or issues. The meeting generally concludes with consensus regarding what is best for their loved one and discussion regarding comfort measures desired by the family and that the care providers feel will best suit the patient. (In some situations more than one meeting may be needed before consensus is reached.)

- All involved frequently join around the patient's bedside following the meeting for prayer and reminiscing, to the extent they are comfortable with this. The family usually has open visitation, and are involved as much as they wish in care for the patient.

- Documentation of the process, participants, content, and outcomes is completed in the patient's record and ongoing follow-up is initiated.

Examples of Potential Dilemmas with Other Technology

In addition to life-sustaining interventions, advances in technology affect nursing and health care in other arenas as well. Examples of a few such technologies are briefly presented here. Nurses who work with patients whose care involves such technologies need to be aware of potential ethical issues associated with their use, as well as the benefits of such interventions. The intention here is to alert the reader to some of the questions and dilemmas that may be associated with these technologies. The reader is encouraged to explore these areas further, reflecting on personal values related to each technology.

Reproductive Technology

Because the inability to conceive and bear children can be a very distressing experience for a couple, any technology that can facilitate the process may be viewed as a life-affirming gift. Such technologies include artificial insemination by donor, in vitro fertilization, and surrogate embryo transfer. While scientists develop and refine these technologies to benefit people, ethicists and others raise questions related to the moral implications of their use. Some questions focus on the potential for changing society's concept of family and parenthood. For example, in the case of surrogacy, is the mother of the baby the woman whose ovum is joined with her husband's sperm, or the woman who donates her body for the baby's development and birth? A question to ponder is whether the use of such technologies might relegate childbearing into little more than the production of a product. Other ethical questions arise regarding who has custody of frozen embryos, and whether these embryos have rights. A related consideration is the potential that women may become more exploited than liberated by the use of these technologies. Because these interventions are expensive, questions arise regarding who should pay for them, and for whom they should be made available. For example, there are racial and ethnic disparities regarding the availability of some of these technologies. Ethical considerations regarding these technologies include attention to societal attitudes about who should or should not have children, and what kind of children should be born.

Genetic Diagnosis, Engineering, and Screening

Advances in molecular biology, new reproductive technologies, and the Human Genome Project have prompted rapid breakthroughs in genetic research. This research has advanced our knowledge of the use of genetic interventions as possible remedies for diseases caused by genetic disorders. The possibilities of these interventions, however, raise ethical as well as legal and social justice questions (ANA, 2006; Anderson & Rorty, 2001; International Council of Nurses [ICN], 2009a, 2009b). **Genetic diagnosis**, which is usually done within an in vitro fertilization program, involves a process of biopsy of embryos to determine the presence of genetic flaws and gender prior to implantation. At present, such diagnosis is aimed at couples who have a high risk of conceiving a child with a serious genetic disorder, with the intent that only embryos that are free of genetic flaws would be implanted. **Genetic engineering** is the ability to alter organisms genetically for a variety of purposes, such as developing more disease-resistant fruits and vegetables, or eventually being able to alter embryos genetically so that the fetus and baby will be healthier. Through **genetic screening** it is possible to determine if persons are predisposed to certain diseases, and whether couples have the possibility of giving birth to a genetically impaired infant. The implications of having such technologies available include the potential for correcting some genetic defects in the embryo, eliminating some very serious genetic diseases, and producing food that is more nourishing and resilient. We must, however, make a distinction between the therapeutic use of these interventions and the possibility that these interventions may be used to modify human characteristics beyond those that are needed to sustain or restore health. The possibility of their use to enhance certain human characteristics has significant social implications. For example, such interventions could offer control over genetic inheritance, including the biological properties and personality traits of our children. They suggest that the ability to discard "undesirable" traits and improve those that are "desirable" may lead to a form of **eugenics**, meaning "good birth." The eugenics movement of the early twentieth century sought to promote traits that proponents felt were desirable for society, while weeding out what they considered undesirable. In the United States and elsewhere around the world, eugenics led to efforts to discourage procreation among people deemed to be "socially inferior" through compulsory sterilization of many people, particularly those who were poor, in prison, or in mental institutions. Another concern that nurses need to be aware of is the potential for these technologies to lead to the imposition of a skewed or harmful definition of what is normal regarding human traits as well as what is considered abnormal or undesirable. Because individuals and societies tend to impose their values and standards on others, this could lead to serious transcultural implications.

Concerns related to these technologies are as varied as their potential benefits, particularly the recognition that relaxing criteria related to a person's value or rights in one arena may lead to abuses or exploitation in other circumstances. Ethicists often speak of these concerns in terms of a *slippery slope* where, for example, one decision based on relaxing criteria supporting the value of human life makes it easy to slide into acceptance of lower standards as ethical guides. For example, one concern is that genetic engineering might produce organisms that could be harmful to humans; another is that employers or insurers might use information gained from genetic screening to exclude people with particular traits from certain jobs or from being insured. Might genetic screening and diagnosis lead to abuses, such as forbidding people with certain traits to have children, insurers refusing to cover expenses if insured mothers give birth to genetically-impaired infants, or prohibiting the birth of babies with particular genetic features deemed undesirable by those in power in a society? These areas include other broad societal implications, such as who pays for the procedures, who determines guidelines for their use, and to whom they are made available.

Controversial Technologies

In spite of their potential benefit for human health, some biotechnologies raise serious ethical concerns even in the research phase. Cloning and stem cell research are examples of technologies that are engendering much debate among ethicists and within the public forum. Ethical concerns related to these technologies are briefly discussed here, and readers are encouraged to deepen their understanding of the scientific and ethical debate surrounding these technologies through further study.

Cloning is the process of creating a cell or an entire organism that is identical in every way to another. Types of cloning include molecular, cellular, and cloning of entire organisms. Techniques of mammalian cloning include embryo twinning and somatic cell nuclear transplantation. The prospect of using somatic cell nuclear transfer to create human beings raises the greatest ethical concern (ANA, 2007). National and international debate on the issue acknowledges that cloning can be both useful and damaging for human health, and that both advantages and disadvantages need to be considered. The overall stance within nursing and other organizations that promote health and human rights is that human cloning is ethically unacceptable and violates the right to one's unique genetic identity, human dignity, and integrity (ANA, 2007, Anderson & Rorty, 2001). The stance of the international nursing community is that vigorous national and international analysis, monitoring, and debate of the ethical, social, legal, scientific, and health concerns related to human cloning are needed, and that there must be mandatory presence of nurses on policy boards examining these issues. Nursing's position includes support for scholarly examination of the implications of core professional nursing values for cloning in humans, and ethical analysis of the possible merits of different techniques of cloning for human health.

The ethical concerns surrounding **stem cell** research vary depending on the origin of the stem cells. Human stem cells used in research are termed *adult, embryonic,* and *germline,* based on how they are obtained (TechNyou, 2012). Adult stem cells (ASC) are cells found in adults that can replace old cells by reproducing new ones. Blood cells and liver cells are two examples. Bone marrow transplants are examples of the use of ASC in therapy. Stem cells retrieved from umbilical cord blood following birth have similar properties to ASC and are also used in treatment for some leukemias. Embryonic stem cells (ESC) are collected from the inner cell mass of an early embryo, thus destroying the embryo. These cells are unspecified (or pluripotent), meaning that they have the ability to develop into any type of cell in the body except the placenta. They also are able to renew themselves indefinitely in the laboratory. Embryonic germline stem cells are immature cells that can become sperm and egg cells. The goal of stem cell research is a relief of human suffering, which, ethically, is good. Potential benefits of interventions developed through stem cell research include therapies for Parkinson's disease, regenerating various tissues that are diseased, and using ESC to develop an entire organ to be used for transplant.

The main controversy surrounding stem cell research focuses on use of ESC, because the process of obtaining these cells results in the destruction of the embryo. There are two main objections to stem cell research (Guenin, 2008; Sandel, 2004). The first focuses on whether the destruction of the human embryo constitutes the killing of a human being. The second objection raises the concern that, if one considers that research on human embryos is not wrong in itself, would it lead to a slippery slope of treating human life as a commodity through practices that are dehumanizing, such as using fetuses for spare parts? Views about when human life begins and whether the early embryo is considered a person with moral status are at the heart of ethical deliberations related to ESC research. Those who believe that human life and personhood begins at conception hold that destruction of a human embryo constitutes killing, thus stem cell research using ESC is never morally allowed. Those who hold the view that the embryo is afforded personhood at the point of viability may consider use of early embryonic tissue permissible for research. Those who suggest that sentience, life history, and memory are requirements for personhood argue that the early embryo does not possess personhood; thus it is morally acceptable to do ESC research using the early embryonic tissue if this may potentially benefit human health.

Other ethical concerns related to stem cell research include issues of obtaining informed consent from donors, the potential of combining embryonic stem cells and cloning technique, the potential development of embryo farms, and issues of ownership of the biologic materials derived from the cells. Because outcomes of stem cell research have the potential to alter human genetics and the human life cycle, there can be social and environmental consequences of extending human life, as well as a shift in our understanding of what it means to be human (Lauritzen, 2005; TechNyou, 2012).

Organ and Tissue Procurement and Transplantation

Organ transplantation is no longer considered as extraordinary or uncommon a health care event as it was in the not-too-distant past. As techniques become more refined, the possibility of a transplant becomes a hope for more and more people afflicted with the failure of a vital organ. Because the demand for organs is great and the supply limited, dilemmas related to allocation of scarce resources emerge. Questions arise regarding eligibility of recipients for organ transplant. Should these determinations be made based on a potential recipient's expectation of survival post-transplant, or ability to pay for the procedure, or power and prestige, or some combination of these and other factors? Transplantation may involve organs from dead or living human donors, animals, or artificial appliances, and there are dilemmas associated with each. This discussion focuses on human donor issues.

Because transplantation requires well-nourished organs, procurement must occur as soon after death as possible. Thus, having criteria for determining when death occurs is imperative. Irreversible cessation of cardiopulmonary functioning is one such criterion. However, until CPR has been attempted, how is one to know if the cessation is irreversible? If CPR is initiated, organs to be donated may be damaged, raising an issue of how to deal with a person's desire to be an organ donor with a consideration for CPR. Questions regarding when and how intensively to initiate CPR become important issues regarding organ donation. If a person has been maintained on life-support technology, brain death is the most likely criteria to be used, which leads to issues regarding what constitutes brain death. Some suggest that current criteria for brain death indicating that all functions of the entire brain must cease are more stringent than necessary, and that irreversible cessation of higher brain functions would be sufficient criteria. Such a change in brain death criteria would open the possibility of harvesting organs from people in persistent vegetative states or in permanent comas, and with this would come questions about the ethics of doing so.

The scarcity of available organs and the long waiting lists of potential recipients raise the possibility that people may be declared dead prematurely. This scarcity of organs also affects organ procurement from living human beings. With living donors, issues related to voluntary informed consent and the buying and selling of organs are of concern. There are places in the world where organs are taken from poor people or prisoners, without their knowledge or against their will, and sold to procurement centers in more affluent countries. Desperate straits have prompted some individuals to sell an organ to raise money for personal or family needs, raising a question about whether there can be true voluntary informed consent under such circumstances.

In cases of sudden accidental death, family members may be asked to consider donation of viable organs. Consider whether there can be true voluntary consent when the family is in the midst of crisis and shock. With the urgency for a decision due to time factors for harvesting organs, coercion could be a factor. In some settings nurses are asked to approach patients or families about considering organ donation. In such situations nurses need to be clear about their own feelings regarding organ procurement and transplantation, and they must remember that attention to family needs takes precedence over the time constraints of organ harvesting.

NURSING PRACTICE IN THE MIDST OF TECHNOLOGY

Nursing practice continues to evolve with expanding knowledge and scientific advances in many arenas. As technology has been developed and refined, related nursing responsibilities have expanded. In the midst of these changes, the essence of nursing remains the human focus of caring for patients and families—being attentive to the needs of persons whose lives are affected by the technology. Integrating caring and technology and juggling the demands of patients and families present challenges for nurses in any area of practice. As new technologies become available, they will bring with them associated issues of concern. Regardless of the technology, important considerations for nursing relate to attitudes and values, communication, and maintaining the human focus of care.

Technology, Privacy, and Confidentiality

Developments in technology related to communication and storage of health care information, while beneficial in many ways, pose concerns related to privacy and confidentiality of personal health information (PHI). The use of electronic medical records, fax machines, e-mail and other Internet transactions, personal digital assistants (PDAs), cellular phones, and telehealth consultation have become commonplace in health care settings. Computerized medical databases, including electronic medical records (EMR), are becoming standard in both private practice settings as well as in large organizations such as hospitals, clinics, and national systems such as the Veterans Health Administration. The benefits of quick access to patient health care information by practitioners and the ability to facilitate communication among health care team members provided by these technologies are evident. However, any method of electronically storing, retrieving, or transferring PHI also poses the possibility of unintentional breeches in confidentiality. Because practitioners, including nurses, cannot completely control access to computerized databases, concern arises that patients may withhold important health information or refrain from seeking care due to fear that their records will not remain private. Although the Health Insurance Portability Accountability Act (HIPAA) regulations are designed to protect the privacy and security of any electronic transactions of PHI, there are loopholes in the regulations (Dudley, 2004). Privacy breeches may occur at the level of the primary user, that is, those who collect, process, and store PHI (such as physicians, nurses, pharmacists); at the level of the secondary user (such as third-party payers and the health information services industry); and at the level of the technology itself through lack of proper encryption techniques or improper disposal of old equipment without purging private information. Other U.S. federal regulations give the Department of Homeland Security the power to bypass HIPAA regulations and access health information for security reasons.

The ethical and legal obligation to protect the confidentiality of patient information directs nurses to implement appropriate safeguards when storing and transferring PHI electronically. Precautions to take to assure privacy and confidentiality include the following (National Association of School Nurses, 2004; Pancoast, Patrick, & Mitchell, 2003):

- Use secure passwords that are changed regularly, and do not share passwords with others.

- Assure that computer systems have programs to thwart hackers, effective virus protection, screen savers or covers that limit visibility of information on the screen for anyone other than the person using the computer, and overwrite protection and multi-level access if multiple persons are entering data.

- When e-mail is used for transmission of health information, include a confidentiality statement, encrypt messages with PHI, take precautions to prevent misdirected e-mail, use password-protected screen savers, and obtain permission from patient, parent/guardian, or health provider before transferring PHI via e-mail and before forwarding messages.

- Assure that virus protection software is brought up to date weekly.

- Include a confidentiality statement on the cover sheet when faxing PHI.

- Assure that any PHI or other health databases stored on notebook computers, PDAs, or other electronic devices comply with institutional policies and state guidelines.

- When storing PHI on electronic devices, use data encryption technology, always maintain careful physical control of the device, use a secure password when turning on the device and a time out to reactivate the password, disable infrared ports except when using the device, do not send infrared transmissions in public areas, and back up any confidential information using approved back-up procedures.

- Assure that all private information is purged from the device when no longer needed for care of the patient and when discarding the device.

Nurses need to be alert to any breach of confidentiality of health records or information related to use of electronic devices and take action to correct the situation, and be involved in developing policies and guidelines aimed at safeguarding the confidentiality of all health information and records.

Attitudes and Values

The importance of self-awareness related to values, beliefs, and reactions is especially significant when dealing with issues related to technology. The process of being more attentive to personal perspectives regarding such issues as quality of life, living, dying, medical futility, and allocation of scarce resources may be facilitated by pondering questions such as those posed throughout this chapter. Such awareness enables the nurse to differentiate personal values from those of patients and others involved in the situation. Principles of self-determination and autonomy counsel the nurse to understand that individuals may judge benefits of an intervention from varying perspectives. Recognizing where personal values may be different enables nurses to be more attentive to fostering good communication, encouraging others to make their own decisions, avoiding judgment about the rightness or wrongness of the decision based on personal values, and accepting those decisions even if they are different from what the nurse would do.

As the various examples presented in this chapter suggest, many dilemmas that emerge surrounding technology relate to differing values among the parties involved. Facilitating discussion of values among patients and families may help them to clarify their own perspectives. Nurses also need to be alert to situations in which there may be differences in values among the patient, family, and physician. Encouraging timely communication may avert a major dilemma, or facilitate more effective resolution of the concern. Nurses who cannot reconcile their values with a particular situation need to take the necessary steps to remove themselves from that situation so as to not compromise patient care or personal integrity. In so doing, it is essential to avoid abandoning the patient by ensuring that there are others who will provide the needed care for the patient.

The Importance of Communication: Who Decides?

As has been noted, there are many factors involved in making decisions about withholding or withdrawing life-sustaining treatments and utilizing other technologies. Nurses need to determine who is involved in making the decision, and how the nurse fits into the scenario. Utilizing the decision-making process described in Chapter 7 may assist in this process. Nurses need to be aware of institutional policies and protocols regarding various technologies. Such policies should include approaches to reaching decisions about particular patients, ways of dealing with conflicts that may arise, protection of patient rights, description of roles of those involved in the decision-making process, and directions for documenting the decision in the patient's chart. In most situations, the patient or the patient's surrogate has the ultimate authority to decide which interventions to use or withhold.

Because nurses are in close and continual contact with patients, they are often perceived as more available and more approachable than physicians. Patients or family members may discuss their concerns about interventions more readily with the nurse, seeking information or advice. It is important to know what they have been told by the physician, determine the patient's and family's level of understanding about the situation, and determine whether they have the necessary information to make an informed decision. If information is needed in such areas as risks, discomforts, side effects, potential benefits, likelihood of success, treatment alternatives, or estimated costs, advocating for the patient in this regard is an expected nursing response. Nurses are in a key position to utilize conversations with patients and families to discover areas of confusion and to elicit information about the patient's wishes regarding interventions.

Sometimes people just need to talk out their concerns and sort through sometimes conflicting messages coming from the head and the heart. Providing a listening presence can help people vent emotions, speak their fears, and clarify their concerns. At times the concern may be such that the nurse must advocate for the patient by facilitating communication with the physician, support people such as family or pastor, or other appropriate persons such as a patient representative or member of the ethics committee. Collaboration among all involved is important to ensure an informed choice. Effective communication can be facilitated by providing an environment that is not rushed; using terms and language that are understood by the other person; allowing time for and encouraging questions; practicing attentive listening; and offering a caring presence.

Caring: The Human Focus

In the context of expanding scientific and technological knowledge, nurses have the responsibility for helping patients and families benefit from what technology offers, while always remembering the human focus of care. Nursing care in its fullest meaning is most essential when medical treatments are no longer effective. This is evident especially in nursing's role in palliative care. However alert, and in whatever stage of living and dying, an individual has a life story that continues to unfold, a story that continues to intertwine with lives of others. In the midst of the technology, nurses can encourage family and loved ones to talk with, touch, and be in touch with the patient. In this way nurses acknowledge the primary importance of relationships, even in a health care setting filled with machines, noises, and other evidences of advanced technology.

Attention to the human focus includes helping patients and families become more comfortable with the sometimes formidable array of machines and equipment, and make sense of the large amounts of clinical data that are generated. Incorporating family members in caring for the patient provides time for connecting and observing the patient in both good and bad moments, and engenders a more realistic view of the patient's condition. Rather than engendering anxiety and mistrust by shutting the family out of the patient's life and experiences at critical moments, nurses should encourage them to share directly in the patient's journey. This provides families more experiences upon which to base hard decisions.

The nursing role of providing care and comfort is paramount in any health care setting, and has many facets. It may take the shape of explaining, as often as necessary, the purpose and problems related to interventions. Caring requires that the nurse see the experience from another's point of view, so that questions, fears, concerns, and frustrations may be addressed appropriately. Providing care and comfort also requires that the nurse support and encourage behaviors that enable patients and families to choose in accordance with their own beliefs and values. Being proficient in technical skills with the intent of doing what is best for the patient is part of human care, as is the ability to be with and wait with persons as they struggle through difficult situations.

SUMMARY

Many of the major ethical dilemmas encountered by nurses and other health care providers today are associated with advances in scientific knowledge and technology. In order to recognize and to deal with such dilemmas, nurses need to clarify their own values and appreciate differences in values among the various people involved in making patient care decisions. The potential of technology has raised very deep questions about life and death that must be addressed on individual, professional, and societal levels. Issues of quality of life, relief of suffering, and futility of interventions are some facets of these questions. Decisions about when to intervene and reasonable goals of interventions are made more difficult because of varying perceptions of the value of such interventions, nondefinitive outcomes, and issues related to availability of interventions. Principles of beneficence, nonmaleficence, justice, and autonomy provide the basis for arguments on different sides of issues related to technology. Nurses must take into account their responsibilities to patients and to the profession, as well as personal integrity, when dealing with ethical dilemmas engendered by technology. Nurses must remember that, in the midst of the technology with its associated dilemmas, there are persons who need the human focus of care that is basic to nursing practice.

CHAPTER HIGHLIGHTS

- The use of technology in health care has prompted the need to address important ethical questions regarding life, death, and allocation of resources.

- Utilization of health care technology may give rise to conflicts between the principles of beneficence and nonmaleficence.

- Appropriate utilization of health care technologies requires that health care providers, patients, and families understand the purposes, benefits, and limitations of specific technologies.

- Attitudes and beliefs concerning life and death affect how health care providers, patients, families, and the legal system approach issues related to health care technology. Ethical dilemmas may arise when there are differing opinions among the parties involved related to the use of technology.

- Determination of medical futility is an important consideration in decisions to withhold or withdraw life-sustaining interventions. Ethical decisions regarding these measures require consideration of whether they are prolonging living or prolonging dying.

- Economics may factor into decisions related to medical futility, availability of technology, and accessibility to many interventions.

- Withholding or withdrawing life-sustaining treatments in situations in which the burden or harm has been determined to outweigh the benefits constitutes allowing a person to die, and is not euthanasia. Dilemmas may arise regarding whether to classify the use of specific interventions as ordinary or extraordinary measures. The courts have sometimes been involved in making this determination.

- Patient self-determination and distributive justice must be considered in decisions regarding technology. Vigilance is required to ensure that people are not harmed, exploited, controlled, discriminated against, or excluded from care by the use of health care technologies.

- Nurses are in a key position to help patients and families articulate their preferences regarding technological interventions, and to facilitate communication with other health team members in this regard. This role requires familiarity with patient and family decisions and institutional policies regarding life-sustaining interventions, and awareness that when medical care is deemed futile, nursing care in its fullest meaning is most essential.

DISCUSSION QUESTIONS AND ACTIVITIES

1. Explore information and resources related to advance directives at the website http://www.wvethics.org. Develop advance directives for yourself, considering interventions you would choose and parameters regarding these choices. Discuss and compare your directives with classmates. Advance directive forms for your state can be found at http://www.caringinfo.org/i4a/pages/index.cfm?pageid=1.

2. Discuss your beliefs regarding determinants of the beginning and end of life.

3. Describe quality of life as it relates to health care decisions.

4. Discuss potential *slippery slope* elements related to reproductive and genetic technologies, cloning and stem cell research, and organ procurement and transplantation. Investigate issues related to stem cell research and cloning at the following websites and discuss with classmates:

   http://www.stemcellresearch.org—Coalition of Americans for Research Ethics

   http://stemcells.nih.gov—Information on stem cells

   http://stemcells.nih.gov/info/ethics.asp—National Institutes of Health

   http://www.icn.ch/images/stories/documents/publications/fact_sheets/6b_FS-Genetics_genomics.pdf

http://www.icn.ch/images/stories/documents/publications/fact_
sheets/6a_FS-Genetics_nursing.pdf

http://www.iom.edu/Reports/2011/Generating-Evidence-for-
Genomic-Diagnostic-Test-Development.aspx

http://www.iom.edu/Reports/2010/The-Value-of-Genetic-and-
Genomic-Technologies.aspx

http://nursingworld.org/MainMenuCategories/EthicsStandards/
Genetics-1

http://www.ornl.gov/sci/techresources/Human_Genome/elsi/elsi
.shtml—Human Genome Project information

http://www.isong.org/ISONG_ethical_legal_social.php—
International Society of Nurses in Genetics

http://education.technyou.edu.au/view/258/310/types-stem-cells

http://education.technyou.edu.au/view/258/270/ethics-stem-cell-
research

5. Plan and engage in a debate in your class focused on economic and justice issues related to health care technologies.

6. Observe several patients who are receiving technological interventions and note how the technology is affecting them and their families, issues surrounding its use, the focus of nursing care, and your reaction to the situation. Describe strengths of the nursing care you observe, and aspects that you might do differently if you were providing care. Talk to nurses and patients regarding the impact of technology on their health and care.

7. Discuss your view about nurses writing DNR orders.

8. Investigate whether your state, province, or hospital has specific policies for determining medical futility. How would you handle a situation where you feel the physician's decision regarding life-sustaining interventions is inappropriate for your patient?

9. Choose one of the topics discussed in this chapter and explore the websites of the ANA, the CNA, and the ICN regarding policies or positions statements on this issue. You may include information from other disciplines as well. Compare and contrast positions of the various organizations. Discuss your views about this issue, and how they compare with the positions of the professional organizations.

ANA—http://www.nursingworld.org

CNA—http://www.cna-nurses.ca

ICN—http://www.icn.ch

10. Explore the following websites regarding issues of confidentiality and privacy and share information with classmates:

http://www.cms.gov/HIPAAGenInfo

http://www.healthprivacy.org

http://wings.buffalo.edu/faculty/research/bioethics/privacy.html— Lists websites for information on privacy

http://www.nasn.org/Portals/0/briefs/2004briefrecords.pdf— School nurse guidelines

11. Role-play a palliative care conference with students in the class, using a real or hypothetical patient case situation, or attend an ethics committee meeting at your hospital. Review and discuss the ethics committee tools available online at http://www.wvnec.org.

REFERENCES

American Nurses Association. (2003). Revised position statement: Nursing care and do not resuscitate (DNR) and allow natural death (AND) decisions. Retrieved March 12, 2012, from http://nursingworld.org/MainMenuCategories/EthicsStandards/Ethics-Position-Statements

AuthorAmerican Nurses Association. (2006). Genetics/genomics: Scope and standards of practice. Silver Springs, MD: Author.

American Nurses Association. (2007). Position statement on stem cell research. Retrieved March 12, 2012, from http://nursingworld.org/MainMenuCategories/EthicsStandards/Ethics-Position-Statements/StemCellResearch.txt

American Nurses Association. (2010). Revised position statement: Registered nurses' roles and responsibilities in providing expert care and counseling at the end of life. Retrieved March 12, 2012, from http://nursingworld.org/MainMenuCategories/EthicsStandards/Ethics-Position-Statements

American Nurses Association. (2011, March 11). Position statement: Forgoing nutrition and hydration. Retrieved March 12, 2012, from http://nursingworld.org/MainMenuCategories/EthicsStandards/Ethics-Position-Statements/prtetnutr14451.pdf

Anderson, G., & Rorty, M. V. (2001). Key points for developing an international declaration on nursing, human rights, human genetics and public policy. *Nursing Ethics, 8*(3), 259–71.

Angell, M. (1990). Prisoners of technology: The case of Nancy Cruzan. *New England Journal of Medicine, 322,* 1226–1228.

Annas, G. J. (1990). Nancy Cruzan and the right to die. *New England Journal of Medicine, 323,* 670–672.

Arraf, K., Cox, G., & Oberle, K. (2004). Using the Canadian code of ethics for registered nurses to explore ethics in palliative care research. *Nursing Ethics, 11*(6), 600–609.

Baily, M. A. (2011). Futility, autonomy, and cost of end-of-life care. *Journal of Law, Medicine & Ethics, 39*(2), 172–182.

Bishop, J. P., Brothers, K. B., Perry, J. E. & Ahmad, A. (2010). Reviving the conversation around CPR/DNR. *The American Journal of Bioethics, 10*(1), 61–67.

Cadogan, M. P. (2010). CPR decision making and older adults. *Journal of Gerontological Nursing, 36*(12), 10–15.

Clark, E. H. (2004). Quality of life: A basis for clinical decision-making in community psychiatric care. *Journal of Psychiatric and Mental Health Nursing, 11*, 725–730.

Clark, P. A. (2007, May). Medical futility: Legal and ethical analysis. *Virtual Mentor, 9*(5), 375–383. Retrieved from http://virtualmentor.ama-assn.org/2007/05/msoc1-0705.html

Day, L. (2009). Medical futility, personal goods, and social responsibility. *American Journal of Critical Care, 18*(3), 279–282.

Devettere, R. J. (1995). *Practical decision making in health care ethics: Cases and concepts.* Washington, DC: Georgetown University Press.

Diem, S. J., Lantos, J. D., & Tulsky, J. A. (1996). Cardiopulmonary resuscitation on television. *New England Journal of Medicine, 334*(24), 1579–1582.

Dudley, G. (2004). Electronic records, patient confidentiality, and the impact of HIPAA. Retrieved July 19, 2006, from http://www.psqh.com/octdec04/dudley.html

Feen, E. (2010). Leave the current system of universal CPR and patient request of DNR orders in place. *The American Journal of Bioethics, 10*(1), 80–81.

Geppert, C. M., Andrews, M. R., & Druyan, M. E. (2010). Ethical issues in artificial nutrition and hydration: a review. *Journal of Parenteral and Enteral Nutrition, 34*(1), 79–88.

Guenin, L. (2008). *The morality of embryo use.* Cambridge: Cambridge University Press.

Hayes, C. (2004). Ethics in end-of-life care. *Journal of Hospice and Palliative Nursing, 6*(1), 36–43.

Hickman, S. E., Nelson, C. A., Moss, A. H., Hammes, B. J., Terwilliger, A., Jackson, A., & Tolle, S. W. (2009). Use of the physician orders for life-sustaining treatment (POLST) paradigm program in the hospice setting. *Journal of Palliative Medicine, 12*(2), 133–141.

International Council of Nurses. (2009a). Fact sheet—Genetics and nursing. Retrieved March 12, 2012, from http://www.icn.ch/images/stories/documents/publications/fact_sheets/6a_FS-Genetics_nursing.pdf

International Council of Nurses. (2009b). Fact sheet—Genetics and genomics in nursing. Retrieved March 12, 2012, from http://www.icn.ch/images/stories/documents/publications/fact_sheets/6b_FS-Genetics_genomics.pdf

Jacobs, B. B., & Taylor, C. (2005). Medical futility in the natural attitude. *Advances in Nursing Science, 28*(4), 288–305.

Lauritzen, P. (2005). Stem cells, biotechnology, and human rights: Implications for a posthuman future. *Hastings Center Reports, 35*(2), 25–33.

Lo, B. (2009). *Resolving ethical dilemmas: A guide for clinicians* (4th. ed.). Philadelphia: Lippincott Williams & Wilkins.

National Association of School Nurses. (2004). *School nurse role in education, school health records* (Issue Brief). Scarborough, ME: Author. Retrieved July 17, 2006, from http://www.nasn.org

Pancoast, P. E., Patrick, T. B., & Mitchell, J. A. (2003). Physician PDA use and the HIPAA privacy rule. *Journal of the American Medical Informatics Association, 10*(6), 611–12.

Pence, G. E. (1995). *Classic cases in medical ethics.* New York: McGraw-Hill.

Plummer, M. & Molzahn, A. E. (2009). Quality of life in contemporary nursing theory: A concept analysis. *Nursing Science Quarterly, 22*(2), 134–140.

Rushton, C. H., Spencer, K. L., & Johanson, W. (2004). Bringing end-of-life care out of the shadows. *Holistic Nursing Practice, 18*(6), 313–317.

Sandel, M. J. (2004). Embryo ethics—The moral logic of stem cell research. *New England Journal of Medicine, 351*(3), 207–209.

Scofield, G. R. (1995). Is consent useful when resuscitation isn't? In J. H. Howell & W. F. Sale (Eds.), *Life choices: A Hastings Center introduction to bioethics* (pp. 172–187). Washington, DC: Georgetown University Press.

TechNyou: Science education resources. (2012). Ethics of stem cell research. Retrieved March 12, 2012, from http://education.technyou.edu.au/view/258/270/ethics-stem-cell-research

Williams, L. S. (2006). Feeding patients after stroke: Who, when, how? *Annals of Internal Medicine, 144,* 59–60.

Chapter

11

PRACTICE ISSUES RELATED TO PATIENT SELF-DETERMINATION

The task set before us is to find the golden mean between moral autonomy and the cooperative action necessary to contemporary life.

(Curtin, 1982)

OBJECTIVES

After completing this chapter, the reader should be able to:

1. Discuss autonomy and paternalism as they relate to patient self-determination.

2. Describe factors that may threaten autonomy in health care settings and situations in which autonomy may be limited.

3. Examine the interaction of justice and autonomy.

4. Discuss informed consent as it relates to patient self-determination.

5. Examine legal and ethical elements of informed consent.

6. Describe the nursing role and responsibilities related to informed consent.

7. Discuss the place of advance directives in health care decisions.

8. Discuss patient autonomy related to choices for life and health.

9. Describe the nursing role and responsibilities related to patient lifestyle and health choices.

10. Discuss the nursing role regarding complementary therapies.

11. Describe confidentiality in relation to health care choices.

INTRODUCTION

The role of the patient and that of the healer, and the implied responsibilities of each, have varied throughout history and in different cultures. In some cultures, decisions regarding "what is best" for the patient are deferred to the healer, who is presumed to know what will bring about healing. Indeed, until recent years, the physician was often viewed in this light. Such paternalism has been challenged in recent years, and greater emphasis has been placed on the role and rights of patients in making health care decisions. This chapter focuses on practice issues related to patient self-determination. Discussion of these issues includes both ethical and legal components, and is intertwined with issues of technology and economics.

AUTONOMY AND PATERNALISM

Self-determination derives from the principle of autonomy. **Autonomy**, which is discussed in detail in Chapter 3, denotes having the freedom to make choices about issues that affect our own lives and to make decisions about personal goals. Autonomy means self-governing and implies respect for persons, the ability to determine personal goals and decide on a plan of action, and the freedom to act on the choices made. The value placed on the primacy of the individual implicit in autonomy is primarily an Anglo-American concept, and may not be fully accepted in other cultures. Autonomy includes an appreciation for the self in relation to others, recognizing that choices are made in the context of community. Implications of this view for health care include viewing patients as members of a social world in which health care decisions affect others and are made in conjunction with trusted persons.

Factors that may threaten autonomy in health care settings include a persisting paternalistic attitude that promotes the dependent role of the patient; assumptions that a patient's values and thought processes are the same as those of the health care provider; failure to appreciate a difference in knowledge level regarding health matters; and a focus on technology rather than caring. Paternalistic attitudes have contributed to increased numbers of patients and families struggling with health care providers over control of health care decisions. **Paternalism**, or acting in a "fatherly" manner, derives from expectations within the patriarchal family structure that the father has the right and responsibility to make decisions on behalf of other family members. In health care, this attitude has historically been the basis for allowing physicians to make unilateral decisions about patient care (Will, 2011). Paternalism (or parentalism, as discussed in Chapter 3) implies well-intended actions of benevolent decision making, leadership, protection, and discipline. In the health care arena, paternalism manifests in the making of decisions on behalf of patients without their full consent or knowledge. Although the principle of beneficence suggests that decisions are focused on the patient's well-being, the power inherent in such a hierarchical arrangement can be abused, and decisions made may reflect the interests of the health care provider more than those of the patient. Consider, for example, many elderly patients in nursing homes who are routinely sedated "for their own protection" because of "agitation and confusion." It is worth pondering whether medication used in this way is for the benefit of the patient, or to make life easier for the staff.

Case Presentation

Determining What Is Best for the Patient

Mr. Zumma, a former butcher who is 84 years old, has had evidence of memory loss and periodic confusion for about 18 months. He has been functional at home, able to do personal care, household chores, and shopping, and has been on no medication. One night he came into the bedroom with two straight razors and told his wife to stay still so he could slit her throat. She was able to escape by exiting through a nearby door and running to a neighbor's house. Reluctant to call the police because "he is not a criminal," she called her son, who came and calmed his father down. On the advice of another family member, Mrs. Zumma contacted a geriatric psychiatrist, who immediately hospitalized Mr. Zumma and started him on Haldol. When he got worse, the physician increased the dose of the medication. Although he was walking and talking when he was admitted, after 1 day in the hospital the patient became incontinent, could not walk, was drooling, and had to be restrained. The decline in his condition throughout the week in the hospital concerned Mrs. Zumma, and she approached the psychiatrist about taking him on a previously planned vacation. The psychiatrist indicated that this would be impossible, and that the patient would need to go to a nursing home. With persistence, however, Mrs. Zumma was able to convince the psychiatrist to discontinue the medications, after which Mr. Zumma's condition improved and he walked out of the hospital and did well on the vacation trip. Although he still gets confused, he remains functional without medication at home, where his wife makes sure that all sharp or dangerous objects are kept hidden.

Think About It

When Interventions Do More Harm Than Good

- *How did paternalism factor into the case of Mr. Zumma?*
- *What ethical issues are evident in this case?*
- *If you were the nurse caring for Mr. Zumma, and his wife approached you with her concerns about his condition, how would you respond?*
- *Describe patient and family values that you believe influenced decisions about Mr. Zumma's care.*

The authoritarian medical model is still encountered within the Western health care system. This model promotes the beliefs that physicians possess the most appropriate skills and capacities to exercise decision-making power and that patients and families do not have sufficient background to make adequate decisions in the face of illness. What this attitude does not address, however, is the reality that decisions about health require more than scientific expertise. Such decisions need to take into account factors such as the patient's values, culture, and spiritual and other beliefs; an evaluation of risks, benefits, and economic considerations; and effects on lifestyle and role. The principle of autonomy directs nurses and others to engage patients in the decision-making process in relationship with others who may need to be part of the process. Respecting autonomy also means appreciating situations in which patients are asking that others have a prominent role in making decisions for them (Leever, 2011; Sakalys, 2010).

How Far Does Autonomy Go?

Although the principle of autonomy has become a key consideration in health care ethics, it does have limits. Practitioners are not obligated to honor requests from patients or families for interventions that, in the best judgment of the practitioner, are outside accepted standards of care or that are contrary to the practitioner's own ethical views. Autonomy may also be limited by availability of resources and economic circumstances.

In discussions of patient self-determination, the principle of justice needs to be considered along with that of autonomy. **Justice** implies fair, equitable, and appropriate treatment in light of what is due or owed to persons, recognizing that giving to some may deny receipt to others who might otherwise have received these things. In determining who deserves what portion of finite health care resources, autonomy and justice may conflict where needs or demands for health care by autonomous patients outweigh available resources. The rights of family members and of society must be considered in relation to the needs of individuals. Hardwig (2000) suggests that the medical and nonmedical impacts of treatment decisions on both the patient and the family need to be considered. He reflects that patient autonomy implies the responsible use of freedom, which means considering the needs of family and society as well as our own desires. He raises the question of whether it is legitimate to ask families to make sacrifices of major resources to meet the needs of one member. The limited availability and expense of many medical interventions bring such questions to the fore. Since people can be maintained on very expensive treatments for prolonged periods of time, justice requires us to ask not only who deserves such an intervention, but also who is expected to pay for it. Although the moral relevance of considering the interests of the family is generally not addressed in current ethical theory, dilemmas faced by patients, families, and practitioners include these issues, and it is well worth pondering their implications.

ASK YOURSELF

Should There Be Limits to Patient Autonomy?

- Can you think of health care situations in which the interests of the family should take precedence over those of the patient? Upon what criteria do you base this decision?
- How would you describe nursing's role regarding patient autonomy?
- How have you experienced paternalism in nursing?
- How do you feel about the suggestion that the physician is most qualified to make health care decisions? What have you experienced in this regard?

INFORMED CONSENT

Informed consent provides legal protection of a patient's right to personal autonomy. The concept of informed consent is one that has come to mean that patients are given the opportunity to autonomously choose a course of action in regard to plans for health care. The choice includes the right to refuse interventions or recommendations about care, and to choose from available therapeutic alternatives. This is usually discussed in relation to surgery and complex medical procedures, but also includes consent to more common interventions that may have undesirable side effects, such as immunizations and contraceptives. Exceptions to informed consent include emergencies in which there is no time to disclose the information, and waivers by patients who do not want to know their prognosis or risks of treatment.

The emergence of informed consent as we know it has been affected by several factors. One factor has been the institutionalization of health care in hospitals, with their associated technologies and life-prolonging techniques over which people have little control and limited understanding. When health providers visited in the home, informed consent was not as necessary, because people had more control and better understanding of traditional remedies (Will, 2011). The courts, however, have exerted the most significant influence on shaping the doctrine of informed consent.

The history of the concept dates back to at least three landmark legal cases. In *Slater v. Baker & Stapleton* (1767), a decision was made that prohibited "unauthorized touching." This decision held that a person has a right to know what is to be done to his or her body. It did not require any participation in the decision-making process. In the 1905 case of *Mobe v. Williams* (Husted & Husted, 2001) and the case of *Schloendorff v. The Society of New York Hospital* (1914), separate rulings established the patient's right to know what was to be done, and also the right to give or withhold consent. These decisions did not address the patient's right to be informed about risks of treatment or nontreatment or about the existence of alternative therapies. In the case of *Salgo v. Leland Stanford, Jr.* (1957), the California Supreme Court ruled in favor of a patient who had not been informed of the risks of aortography and subsequently became paralyzed. This ruling established a patient's right to be advised of the risks involved in any proposed treatment (Husted & Husted, 2001).

Ethical and Legal Elements of Informed Consent

Although the informed consent doctrine has foundations in law, it is essentially an ethical imperative based on respect for persons as autonomous agents. Informed consent is more than simply a legal document and a process of having a patient sign a form. Consent is a process of shared decision making flowing from communication between patient and health care provider that is based upon mutual respect and participation. The two major legal elements of informed consent that are inherent in the ethical imperative are *information* and *consent*.

Information

The information component of informed consent includes both disclosure and understanding of the essential information. Figure 11–1 lists the information that must be included in an informed consent. People need access to sufficient information to help them understand their health concerns and make decisions regarding treatment. The information provided need not be in "textbook" detail, but does need to offer enough explanation for the person to have a clear picture of the situation, what is being offered,

- The nature of the health concern and prognosis if nothing is done
- Description of all treatment options, even those that the health care provider does not favor or cannot provide
- The benefits, risks, and consequences of the various treatment alternatives, including nonintervention

FIGURE 11–1   Content of Informed Consent

and the alternatives as well as their risks, benefits, and consequences. Determining the adequacy of information disclosed in an informed consent is based on one or more standards: (1) *the professional practice standard*—the disclosure is consistent with the standards of the profession; (2) *the reasonable person standard*—the disclosure is what a reasonable person in similar circumstances would need in order to make an informed decision; and (3) *the subjective standard*—the disclosure is what the particular person wants or needs to know. Informed consent implies that the person has received the information and understands what is provided. Verification of understanding can be accomplished through discussion in which patients have an opportunity to ask questions and are asked to describe their understanding of the nature of the intervention, alternatives, risks, and benefits.

Consent

Consent to something implies the freedom to accept or reject it. This means that consent to health care interventions must be voluntary, without coercion, force, or manipulation from health care providers or family. Force entails making someone do something against his or her will. Coercion and manipulation may be overt or subtle, and may include threats, rewards, deception, or inducing excessive fear. The voluntary nature of consent does not prohibit health care providers from making recommendations or attempting to persuade patients to accept their suggestions. However, we must be alert to situations in which persuasion takes on qualities of coercion or manipulation.

Nursing Role and Responsibilities: Informed Consent

While the practice of documenting informed consent for a procedure usually ends with the signing of a consent form, the process is much more complex. Following the rules laid out previously, informed consent must include explicit verification that the patient is aware of all options, the possible outcomes of each option, and the likely outcome with nontreatment. The patient must also recognize the implications that each option will have upon his or her lifestyle. The nurse must be sensitive to the fact that the very act of asking a patient to sign a form giving permission for a particular

Case Presentation

Language and Informed Consent

Mohano is a 67-year-old deaf man who was admitted to the hospital with atrial fibrillation. The nurse notes that he is alert, apparently oriented, and able to follow simple directions that she acts out, although he does look apprehensive as she cares for him. Mohano's social history indicates that he was brought into the hospital by a community worker who looks in on him because he is deaf and illiterate and has no family in the area. She has indicated that he came to the area as a migrant worker a number of years ago, along with a brother who died the previous year. She has also noted that two of his five siblings were also deaf, and they had developed a type of sign language that was understood only by family members. At the interdisciplinary care conference, the medical resident who is in charge of his case voices frustration because of the need to get the patient's permission to do a stress test and to talk to him about medications and risk for stroke. He suggests that they should just get the patient to make an X on the form so they can go ahead with the treatment protocol, because it is in the patient's best interest to do so. The social worker suggests that they get an interpreter for the deaf to come in and try to talk to him through sign language, although she is not sure he will understand.

Think About It

Obtaining Informed Consent When There Is No Common Language

- *What ethical dilemmas are evident in this case?*

- *What do you think about Mohano's decision-making capacity?*

- *Do you think it is possible to obtain an informed consent from Mohano? Support your position with discussion of elements of informed consent and decision-making capacity.*

- *In a situation such as this, it is evident that the patient has a language, although it is not understood by the health care providers, and that he has been able to care for himself with some assistance. How would these factors enter into determination of his decision-making capacity?*

- *How does the inability of the health care provider to communicate with a patient affect determination of the patient's decision-making capacity?*

- *What are the implications of denying Mohano important services because of lack of common language and subsequent inability to ensure informed consent?*

treatment may constitute a form of coercion. It is the nurse's responsibility as advocate for the patient to ensure that all criteria for autonomous decision making are met. If the nurse believes that the patient does not understand the implications of any part of the process, including nontreatment and alternative options, or that the patient is unable to deliberate and to reason on the various choices, it is the responsibility of the nurse to intervene. Legally the nurse must act if it becomes apparent that the patient is not informed. Actions may include notifying the physician and requesting further information for the patient, or stopping the process until it is ensured that the decision can be made autonomously. Although the mechanics of the process usually require the nurse to obtain the patient's signature on a consent form, the primary concern of the nurse is to ensure that all criteria for autonomous decision making are met.

Federal, state, and institution policies govern expectations regarding a properly executed informed consent (including who can legally obtain this consent), and nurses need to be familiar with these policies. Merely witnessing a patient's signature on a consent form that has previously been discussed with the patient by the physician is not considered obtaining informed consent (Petersen, 2010). However, witnessing a patient's signature implies accountability on the part of the nurse to assure that the patient is giving consent willingly, is competent in that moment to give consent, and that the patient's signature is authentic. An important part of the nursing role is to verify the patient's understanding of the procedure, to determine whether there are any questions that need to be discussed with the physician, and to be alert for any indication of coercion (Plawecki & Plawecki, 2009). Nursing documentation of communication with the patient and with the physician regarding any questions, concerns, or teaching related to the informed consent is of utmost importance. Any special circumstances should also be documented, such as the patient's inability to read or write, or the use of an interpreter if the patient speaks a different language.

Nurses in advanced practice roles are accountable for providing information and obtaining informed consent for interventions that they initiate under their scope of practice. The question of the nurse's right to inform a patient of the risks inherent in a certain procedure or alternative courses of action in other settings is not as clear. In 1977, in the course of initiating chemotherapy, Jolene Tuma, a nursing instructor, answered an elderly patient's questions about cancer treatment alternatives. The patient indicated that she did not want to question the physician because he was not open to considering other therapies. Tuma was also asked to describe the therapies to the patient's son, who was upset by this. Although the patient decided to continue chemotherapy, she died 2 weeks later. After the patient's death, the son told the physician of Tuma's action. The physician subsequently brought charges against Ms. Tuma for disrupting the physician-patient relationship. She was fired from her job and lost her nursing license as a result. Ms. Tuma pursued an appeal of the decision. In 1979 the Idaho Supreme Court ruled that she could not lose her license for "unprofessional behavior" because there was no statutory description of this offense. The court did not address, however, the nurse's right to inform the patient (*Tuma v. Board of Nursing of the State of Idaho*).

Unfortunately, this leaves the nurse in a sort of limbo in regard to ensuring informed consent. Although the nurse is legally required to act on behalf of the patient to guarantee true informed consent, there is no clear course of action when a nurse believes that the patient has not been informed or does not understand the information, and the physician is uncooperative in remedying the situation. Institutional and legal constraints may impede the nurse from following the ethically correct course of action.

ASK YOURSELF

What Is the Nurse's Responsibility Regarding Informed Consent?

- In the case described previously, do you feel that Jolene Tuma's actions were appropriate? Support your position.
- What ethical issues are apparent in situations such as this?
- How does the nurse-patient relationship factor into such a situation?

ADVANCE DIRECTIVES

Given the dilemmas that can arise regarding the use of technology, an important nursing role is to encourage and assist people to make their wishes known concerning the use of such interventions. For those who are mentally alert and capable of making decisions, informed consent is needed prior to initiating any life-sustaining interventions. To ensure that our wishes regarding treatment are followed in the event that we have lost decision-making capacity, advance directives are needed. **Advance directives** are instructions that indicate health care interventions to initiate or withhold, or that designate someone who will act as a surrogate in making such decisions in the event that we lose decision-making capacity. Such directives can be considered as a kind of informed consent for future interventions. Advance directives support people in making decisions on their own behalf, and help to ensure that patients have the kind of end-of-life care that they want. In order to help patients be as clear as possible about their choices, the various life-sustaining measures that may be considered in end-of-life care should be discussed openly and clearly. Patients should be encouraged to express verbally, or in writing, their wishes about tube feedings, breathing machines, cardiopulmonary resuscitation, and dialysis. Consideration of interventions should include how long they might want to stay on an intervention if it is initiated and their condition continues to decline or is not improving. In addition to enabling people to have choices in their dying process, the presence of clearly understood advance directives can alleviate stress on family and clinicians when dealing with end-of-life concerns.

Perhaps the most important factor in decision making regarding end-of-life care is clear and open communication between the patient or the surrogate and health care providers. We need to do more than merely seek to know which potential life-sustaining technology a person does or does not want. We need to see and get to know the person who is making these decisions. Eliciting a clear statement of personal values is basic to this process. What does the person value in life? What constitutes quality of life for the person? What are his or her personal beliefs and concerns about dying? We must recognize the influence of cultural, societal, spiritual, and family norms and perspectives on personal values. For example, in some cultures, speaking of death and dying is believed to bring bad luck. Family wishes may influence personal choices, and in some cultures the patient may defer decisions about end-of-life care to the family. When discussing different interventions, we need to ensure that patients understand what the procedure is and what it involves. They also need to appreciate that risks and benefits of life-sustaining interventions vary with age, health condition, and circumstances that prompt the consideration of the intervention. For example, the literature shows no evidence that tube feedings prolong life or improve quality of life for patients with dementia or multisystem illness (American Nurses Association [ANA], 2011; Geppert, Andrews, & Druyan, 2010; Williams, 2006). We need to understand why the patient or family wants a particular intervention, and what it is that they think it will do for them.

Advance directives include living wills and durable powers of attorney. **Living wills** are legal documents giving directions to health care providers related to withholding or withdrawing life support if certain conditions exist. Statutes regulating living wills vary from state to state, so nurses must be familiar with their own state laws. Living wills guide decisions by indicating a person's desires regarding life-sustaining interventions; however, they also raise issues of concern. Directives in living wills may be vague, and can address only the interventions a person does not want. In some states, only persons who are terminally ill or whose death is imminent are allowed to make living wills. Particularly in emergency situations, there may be a concern that a document that had been developed when a person was in good health may not reflect the patient's current desires.

A **durable power of attorney** allows a competent person to designate another as a surrogate or proxy to act on her or his behalf in making health care decisions in the event of the loss of decision-making capacity. Although there is no particular legal form required, the designation must be in writing and must be signed and dated by the person making the designation and two witnesses other than the designated surrogate. The designating person may revoke the designation at any time by changing the person named as surrogate, or by destroying the document. The authority of the surrogate does not become effective until it has been determined that the person has lost decision-making capacity. The authority of the surrogate is effective only for the duration of the loss of decision-making capacity. For example, in the case of a person who has a temporary loss of consciousness, the surrogate's authority to make decisions would end once the person regained consciousness and the ability to make decisions for self.

The presence of a living will or durable power of attorney and surrogate designation should be documented in a patient's health record. Nurses can seek opportunities to explore with patients whether they have such documents and to discuss the importance of such directives with patients and families. Discussion can begin with providing materials on advance directives to patients and families, or by asking patients whether they have discussed end-of-life choices with their family or health care provider and by asking whether they have, or would like to develop, an advance directive.

It is well known that patients may indicate concerns to nurses that they have not discussed with their physicians. Issues related to advance directives may be one such concern.

Decision-Making Capacity

Informed consent requires that the patient or surrogate have the ability to make a reasonable decision regarding health care concerns. A surrogate or health care proxy is someone who makes medical decisions on the patient's behalf if the patient is incapable of doing so. Conscious adults are presumed to have decision-making capacity, unless there is evidence to the contrary. **Decision-making capacity** is a medical determination relating only to the issue at hand, as people may have the ability to make decisions about some areas but not about others. For example, a person may be able to make decisions about health, while unable to make reasonable decisions about household matters. Persons may have decision-making capacity at some times and not others, and in each specific situation, there must be a determination that they have, or do not have, the capacity. The fact that a person makes a decision that seems unreasonable to the health care provider does not necessarily mean a lack of decision-making capacity; it may merely reflect a difference in values. If the decision seems unreasonable, however, it is wise to explore the patient's capacity regarding decision making.

Elements of Decision-Making Capacity

When evaluating a patient or surrogate for decision-making capacity, several elements must be present. These are listed in Figure 11–2. First, the patient must be able to understand all relevant information, including the nature of the health care problem; the prognosis; treatment options and recommendations; and the risks, benefits, and consequences of each. Second, the patient must be able to communicate this understanding and her or his choices. Third, the patient must possess a set of values and goals that enable evaluation regarding whether this health care decision will be of benefit in terms of personal goals. Fourth, the patient must have the ability to reason and to deliberate about available choices, which includes the ability to grasp notions such as risk and percentage, cause and effect, and chance and probability. Although it is not unreasonable to see some indecision, or even a change of mind once a choice has been made, a great deal of vacillation between choices suggests the need to re-evaluate decision-making capacity. Nurses are in a key position to observe patients and families for the presence of these elements of decision-making capacity. As patient advocates, nurses need to assess, document, and communicate to appropriate members of the health care team any concerns in this regard.

Physicians usually have legal authority and responsibility to determine decision-making capacity. In at least one state, however, an advanced practice nurse or a psychologist can also legally certify incapacity (West Virginia Health Care Decisions Act, 2002/2007). Determining incapacity is best done in consultation with family or others who have the patient's best interest in mind. There is a distinction between decision-making capacity and competence. Decisions about competence, which is the ability to make meaningful life decisions, require a legal action. Legally, persons are considered competent unless there is a ruling by a judge that they cannot make meaningful life decisions. Legal declarations of incompetence generally stay in effect for the remainder of the person's life, and include a court-appointed guardian to be the surrogate decision maker for the person.

When a patient lacks decision-making capacity, someone else must be identified as a surrogate to make decisions for the patient. In the case of children, the surrogate is usually a parent or legal guardian. With adults, the

---

The patient must
- Have the ability to understand all information.
- Have the ability to communicate understanding and choices.
- Have personal values and goals that guide the decision.
- Have the ability to reason and deliberate.

FIGURE 11–2 Elements of Decision-Making Capacity

surrogate may be a spouse, parent, adult children, other relatives, or other person named as surrogate in the patient's advance directives. In situations where a patient has no advance directives or has not named a surrogate to make decisions in the event of incapacity, health care providers should work with family and others to identify a surrogate. The legal process for choosing a surrogate varies from state to state, and you need to be familiar with the process in your state. The person chosen as surrogate should be someone willing to serve in this role and who can make health care decisions that are in accordance with the patient's wishes, or that are consistent with the patient's best interest if these wishes are not known or cannot be reasonably discerned. The surrogate should demonstrate care and concern for and have regular contact with the patient. In addition, the surrogate should be willing and able to participate fully in the decision-making process and to engage in face-to-face contact and communication with caregivers. Close family members such as parents, adult children, adult siblings, and adult grandchildren are often considered first if the patient has not designated a surrogate. However, close friends or neighbors may at times be better qualified to make these decisions. The decisions made by the surrogate should reflect the patient's values, including the patient's cultural and spiritual perspective, to the extent that these are reasonably known.

Patient Self-Determination Act

The **Patient Self-Determination Act** (PSDA), which went into effect December 1991, is a federal law requiring institutions such as hospitals, nursing homes, health maintenance organizations, and home care agencies receiving Medicare or Medicaid funds to provide written information to adult patients regarding their rights to make health care decisions. Such decisions include the right to refuse treatments and the right to write advance directives for guiding decisions should they become incapacitated. The ANA (2010a, 2010b) notes that nurses have a responsibility to support patients in making informed decisions. This is especially important regarding end-of-life care. Nurses have a critical role in implementing the PSDA within all health care settings.

In spite of the PSDA, only a small percentage of patients have advance directives, and many clinicians are not aware of the wishes of the seriously ill patients for whom they care (Rodriguez & Young, 2006). Paternalistic attitudes of some clinicians may result in their disregarding advance directives because of their belief that they know what is best for the patient in the current circumstances. Developing advance directives is part of the ongoing process of communication between patients or their surrogates and clinicians (ANA, 2010a; Canadian Nurses Association [CNA], 1998; Dunn, 2005; Levi & Green, 2010). Open discussion of end-of-life decisions should occur routinely within primary care settings, before the physical and emotional stress of serious illness or hospitalization.

Case Presentation

Terri Schiavo

The well-publicized case of Terri Schiavo illustrates a number of ethical issues regarding end-of-life care decisions made in the absence of advance directives. It is an example, as Quill (2005) notes, of medicine, ethics, law, and family working together poorly to meet the needs of a patient in a persistent vegetative state. Terri Schiavo had a cardiac arrest in 1990, reportedly triggered by severe hypokalemia related to an eating disorder, and was left paralyzed and severely brain damaged. For 15 years she was sustained by artificial nutrition and hydration via feeding tube. Reports of her neurological exams indicated that she was in a persistent vegetative state, which includes some reflexive response to noise and light, basic gag response, and periods of alternating sleep and wakefulness, without signs of cognition, emotion, or willful activity. In the absence of advance directives, her husband was made her legal guardian and health care surrogate. Reports indicate that the relationship between Ms. Schiavo's husband and her family (parents and siblings) had been strained since around 1993, and that they held vastly different opinions about what Ms. Schiavo would want and should have. Based on reports of medical experts and diagnostic tests, the state court of appeals ruled that there was clear and convincing evidence that supported the diagnosis of a persistent vegetative state. Stating that his wife would not want to be kept alive indefinitely in this condition (because of a reported statement she had made when she was cognizant that she would not want to be kept alive on machines), her husband requested that the feeding tube be discontinued. Ms. Schiavo's family, however, found other medical practitioners who believed that her condition could improve with therapies (for which there was no research evidence), and they would not accept the diagnosis of persistent vegetative state. Between 2001 and 2003 the courts authorized removing the feeding tube two different times, ruling that the evidence showed that she would not have chosen life-prolonging interventions given her condition. Because of legal action initiated by her family, the tube was reinserted each time. In the midst of an ongoing legal battle (during which a guardian *ad litem* was appointed) and massive media attention, public debate, and political and religious rhetoric, her feeding tube was again removed March 18, 2005. Multiple legal appeals to reinsert the tube were denied, and she died 13 days later.

Think About It

- *What do you see as the ethical issues in this case?*
- *Because of the media coverage of this case you may already have an opinion of the ethical nature of the decisions made. What values, beliefs, and information have shaped your opinion?*
- *The media brought up many more issues regarding Terri Schiavo's situation and family disagreements than mentioned in the Case Presentation. Explore some of these issues and ethical discussion at the following websites and one or two others of your choosing.*

  Article: "Terri Schiavo–A tragedy compounded":
  http://www.nejm.org/doi/full/10.1056/NEJMp058062

(continued)

"Exploring the Terri Schiavo ethics meltdown":
http://www.ethicsscoreboard.com/list/schiavo2.html

University of Miami Terri Shiavo Case Resources:
http://www.miami.edu/index.php/ethics/projects/schiavo

Article regarding public discussion of the Terri Schiavo case:
http://www.csmonitor.com/2005/0325/p01s04-wogi.html

Bioethics resources on the Web:
http://bioethics.od.nih.gov/endoflife.html

- *What ethical considerations were posed by various parties vocal in the public and media discussion about this case? Based on your understanding of the case, if you were appointed guardian ad litem for Ms. Schiavo, what would you recommend regarding life-sustaining measures? Support your position with what you understand to be the facts in the case and the ethical reasoning that would guide your recommendation.*

- *How might have Ms. Schiavo's end-of-life care been different if she had completed advance directives?*

- *Quill (2005) notes that the media coverage, distortion by interest groups, and emotional overtones associated with this case show what can happen when someone becomes more of a precedent-setting symbol than a unique human being. How do you feel about the public treatment and discussion of Ms. Schiavo's situation? Describe ethical considerations inherent in the public discussion of this case. How do you think you would have felt if she were your family member?*

- *How might you deal with a situation in which family members of a patient who is terminally ill (and unable to make decisions for self) or in a persistent vegetative state hold vastly different views of both the patient's condition and of what the patient would want regarding end-of-life care?*

- *How might the health care system, ethics, law, and the family work more effectively together to preserve the dignity and meet the needs of a patient in Ms. Schiavo's condition?*

Nursing Role and Responsibilities: Advance Directives

What is the nursing role and responsibility regarding advance directives? Whatever the work setting, nurses have a key role and responsibility in ensuring that patients have an opportunity to complete advance directives, and in interpreting and following through with patient's wishes as expressed through these directives. As nurses, we need to know our state's statutes that guide and govern advance directives. We also need to be aware of the policies and procedures regarding advance directives where we work. Completing our own advance directives helps us to reflect on our own values, beliefs, and concerns associated with end-of-life issues, to learn more about the specific forms and

Case Presentation

The Absence of Advance Directives

Ninety-year-old Mr. Moshe did not have advance directives when he was admitted to the hospital with Alzheimer's disease and renal failure. Although he was coherent at times and could converse with caregivers, the doctor determined that Mr. Moshe did not have decision-making capacity and named his daughter Zelda, with whom he had been residing, as his surrogate. The nursing staff questioned this choice because of their concerns about the quality of care Mr. Moshe had been receiving from Zelda and her husband Josh. As Mr. Moshe's health began to deteriorate rapidly, the nurses inquired about his DNR status. Josh replied he wanted Mr. Moshe kept alive, and that this was what Mr. Moshe wanted also. Zelda concurred with this. Although Zelda's four siblings called frequently inquiring about their father, Zelda would not inform them about their father's condition nor allow them access to him. Because of this conflict and their concerns regarding the motives for his DNR status, the nurses notified the physician about the family issues and requested an ethics committee consultation to determine the best interests of the patient. The nurses also noted that the physician had not signed the surrogate form as required by their state law, so legally there was no surrogate. The ethics committee representative convened a family meeting that included all five siblings, the physician, the primary nurse, and a member of the pastoral care team. After explaining that the purpose of the meeting was to discuss the type of care that would be in the best interests of their father, not to resolve family issues, the physician was asked to discuss Mr. Moshe's current health status and prognosis. All of the children were given the opportunity to ask questions of the physician and primary nurse. Then each family member was asked to voice what their father valued in life, and what they believed to be his wishes regarding end-of-life care. Even though some of the siblings had not spoken to each other for nearly 10 years, they each stated that their father had told them he would never want to be on life support. Zelda, who was asked to speak last, agreed, much to the dismay of her husband, that her father would not want to be placed on life support. The siblings also requested that they be allowed to visit their father and to call and check on him. When they were informed that there currently was no legal surrogate for their father, they all agreed to have Zelda continue in that role, providing that she allow them access to him. They stated that even though they were upset with her, they believed she loved him and provided good care for him. To close the meeting all family members were invited to go join together at their father's bedside, where they shared prayer and family stories. Mr. Moshe died that night.

Think About It

Considering the Patient's Best Interests

- *Because Mr. Moshe was coherent at times, do you think the physician should have asked him what he would want regarding life support?*

- *What do you think of the physician's choice of a surrogate for Mr. Moshe? What factors do you think he considered in appointing Zelda as surrogate? Are there factors you think he should have considered that he may not have?*

(continued)

- *As the nurse caring for Mr. Moshe, what would be your concerns regarding his situation? How do you think you would have responded in this situation?*

- *How did the process of the family meeting address the communication that is needed for making end-of-life decisions?*

processes involved, and ultimately to have more empathy with patients going through this process. Information concerning advance directives is often provided to patients on admission to a facility by a clerical worker. Because there may be limited explanation of this information to patients or limited opportunity for questions, we need to explore patient and family understanding of the information received. We can use this as an opening to stress the importance of having such directives, and to advocate for patients who may need assistance in developing advance directives. This is also a beginning opportunity for us to help patients explore personal values, their understanding of themselves in the context of their current situation, and significant cultural or other issues that may influence decision making. As nurses, we need to be familiar with our patients' directives for care, and ensure that care is consistent with the patient's wishes as expressed in the advance directives. Nursing's advocacy role in this regard includes informing other health team members of the presence and content of advance directives, alerting appropriate team members to changes in patient wishes or to evidence of changes in the patient's decision-making capacity, and intervening on behalf of the patient when wishes expressed in advance directives are not being followed. Nurses have an important role in increasing public awareness about advance directives through patient and community education, through research, and through education of nurses and other health care providers.

CHOICES CONCERNING LIFE AND HEALTH

Although discussion of patient autonomy frequently focuses on issues of informed consent and end-of-life decisions, issues related to self-determination can arise in any area of nursing practice. In every area of practice, nurses must deal with the effects of lifestyle choices on patients' health and healing. Many people who come into our care are suffering from ill effects of such things as overeating; tobacco, drug, or alcohol use; sexual activity; or work-related stress. Our job is to deal with the present health concern while encouraging change toward healthier living. However, patients are often not willing to follow the treatment plan and make the changes needed for healthier living. Dealing with patients whose health problems are clearly related to lifestyle choices, yet who are not willing to change their behaviors, may present dilemmas for nurses. Although nurses may acknowledge that the autonomous person has the right to choose healthy or unhealthy behaviors, it may be difficult to be as caring toward those who are perceived to have brought problems on themselves.

This is another area where the principle of justice may temper the bounds of autonomy. In situations where resources are limited, questions arise regarding whether it is ethical to put resources into treatments for people whose health problems are brought on by unhealthy life choices. This is countered by the question of whether it is ethical to refuse treatment or provide a lesser level of care to someone because the provider does not agree with that person's lifestyle choices.

Choices Regarding Recommended Treatment

What are nurses to do when patients are well informed and apparently able to follow plans of care, yet do not? Certainly one hears of physicians who refuse to continue to care for patients who do not comply with instructions—smoking cessation, for example. In a climate of limited resources, this is a question worthy of contemplation. The first tenet of ANA's revised *Code of Ethics for Nurses* (2001) states that nurses in all professional relationships practice "with compassion and respect for the inherent dignity, worth, and uniqueness of every individual, unrestricted by considerations of social or economic status, personal attributes, or the nature of health problems." Further, the nurse must not be affected by the patients' individual differences in background, customs, attitudes, and beliefs. Health care practices are an integral part of patients' backgrounds, customs, and beliefs. Therefore, it is clear that refusal to participate in a plan of care, regardless of the outcome, is the prerogative of the patient, and must not affect the caring attitude of the nurse. Unhealthy life practices are part of the whole person, and should be taken into consideration when revising plans of care.

Ultimately, choices about health care practices belong to patients. If allowed to choose, patients should not be labeled in a negative way for choices with which nurses do not agree. It is not appropriate for professionals who express the belief that all competent patients have the right to autonomous choice to then make value judgments about the choices made, and subsequently label patients as noncompliant. In fact, it is worth pondering whether the term *noncompliant* even belongs in nursing vocabulary. The notion of compliance relates to a paternalistic view that health care providers know what is best for patients and that, providing patients follow these directions, they will get well. Nurses should speak more appropriately in terms of motivation to follow a mutually agreed-upon plan of care that incorporates patient and family values and beliefs. We must remember that patients have a right to refuse interventions, and they have a right to seek therapies other than those offered by conventional Western medicine.

ASK YOURSELF

Who Should Pay for Ill Effects of Unhealthy Lifestyles?

It is interesting that in the time of Hippocrates, physicians were taught that they should not treat persons whose bodies were overmastered by their disease because it was an inappropriate use of medical resources.

- How do you feel about this?
- Would this same stance be considered ethical today?
- To what extent do personal lifestyle choices impinge on the rights of others if significant health care resources are needed to pay for the ill effects of these choices?

Autonomy implies that persons have the right to make choices about things that affect their lives, whether these choices have a positive or negative effect, unless these choices impinge on the rights of others.

- Is it just to expect society to pay for the health care services required for treating the effects of unhealthy behaviors?
- How would you go about allocating health care resources in relation to unhealthy lifestyle choices?

Case Presentation

A Challenging Patient

Rochelle, a 36-year-old woman who is a known cocaine addict, presented to the emergency room (ER) with severe left leg pain and swelling. The triage nurse reviewed her chart and presenting problem, noting that she had been seen 2 days prior for chest pain and left leg pain. Assuming these complaints were evaluated then, the nurse sent her to the "fast track" area to be seen by the nurse practitioner (NP). The NP noted that her chart was flagged regarding her cocaine addiction and that the physician who had seen her at the previous visit, after doing an EKG, CBC, electrolytes (which were normal), and a urine drug screen (which was positive for cocaine), discharged her with diagnoses of chest pain and illicit drug use. The NP's assessment revealed no shortness of breath, cough, or chest pain. Severe swelling and skin tightness of the left leg, with exquisite tenderness and positive Homan's sign, were suggestive of deep vein thrombosis. When the NP went to the ER physician saying that the patient needed to be evaluated by him, she was told to keep the patient over there and do the work-up because he had a patient with a similar problem in the ER.

When the ultrasound confirmed extensive deep vein thrombosis, the NP told the patient the situation and that she needed to be hospitalized. The patient immediately said that she could not stay because she had no one to watch her 9-year-old daughter, and she began to put on her shoes to leave. The NP told her that she could choose to leave but that the reason she (the NP) wanted her to stay was that this was a very serious problem from which she could die. Rochelle's response was to start crying, saying that she thought she would go home anyway because she had nothing to live for since her husband had died, so she would go home to die. When the NP called Rochelle's primary physician to alert him to the situation, he responded that he would come in to see her only if Rochelle agreed to stay; otherwise, it would be a waste of his time. After considerable effort, the NP contacted Rochelle's mother, who reluctantly agreed to keep her granddaughter when the NP explained the situation, and Rochelle agreed to stay.

Think About It

Dealing with Patients Who Make Apparently Unhealthy Choices

- *What issues of patient self-determination are evident in this case?*

- *How do you see lifestyle choices affecting Rochelle's care? What ethical issues must be considered here?*

- *Take an honest look at how you think you might react to Rochelle, knowing that she frequently shows up in the ER and is a cocaine addict.*

- *As the nurse in this situation, how would you deal with the patient's saying she could not stay? What do you think of the way the NP handled it?*

- *Evaluate ethical issues involved in the responses of the various health care practitioners in this case.*

- *Interestingly, Rochelle was indigent, African-American, and without health insurance, and the woman in the ER with similar complaints was middle class, Caucasian, and had health insurance. Discuss the implications of these factors in this case.*

Complementary Therapies

Many people utilize therapies that may be termed complementary, alternative, or integrative in regard to Western allopathic medicine. Examples of **complementary therapies** include acupuncture, herbal and nutritional interventions, energy healing modalities, biofeedback, tai chi, yoga, relaxation techniques, massage, and guided imagery. Most people tend to use such therapies along with conventional modalities, but some will choose to use them in lieu of what is offered by medical practitioners. Most people do not inform their medical practitioner that they are using these therapies.

Several issues regarding the use of complementary therapies need to be considered. First, people have a right to use modalities other than conventional medicine to address their health care needs. Second, nurses and other health care practitioners need to develop at least a talking knowledge, and better yet a working knowledge, of such therapies in order to be better able to discuss their use with patients. Many therapies work as an adjunct to medical interventions, some may interact in unhealthy ways, and the efficacy of many modalities is not yet known. Nurses need not be practitioners of other modalities in order to discuss them with patients any more than they need to be able to do surgery in order to discuss it. Nurses should create an atmosphere that encourages nonjudgmental discussion of all modalities being considered or employed, with a goal of using whatever is beneficial for the particular patient. Transcultural considerations (which are discussed in Chapter 18) may influence a person's choice of treatment modalities. Third, complementary modalities should not be discounted merely because they are not understood within the Western medical framework; however, it is important to counsel patients to explore the validity of claims made about a particular therapy. Fourth, as research continues and expands in the area of complementary therapies, the question of whether informed consent will need to at least acknowledge these therapies as treatment options must be addressed. Fifth, nurses who are skilled in complementary therapies need to be clear about what is within their scope of practice according to their state's nurse practice act. The ethical stance with complementary therapies, as with other interventions, requires offering an explanation of the intervention and receiving permission from the patient or family prior to initiating the therapy. Because these therapies can affect conventional interventions, practitioners should apprise other health team members of their use and document both treatments and their effects. The reader is encouraged to explore the website of the National Center for Complementary and Alternative Medicine (http://nccam.nih .gov) to learn more about research and other considerations regarding complementary therapies.

Controversial Choices

The value of patient self-determination is cited to support two decisions that have been the focus of much controversy in this country for many years: abortion and active euthanasia. Both of these choices are surrounded by ethical and religious opinion and debate. Abortion in particular is an example of an issue in which legal answers have been sought for ethical dilemmas. The potential for transmission of HIV infections within health care settings raises controversial issues regarding testing and disclosure. This discussion presents some of the arguments on both sides of these issues.

Nurses need to be very clear about their own values regarding each of these issues and need to find a balance between personal values and professional obligations to patients and families. Through understanding their own beliefs about what is right and wrong, nurses can differentiate between tasks and roles that are consistent with their ethical stance and those that are not, and make responsible practice decisions accordingly. Decisions regarding care are guided by professional ethical codes that include the directives to respect the rights of others and to not abandon patients, yet to practice within the integrity of one's own values and beliefs. If a nurse feels a strong ethical conflict in caring for a particular patient, it is appropriate to ask that the patient be assigned to another nurse. Aligning one's care with the Golden Rule of "do unto others as you would have them do unto you," even when there is disagreement with patient choices, is a good practice.

Abortion

The abortion debate sparks passionate, emotion-laden arguments in political, social, legal, religious, and moral arenas. Issues of self-determination arise regarding the mother's right to control her body and her life (right to choose) in contrast to rights of the unborn fetus to a chance at life (right to life). Those in the right-to-life camp believe that abortion constitutes murder of an unborn person, suggesting that it is a legal as well as an ethical matter. This has raised questions about the role of government in dealing with this ethical concern. Those who hold to the right to choose maintain that the right to privacy regarding health care decisions includes a woman's reproductive choices, implying that governmental regulation is an infringement on this privacy.

Values in relation to life are fundamental considerations in regard to abortion. Such values include beliefs about when life begins, considerations regarding quality of life for children who are unwanted, and concerns about the mother's life and health. Some believe that life starts at conception, while others hold that life begins only when a fetus is viable outside the womb. Discussions regarding viability continue to change as technology enables the survival of babies of lower and lower birth weights, resulting in saving some imperiled newborns of the same gestational age as some aborted fetuses.

Opponents of abortion hold the position that because a fetus possesses humanity, it must be accorded all human rights, including the right to life. Proponents of abortion argue that, based on autonomy, a woman has a right to her own body, and that no woman should be forced to bear a child that she does not want. Because abortion is a situation in which two lives are involved, dilemmas arise regarding who has rights, and whose rights take precedence.

> Some take the position that pregnant women, no matter what the circumstances of conception, have obligations toward the life and well-being of the fetus that overshadow any discussion of the woman's rights. . . . So we have a moral argument, where the stakes are high, in which some people support abortion on demand based on the woman's autonomy. At the same time we have people who oppose abortion perhaps except to save the life of the mother or not at all, based on the sanctity of life principle and the personhood of the fetus. To think in a simple way about this ethical dilemma, on the one hand the fetus is viewed as an object or thing while on the other, the woman is viewed as an object or thing. (Davis & Aroskar, 1991, pp. 130–131)

From either perspective, the consideration of abortion presents a dilemma for those involved.

There is no agreement about the morality of abortion in our society. It is a complex issue with many facets to consider. Although debate generally focuses on areas related to the rights of the woman or the fetus, Mahowald (2000) suggests that it is also important to consider the morality of circumstances that provide fertile ground for abortion. She notes that immoral conditions that sometimes occasion abortion include: poverty, lack of social and medical supports for pregnancy and parenthood, stereotypic views of sex roles and biological parenthood, and a eugenic mentality that welcomes only those babies that meet the parents' desired specifications. She stresses the need for society to direct more effort into rectifying these conditions.

A Broader Look at Reproductive Rights

Roberts (2000) addresses ethical concerns related to reproductive rights that extend beyond abortion to such areas as contraceptive choices, decisions about cesarean sections, and reproductive-assisting technologies. She discusses in particular how race and gender affect the ethics of policies and practices in these areas. She reflects that the early birth control movement in the United States became tied to the **eugenics** movement, which advocated policies encouraging so-called "genetically superior" people to have children, while discouraging so-called "genetically inferior" people from having children—even through forced sterilization. She points to the historical example of the first public birth control clinics in the United States that were established in the South and directed toward poor black women. Another example is a class action lawsuit in Alabama that uncovered that hundreds of thousands of women in the United States, the majority of whom were black, were being coercively sterilized through government welfare programs that conditioned health care and benefits on sterilization. This lawsuit prompted the 1970's federal regulation requiring informed consent and a waiting period before sterilization.

Roberts (2000) suggests that while the abortion debate relates to compulsory motherhood, where women's value is linked to their ability to reproduce, contraceptive policies often devalue poor women and women of color as mothers in that such policies are aimed at preventing these women from having children. She cautions that various societal norms can lead to reproductive regulation of women, and that we need to expand the meaning of reproductive freedom to include the right to have a child—the right to decide to be a mother. She notes that there are as many policies that have sought to deter women from having children as there are those that have sought to force women to have children.

Roberts raises some very important questions regarding the dangers of eugenics in population control, such as deciding that some people are unfit to have children because of their biology or socioeconomic status, and suggesting that reproduction is the cause for social problems. A very important ethical issue that she points out is the racial disparity in reproductive policies and practices. Technologies that help women to have children are more available to white women, in contrast with policies and practices aimed at deterring women from having children that are being targeted toward poor women, particularly women of color. Such policies raise questions about who is valued in society, and how we use reproductive technologies to encourage the birth of certain "valued" children versus those perceived to be of less value. Reproductive policies that flow from such attitudes, she asserts, affect not just individuals, but group status and social structure. Dealing with issues regarding the ethics of reproduction then requires social justice and addressing power relationships in the broader society.

Active Euthanasia

As noted in Chapter 10, technology has caused death to become an unnatural event in the lives of many people. Public dissatisfaction with end-of-life care has prompted efforts to legalize active euthanasia and assisted suicide and has fueled much public debate surrounding these efforts. Because of the concern that health care providers will not adhere to personal wishes regarding end-of-life issues, fears about prolonged suffering resulting from prolongation of dying, and the lack of control that each of these engenders, many people consider the possibility of active euthanasia or assisted suicide. **Active voluntary euthanasia** is an act in which the means of death, such as a lethal dose of medication, is administered by a health professional, family member, or friend. With **assisted suicide** the patients receive the means of death from someone, such as a physician, but activate the process themselves. Justification offered by proponents of these acts include respect for the person's autonomy in choosing to end his or her life if it is deemed intolerable due to conditions of a lingering terminal illness, and compassion exhibited in relief of the patient's suffering. Opponents argue from a stance of the sanctity of life, saying that any such act violates the prohibition against killing human beings. They hold that suffering can almost always be relieved, and they voice concerns about potential abuses, such as involuntary euthanasia to contain health care costs, if such acts were permitted (ANA, 1994; Lo, 2009; Zerwekh, 2006).

It is particularly important to consider the reason for a patient's request for assisted suicide or euthanasia. When the patient indicates that life has become intolerable, we must determine why this is so. Often, inadequate pain management and depression are factors that enter into this perception, which, when treated appropriately, can change the patient's perspective. This may not always be the case, however, and nurses need to be able to support patients and families as they struggle with questions regarding whether natural death is always the best and most loving choice (ANA, 1994, 2010a; Baumrucker et al., 2009; Hayes, 2004; Zerwekh, 2006).

Attending to the nature and cause of a person's suffering and providing comfort care throughout the dying process are important components of the nursing role that may influence choices regarding active voluntary euthanasia or assisted suicide.

Issues Related to HIV/AIDS

We know that human immunodeficiency virus and acquired immunodeficiency syndrome (HIV/AIDS) is a major worldwide health concern, and that the virus is generally contracted through sexual contact. Although most cases of HIV/AIDS have resulted from a choice to have unprotected sexual relations, not all HIV/AIDS results from lifestyle choices. The ANA *Code for Nurses* directs nurses to care for patients regardless of their values or lifestyle; thus, nurses need to be aware of potential judgmental attitudes toward persons with HIV/AIDS, and be alert to how these attitudes may affect the quality of their care.

Because of the risk of exposure to HIV in health care settings, questions arise regarding issues of autonomy and confidentiality in relation to HIV testing and status. One issue relates to whether patients can be required to submit to HIV testing in situations of potential or actual percutaneous exposure of health care workers to their blood. In order to protect persons from potential discrimination, confidentiality of HIV testing and status is generally assured by law. Although prior written consent to HIV testing has been the general norm, revised CDC (2006) guidelines recommend that prevention counseling not be required with HIV testing in busy health care settings due to concern that it can present a barrier due to time constraints. These guidelines also include recommendations to incorporate HIV screening into the general consent for medical care rather than requiring a separate written consent, to do screening on patients ages 13–64 in health care settings after notifying that testing will be performed (unless the patient declines), to test people at high risk for HIV yearly, and to include HIV screening as part of routine prenatal screening (unless the patient declines). Because testing for HIV without the patient's consent violates the patient's autonomy and privacy, the CDC recommendations continue to emphasize voluntary testing.

There are concerns on both sides of the recommendation for separate informed consent. Some argue that not requiring a separate informed consent might lead to some patients being tested without their knowledge. Others argue that removing this requirement eliminates a barrier to HIV testing and opens the possibility for more widespread screening of HIV. The recommendation to screen more routinely for HIV is based on the awareness that nearly one-quarter (about 250,000) of the people living with HIV in the United States do not know they are infected; thus they unknowingly continue to spread the disease. These people could receive counseling and treatment, and their prognosis would be better with earlier diagnosis.

Concerns about potential stigma and discrimination in work or home settings related to having a documented HIV test, regardless of its result, may lead patients to refuse a test even if they are sure it will be negative. Considerations of routine screening of all patients for HIV may reduce this stigma. Newer testing options that use oral fluids or saliva may make routine screening easier and more cost effective. In order to ensure confidentiality and to encourage patient agreement to testing in the event of exposure of a health care worker to a patient's blood, anonymous testing of the patient may be a consideration. Patients may also be more willing to be screened using the oral fluids or the saliva HIV test. Anonymous testing would necessitate paying for the test by a source other than the patient's insurer (such as an employee health fund), recording the results in a location other than the patient's medical record (such as a special occupational health file), and labeling the specimen with a code rather than the patient's name. In this way the health care worker could know if he or she is at risk, while protecting the patient from potential stigma resulting from the test.

Another issue that has become a public concern relates to potential exposure of patients to the blood of a seropositive health care worker. Questions arise whether HIV testing among health care workers, or at least those involved in certain invasive procedures, should be mandatory; whether seropositive health care workers should have restrictions on their practice; and whether the HIV status of health care workers should be made known to patients. Some argue that if it is mandatory for health care workers to be tested, then it should be mandatory for all patients as well. Principles of autonomy, confidentiality, and nonmaleficence become part of this discussion. Health care workers, as well as patients, have a right to autonomy and confidentiality regarding health matters, particularly where discrimination could result from disclosure. At the same time, nonmaleficence directs them to do no harm to patients, and the doctrine of informed consent requires advising patients of potential risks related to interventions being considered. Economic factors enter into the discussion as well. At the present time, presuming health care workers follow universal infection control precautions, the risk of a patient contracting HIV from a seropositive health care worker is low, in contrast to the cost of mandatory testing.

Current issues related to HIV/AIDS may become less of a concern as technology advances toward more effective prevention and treatment of the disease. However, ethical concerns surrounding these issues apply to other health problems of similar nature. Nurses and other health care workers must be aware of any factors in their own health that might put their patients at risk, and take necessary precautions to protect patients from harm. It is also essential that nurses follow universal precautions aimed at protecting themselves and others from harm. If behaviors on the part of health care workers are observed that might put patients at risk, the imperatives of beneficence and nonmaleficence direct nurses to do what is necessary to protect the patient. Actions may include approaching the person involved, reporting the situation to appropriate persons within the agency, and working with groups to institute changes to prevent similar situations from occurring.

Although cases of HIV/AIDS must be reported, as with other infectious diseases, caregivers cannot disclose a person's HIV status without consent. The legal and ethical right to confidentiality regarding HIV/AIDS raises an ethical issue related to protection of others when the infected individual continues behaviors that may expose others to the infection. In some circumstances, physicians are allowed limited disclosure without consent, such as to the patient's spouse. In such situations the imperative of confidentiality must be weighed against the duty to warn others in order to protect them from potential harm. At the present time there are no clear directives in this area for health care providers.

Confidentiality

The imperative of **confidentiality** in health care, which is discussed in Chapter 3, can be traced at least as far back as the Hippocratic vow not to reveal secrets. In order to care for people with health concerns, nurses must be privy to very personal, and sometimes secret, information. Without assurance of confidentiality, many people would not disclose information that is important in diagnosis and treatment of, and caring for, health concerns. This is especially true in situations where there is stigma attached to, or other risks for social repercussions from, the information disclosed. Nurses need to remember that a patient's trust is sacred, and any breach of confidentiality, no matter how small it might seem to the nurse, is a violation of this trust. Special considerations related to privacy and the growing use of electronic methods of storing, transferring, and retrieving personal health information is discussed in Chapter 10. As with so many other areas, there are situations where other factors override confidentiality. In circumstances such as court cases, the law might require disclosure. In situations where secrets entrusted to the nurse suggest potential harm for the patient or others, the duty to warn may take precedence over confidentiality. For example, if a patient tells a nurse about suicide plans that the nurse believes are genuine, and the patient is not willing to be hospitalized, protection of the patient may require the nurse to initiate the process of involuntary hospitalization. In addition to the ethical imperative, confidentiality is also a legal mandate. Nurses must be familiar with and adhere to guidelines of the Health Insurance Portability and Accountability Act (HIPAA), which is discussed in Chapter 3.

SUMMARY

This chapter discusses considerations for nursing practice related to patient self-determination. The concept of self-determination derives from the principle of autonomy, and denotes the right and freedom to make choices about issues that affect one's life. Principles of justice, beneficence, and nonmaleficence may temper the bounds of autonomy in some circumstances. The doctrine of informed consent is both a legal and ethical imperative for protecting a person's right to self-determination in health care decisions. Informed consent implies the right to accept or reject recommended treatment plans. As patient advocates, we need to be alert for situations in which patient autonomy may be limited, or in which there is a lack of sufficient information for the patient or family to make informed decisions. Nurses have a particular responsibility for facilitating informed decision making regarding patient choices for end-of-life care. Nursing's professional code directs nurses to provide services with respect for the rights and dignity of the patient regardless of a person's background or the nature of the health concern. If professional responsibilities expected of a nurse in a patient care situation are inconsistent with the nurse's ethical stance, integrity, and accountability, she should remove herself from that situation after ensuring that there are others to assume care for the patient. A nurse's attention to the many-faceted issues surrounding patient self-determination may be the factor that ensures the patient's involvement in important health care decisions.

CHAPTER HIGHLIGHTS

- Self-determination derives from the principle of autonomy, and implies having freedom to make choices about issues affecting one's life, an ability to make decisions about personal goals, and an appreciation for self in relation to others.

- Autonomy may be threatened by factors such as paternalism; presumptions that a patient's values, knowledge level, and ways of dealing with issues are consistent with those of health care providers; and greater attention to technology than caring. In some situations, principles such as justice or nonmaleficence may temper the bounds of autonomy.

- Decisions about health care require attention to patient values, culture, and beliefs; effects of lifestyle and role; and others who are affected by a patient's choices; as well as evaluation of risks, benefits, and economic considerations.

- Practitioners are not required to honor requests for interventions that are outside accepted standards of care or contrary to the practitioner's ethical views.

- Informed consent provides legal and ethical protection of a patient's right to personal autonomy regarding plans for health care, including the right to refuse interventions and to choose from available alternatives. Information necessary in an informed consent includes: the nature of the concern and prognosis if nothing is done; description of treatment options; and benefits, risks, and consequences of treatment options or nonintervention.

- Decision-making capacity, which is a medical determination and essential for informed consent, includes evidence of the ability to understand information, to communicate understanding and choices, to evaluate decisions in relation to personal values and goals, and to reason and to deliberate. Conscious adults are presumed to have decision-making capacity, unless there is evidence to the contrary.

- Nursing responsibility regarding informed consent includes verifying that the patient is aware of options and the implications of each, and advocating for patients to ensure that criteria for autonomous decision making are met in situations where the physician has not attended to these criteria. Nurses in advanced practice must obtain informed consent for interventions that they initiate within their scope of practice.

- Advance directives, which include living wills and durable powers of attorney, provide instructions regarding health care interventions in the event that one loses decision-making capacity. The PSDA provides legal support for ensuring that patients are informed of their rights regarding health care decisions.

- In dealing with patient lifestyle choices, nurses must remember the instructions in the ANA *Code for Nurses* to provide services with respect for human dignity and to avoid value judgments related to differences in background, customs, attitudes, and beliefs.

- Nurses need to be aware of their own values and beliefs regarding various lifestyle and health care choices, and know how these affect their care with patients.

- Nurses must recognize the patient's right to use complementary therapies, become more knowledgeable about other modalities, and create an atmosphere encouraging of nonjudgmental discussion of such interventions.

- Ethical codes direct nurses to maintain confidentiality regarding patient health status and choices, except in special circumstances in which the "secrets" revealed suggest potential harm for the patient or another.

DISCUSSION QUESTIONS AND ACTIVITIES

1. Discuss your understanding of patient self-determination, including its ethical and legal basis, and nursing practice considerations.

2. Describe dilemmas that nurses may face related to patient self-determination and suggest approaches for dealing with such dilemmas.

3. Explore how nurses in your institution perceive their role regarding informed consent. What dilemmas related to consent have they encountered, and how did they deal with these issues?

4. Analyze your own values regarding abortion and active voluntary euthanasia. How would you respond to a patient under your care who was deliberating such a choice?

5. Explore your state's statutes regarding advance directives, HIV testing and disclosure, euthanasia, assisted suicide, and abortion. What are the implications of these regulations for nursing practice in your state? Advance directive forms for your state can be found at http://www.caringinfo.org/i4a/pages/index.cfm?pageid=1.

6. What are your views on mandatory HIV testing for health care professionals? What about limiting the practice of seropositive health care workers? Review current literature to determine recommendations by professional organizations concerning these issues.

7. Determine how your institution meets requirements of both the PSDA and HIPAA. Discuss the adequacy of each process and nursing's involvement.

8. What is the process for obtaining support and guidance for dealing with ethical concerns and dilemmas in your institution? If there is an ethics committee, how are referrals made? Who is on the committee, and how are members chosen? Talk with a member of an ethics committee, and discuss how that person sees his or her role and the effectiveness of the committee. Review and discuss the ethics committee tools available online at http://www.wvnec.org.

9. Select a case situation in which there are ethical concerns that warrant referral to the ethics committee. With classmates, role-play the

ethics committee discussion, decisions, and actions regarding the case. Explain why you take your position, and how you feel about the outcome.

10. Choose one of the issues discussed in this chapter and explore the websites of the ANA, the CNA, and the ICN regarding policies or positions statements on this issue. Compare and contrast positions of the various organizations. Discuss your views about this issue and how they compare with the positions of the professional organizations.

> ANA—http://www.nursingworld.org
>
> CNA—http://www.cna-nurses.ca
>
> ICN—http://www.icn.ch

Explore the issue as well at http://bioethics.od.nih.gov.

REFERENCES

American Nurses Association. (1994). Position statement on active euthanasia. Retrieved July 19, 2006, from http://www.nursingworld. org/readroom/position/ethics/

American Nurses Association. (2001). *Code of ethics for nurses.* Kansas City, MO: Author.

American Nurses Association. (2010a). Revised position statement: Registered nurses' roles and responsibilities in providing expert care and counseling at the end of life. Retrieved March 12, 2012, from http://nursingworld.org/MainMenuCategories/EthicsStandards/ Ethics-Position-Statements

American Nurses Association. (2010b). Revised position statement: The nurses' role in ethics and human rights: Protecting and promoting individual worth, dignity, and human rights in practice settings. Retrieved March 12, 2012, from http://nursingworld.org/ MainMenuCategories/EthicsStandards/Ethics-Position-Statements

American Nurses Association. (2011, March 11). Revised position statement: Foregoing nutrition and hydration. Retrieved March 12, 2012, from http://nursingworld.org/MainMenuCategories/EthicsStandards/ Ethics-Position-Statements

Baumrucker, S. J., Sheldon, J. E., Stolick, M., Oertli, K. A., Morris, G. M., Harrington, D., & VandeKieft, G. (2009). Comfort care versus euthanasia. *The American Journal of Hospice and Palliative Care, 26*(2), 119–128.

Canadian Nurses Association. (1998, May). Advance directives: The nurse's role. *Ethics in Practice.* Retrieved March 12, 2012, from http://www2.cna-aiic.ca/cna/documents/pdf/publications/Ethics_ Pract_Advance_Directives_May_1998_e.pdf

CDC. (2006). CDC HIV/AIDS Science facts: CDC releases revised HIV testing recommendations in health care settings. Retrieved March 12, 2012 from http://www.cdc.gov/hiv/topics/testing/resources/factsheets/ healthcare.htm

Curtin, L. (1982). Autonomy, accountability, and nursing practice. *Topics in Clinical Nursing, 4,* 7–14.

Davis, A. J., & Aroskar, M. A. (1991). *Ethical dilemmas and nursing practice* (3rd ed.). Norwalk, CT: Appleton & Lange.

Dunn, H. (2005). *Hard choices for loving people* (4th ed.). Herndon, VA: A & A Publishers.

Geppert, C. M., Andrews, M. R., & Druyan, M. E. (2010). Ethical issues in artificial nutrition and hydration: A review. *Journal of Parenteral and Enteral Nutrition, 34*(1), 79–88.

Hardwig, J. (2000). What about the family? In J. H. Howell & W. F. Sale (Eds.), *Life choices: A Hastings Center introduction to bioethics* (2nd ed., pp. 145–159). Washington, DC: Georgetown University Press.

Hayes, C. (2004). Ethics in end-of-life care. *Journal of Hospice and Palliative Nursing, 6*(1), 36–43.

Husted, G., & Husted, J. (2001). *Ethical decision making in nursing* (3rd ed.). New York: Springer.

Leever, M. G. (2011). Cultural competence: Reflections on patient autonomy and patient good. *Nursing Ethics, 18*(4), 560–570.

Levi, B. H., & Green, M. J. (2010). Too soon to give up: Re-examining the value of advance directives. *American Journal of Bioethics, 10*(4), 3–22.

Lo, B. (2009). *Resolving ethical dilemmas: A guide for clinicians* (4th ed.). Philadelphia: Lippincott Williams & Wilkins.

Mahowald, M. B. (2000). Is there life after *Roe v. Wade?* In J. H. Howell & W. F. Sale (Eds.), *Life choices: A Hastings Center introduction to bioethics* (2nd ed., pp. 188–203). Washington, DC: Georgetown University Press.

Petersen, C. (2010). Clinical issues: Responsibility for obtaining the surgical informed consent. *AORN Journal, 92*(5), 585–586.

Plawecki, L. H., & Plawecki, H. M. (2009). Simply stated: Obtaining informed consent can be a very complex task. *Journal of Gerontological Nursing, 35*(2), 3–4.

Quill, T. E. (2005). Terri Schiavo—A tragedy compounded. *New England Journal of Medicine, 352*(16), 1630–1633.

Roberts, D. (2000). Race, gender, justice, and reproductive health policy. Presentation at New Century, New Challenges: Intensive Bioethics Course XXVI. Kennedy Institute of Ethics, Georgetown University, Washington, DC.

Rodriguez, K. L., & Young, A. J. (2006). Patients' and healthcare providers' understandings of life-sustaining treatment: Are perceptions of goals shared or divergent? *Social Science and Medicine, 62*(1), 125–133.

Sakalys, J. A. (2010). Patient autonomy: patient voices and perspectives in illness narratives. *International Journal for Human Caring, 14*(1), 15–20.

Salgo v. Leland Stanford, Jr. (1957). 317 P. 2d 170 (Cal. Dis. Ct. App; 1951).

Schloendorff v. The Society of New York Hospital. (1914). 211 NY125, 105 N.E. 92 (1914).

Slater v. Baker & Stapleton. (1767). High Court of Justice, King's Bench Division. English Reports (Vol. 95, pp. 860–863).

Tuma v. Board of Nursing of the State of Idaho. (1979). 593 P 2d 711 (1979).

West Virginia Health Care Decisions Act. (2002/2007). Retrieved March 12, 2012, from http://www.wvendoflife.org/MediaLibraries/WVCEOLC/Media/laws/WV_HCDA_3-13-07.pdf

Will, J. F. (2011). A brief historical and theoretical perspective on patient autonomy and medical decision making: Part II: The autonomy model. *Chest, 139*(6), 1491–1497.

Williams, L. S. (2006). Feeding patients after stroke: Who, when, and how. *Annals of Internal Medicine, 144*(59–60).

Zerwekh, J. V. (2006). *Nursing care at the end of life: Palliative care for patients and families*. Philadelphia: F.A. Davis.

Chapter

12

SCHOLARSHIP ISSUES

My experience tells me that people instinctively trust those whose personality is founded upon correct principles.

(Covey, 1992, p. 18)

OBJECTIVES

After completing this chapter, the reader should be able to:

1. Describe scholarship issues encountered by nurses in academic and clinical settings.

2. Discuss principles basic to academic honesty and the ethical treatment of research data.

3. Describe principles and nursing standards undergirding the protection of human rights in research.

4. Explain why informed consent is mandated for research involving human subjects, and describe the elements required for this consent.

5. Discuss the nursing role regarding protection of human rights in research.

6. Describe principles guiding personal response to dilemmas regarding nursing scholarship.

INTRODUCTION

Scholarship issues face students, teachers, researchers, and clinicians from the moment a person enters a nursing program and throughout that person's professional career. This chapter discusses principles that undergird ethical behavior in academic matters, in conducting research, and in the treatment of data both during the research process and in presentations or publication. Respect for all persons, including ourselves, is basic to ethical behavior regarding scholarship. Personal values affect how we approach situations that present ethical dilemmas. It is essential that nurses be knowledgeable about principles guiding ethical conduct, whether dealing with academic assignments, research data, or research with human subjects.

ACADEMIC HONESTY

Integrity in upholding the principles of veracity and fidelity is expected of nurses in any setting and is at the core of academic honesty. Veracity refers to truth telling, which is an essential ingredient for trust among humans. True interaction and communication cannot occur where there is no trust (Husted & Husted, 2007). These authors describe fidelity as promise keeping, suggesting that it is the form that truth takes in an agreement between persons, such as nurse-patient, researcher-participant, or student-teacher. Integrity implies respect for self and others, and a personal commitment to principled behavior over time in our personal and professional lives. When integrity is present, there is no need for monitoring a person's behavior; rather, there is an implicit trust that we represent ourselves in a truthful way. Honesty and integrity are key considerations in both academic and clinical situations. Personal values such as honesty serve as the basis for professional integrity.

Students at all levels face many stresses in regard to academic performance, and nursing students are no exception. Pressures may come from many areas, such as family expectations, personal goals of being accepted into graduate school, needing a certain grade to receive tuition reimbursement, or self-expectations that say "I always get good grades." When pressures become intense, values such as honesty and integrity may become challenged.

Academic institutions provide written policies that address issues of academic honesty. These issues include plagiarism, cheating, and forgery. **Plagiarism** is taking another's ideas or work and presenting them as our own. Examples include submitting written, oral, or visual materials (such as a paper, a report, PowerPoint slides, a speech, or a thesis) that have been knowingly copied or obtained, in whole or in part, from another's work without appropriate acknowledgment. This includes materials found on the Internet such as portions of books, journal articles, or content from websites. The Office of Research Integrity (ORI) of the U.S. Department of Health and Human Services offers a free module on ethical writing that includes guidelines for avoiding plagiarism. Students are encouraged to review these guidelines, found on the ORI website (http://ori.hhs .gov/avoiding-plagiarism-self-plagiarism-and-other-questionable-writing-practices-guide-ethical-writing). **Cheating** refers to dishonesty and deception regarding examinations, projects, presentations, or papers. Examples include receiving help from or giving help to another student during an exam, allowing another to copy our work, doing work for another student that is to be submitted by that student, or unauthorized use of notes or other materials (including electronic devices) during an exam. The academic policy regarding use of (and restrictions on) handheld electronic devices in both class and clinical settings may vary in different academic settings, and students are advised to be familiar with the policy at their school. **Forgery** includes fraud or intentional misrepresentation—for example, altering or causing a grade to be altered in an academic record or presenting false data on admission records.

Implicit in academic honesty is a trust that work submitted by a student, whether papers, projects, presentations, or exams, is indeed that of the student. When material from another source is included in a student's work, the student must appropriately reference the material to avoid plagiarism. Academic dishonesty engenders an atmosphere of mistrust, disrespect, and insecurity. The breach of trust and potential consequences within a student-teacher relationship that academic dishonesty creates are self-evident. Litigation is another potential consequence in severe situations. Because of the value of honesty, academic dishonesty may carry consequences as serious as the student's being suspended, failed, or expelled for dishonest practices.

ASK YOURSELF

What Are Your Perspectives on Academic Honesty?

- One of your closest friends is in a different section of the same course, and his section meets 2 days after yours. You know he has been very stressed because of his mother's illness and the fact that he needs good grades to keep his scholarship. You have just taken the midterm exam, and he asks you to give him an idea of the topics covered so he can focus his studying. What would you do? How do you feel in this situation? What principles would guide your decisions?

- During an exam you notice two students passing what appear to be notes between them. You also notice another student texting on her cell phone. You are fairly sure that the instructor has not seen these activities. How do you feel in response to these situations? What would you do, and why?

- You are struggling with an assignment that is due in just a few days. A classmate says she has a paper that her cousin did for this same course 3 years ago that she is using as a guide, changing the text so that it seems like her own writing. She offers to let you see her cousin's paper to do the same. What do you think about her plan? How would you respond? What would guide your decision?

Case Presentation

Suspicions of Dishonesty

Sabrina and Jude have been close friends and study partners throughout their nursing program. They discuss their readings and class notes and frequently choose the same topic, sharing articles between them when writing papers. After a recent submission of papers, the instructor called them in and noted that their papers were almost identical, including mistakes in grammar, and said that it appeared that one had copied the other's paper. They each denied copying from the other.

Think About It

Considering Consequences for Academic Dishonesty

- *What ethical issues are involved in this situation?*
- *How do you feel about incidences of academic dishonesty?*
- *How do you think this situation should be handled? What consequences would you consider?*
- *In light of the standards that guide nursing practice, what is your position on allowing a student who has violated academic honesty through plagiarism, cheating, or forgery to continue in a nursing program?*

RESEARCH ISSUES AND ETHICS

Nurses must be accountable for the quality of care they deliver, and research is one way of documenting the efficacy of nursing practice. Both the art and science of nursing are expanded through research. Research is necessary for the ongoing development of the unique body of knowledge that undergirds the discipline of nursing, and provides an organizing framework for nursing practice.

Participating in research can be exciting and encourage professional growth. It can also present some dilemmas for the nurse and nurse researcher in the academic and clinical realms. Seeking new knowledge and understanding is the expected motivation for conducting research. However, personal or institutional gains related to rewards such as grant funds, prestige, the need to succeed, or promoting a product can be other motivating factors that may challenge principled behavior in regard to research.

A nurse who works in clinical areas where research is being conducted must be aware of principles for the conduct of research, regardless of whether the nurse has an active role with the research project. In this regard, guidelines from the American Nurses Association (ANA) state:

> A relationship of trust between nurse and patient has always been an essential element of the professional code of ethics. In research, a relationship of trust between subject and investigator requires that the investigator assume special obligations to safeguard the subject.... The individual has the right of self-determination concerning what will be done to his person. Each practitioner of nursing has an obligation to endorse and support self-determination as a moral and legal right of the individual. The responsibilities of safeguarding the rights of others must be fully accepted by nurses whether their roles are as practitioners, educators, or researchers. (1985, p. 3)

Ethical Issues in Research

Many research texts focus their discussions of ethical issues in research primarily on protection of human rights. This emphasis is understandable because of violations that have occurred. The most cited violations of human rights in research are those that were perpetrated by the Nazis during World War II and that came to public awareness during the Nuremberg trials. International efforts to provide guidelines for protection of human rights have been documented in the **Nuremberg Code** and the **Declaration of Helsinki**. The Nuremberg Code was developed as a set of principles for the ethical conduct of research against which the experiments in the Nazi concentration camps could be judged. The Declaration of Helsinki was issued by the World Medical Assembly in 1964 to guide clinical research and was revised in 1975 and in 2008. Included in the **Belmont Report**, the principles set forth in these codes serve as the basis for policies developed by the United States National Commission for the Protection of Human Subjects of Biomedical and Behavioral Research (1979).

In spite of these policies and guidelines, ethical lapses continue to occur in research with human subjects (Lafleur, Bohme, & Shimazono, 2007; Shrader-Frechette, 2007; Wynia & Boren, 2009). Ongoing concerns prompt questions about whether current regulations adequately protect the rights and welfare of research subjects. In order to oversee and enforce federal regulations pertaining to research with human subjects, the U.S. Department of Health and Human Services formed an Office for Human Research Protection. Efforts to bolster protections for human research subjects focus on education and training of clinical investigators and institutional review board members; auditing records for evidence of compliance with informed consent; improved monitoring of clinical trials; managing conflicts of interest so that research subjects are appropriately informed; and imposing monetary penalties for violations of important research practices, such as informed consent (U.S. Department of Health and Human Services, 2012).

Principles of beneficence, respect for human dignity, and justice underlie the ethical conduct of research (ANA, 1985; Childress, Meslin, & Shapiro, 2005; United States National Commission for the Protection of Human Subjects of Biomedical and Behavioral Research, 1979). The principle of **beneficence** implies the right to protection from harm and discomfort, including a balance between the benefits and risks of a study. The principle of **respect for human dignity** implies the rights to full disclosure and self-determination or autonomy. The principle of **justice** implies the rights of fair treatment and privacy, including anonymity and confidentiality. A brief discussion of each principle follows. The ANA guidelines for the protection of human rights are summarized in Figure 12–1.

Beneficence

This principle derives from the maxim that says "above all, do no harm." In research situations this means that researchers need to design and conduct studies so as to protect the participants from physical, mental, emotional, spiritual, economic, and social harm. Discomfort can range from no anticipated effects to certainty of permanent damage, and includes such things as fatigue, physical pain, anxiety, embarrassment, confronting meaning and purpose in life, threats to self-esteem or to values, lost earnings for time given to participate in research, and social stigma (Burns & Groves, 2009). If discomfort is anticipated as part of the research protocol, the participant must be willing to experience the discomfort after being given all relevant information, and the risk for harm must be balanced with anticipated benefits. In general, a minimal risk is that which is no more than would be expected within the context of routine life activities. When risks are greater than minimal, the researcher's aim must be to minimize risks while maximizing the benefits to participants. Since our role as nurses impels us to

---

Right to Freedom from Intrinsic Risk of Injury

- When an individual participating in research is exposed to increased risk for social, emotional, or physical injury, the investigator must specify the degree of risk and estimate how the risk to the individual compares to the benefit to humanity through knowledge gained.

- All relevant information concerning activities that go beyond established and accepted procedures for meeting personal needs must be given to a prospective participant prior to that person's participation in the study.

- Nurses must be vigilant in their concern for persons who are unable to effectively protect themselves from harm or injury due to illness or other condition and be aware of potentials for exploiting captive populations, such as persons in institutions, students, or prisoners.

Right to Privacy

- Since an investigator cannot decide for another person what is considered an invasion of privacy for that person, all proposals, protocols, investigative instruments, and procedures to be used in research activities must be specified and discussed with the prospective participant.

- The above must be discussed as well with any workers who are expected to take part in the research as data gatherers or research participants.

Right to Anonymity

- There must be safeguards against unanticipated physical, psychological, or social disadvantages occurring to participants because of their role in the research, either during the study or from dissemination of findings.

- Assurance that a participant's anonymity will be protected must be provided when the participant agrees to share personal information that might not be divulged to others in another context.

- When collected data is not to remain under the control of the investigator, mechanisms for protecting the identity of the participant and safeguarding confidentiality must be established.

- When the plan of the study or the report of the findings will sacrifice the participant's anonymity or confidentiality, specific prior consent must be obtained.

- Potential violations of human dignity from demeaning or dehumanizing situations in the research protocol require special consideration, recognizing that such violations can have long-range repercussions when significant values of the individual are involved.

Adapted from American Nurses Association. (1985). *Human rights guidelines for nurses in clinical and other research* (p. 67). Kansas City, MO: Author.

FIGURE 12–1   Protection of Human Rights

protect those in our care from unnecessary physical or mental suffering, if the risks of research outweigh the benefits, the study should be redesigned or discontinued. A well-publicized example of this occurred with the National Institutes of Health, Women's Health Initiative (WHI) study. When preliminary findings of the study indicated that long-term use of hormone replacement therapy (HRT) was associated with increased health risks among the participants, the HRT arm of the WHI study was discontinued.

Respect for Human Dignity

Implicit in this principle is the right to self-determination, which acknowledges the autonomy of the potential participant in research. This means that persons have the right to choose whether they wish to participate in the research; that is, participation is voluntary and free from coercion of any type. **Coercion** includes threat of harm or penalty for not participating in the research, or offering excessive rewards for participation. The right of self-determination means that the person has the right to withdraw from participation in the study at any time without imposed consequences, such as denial of health care or benefits. Voluntary participation requires **full disclosure**, that is, that the potential participant be fully informed of the nature of the study, the anticipated risks and benefits, time commitment, what is expected of the participant and the researcher, and the right to refuse to participate. This is addressed through the process of informed consent, which is discussed later.

Justice

The principle of justice includes the rights to privacy and to fair treatment. The nature of research is to gather information about that which is being studied. When persons are the focus of study, the **right to privacy** is a critical issue. Attentiveness to privacy means the participant determines when, where, and what kind of information is shared, with an assurance that information, attitudes, behaviors, records, opinions, and the like that are observed or collected will be treated with respect, kept secure, and kept in strict confidence. Privacy is maintained through anonymity, confidentiality, and informed consent. Because the concept of privacy may vary in different cultures, the kinds of information participants feel comfortable in allowing to be shared may also vary (Calloway, 2009; DuBois, 2004; Monshi & Zieglmayer, 2004). If even the researcher cannot link information with a particular participant, then **anonymity** exists. **Confidentiality** refers to the researcher's assurance to participants that information provided will not be made public or available to anyone other than those involved in the research process without the participant's consent. Confidentiality is maintained by using codes rather than personal identification on data collection forms and restricting access to raw data to those on the research team who need to use the data.

The **right to fair treatment** is related to the right to self-determination. Equitable treatment of participants in the selection process, during the study, and after the completion of the study is the foundation of this right. Factors to consider in fair treatment include the following:

- Selecting participants based on the research needs, not on the convenience or compromised position of a group of people

- Equitably distributing the risks and benefits of the research among participants, regardless of age, gender, socioeconomic status, race, or ethnic background

- Honoring any agreements made or benefits promised

- Treating participants with respect, providing access to research personnel or other professionals as needed

- Treating persons who decline to participate or withdraw from the study without prejudice

- Debriefing as needed to clarify issues or when information had been withheld prior to the study

Case Presentation

Protecting Patients Who Are Research Subjects

Annissa, a nurse in a primary care clinic, talked with her coworker, Bill, about his non-nursing graduate program. Bill said he plans to study the emotional attitudes of patients using a standardized instrument for his required research project. When Annissa asked about recruiting participants, he said he will have all his patients complete the instrument when he sees them for routine visits over the next few weeks. In response to Annissa's questions about the possibility of patients not wanting to participate, Bill said that he will just tell them it is for a student project, and he is sure they will fill out the form to help him out and keep on his good side. Annissa asked which institutional review board (IRB) reviewed his proposal, and Bill replied that his school does not have an IRB, so only his advisor had to give approval.

Think About It

What Principles Guide Ethical Conduct of Clinical Research?

- *What principles are involved in this situation?*
- *What dilemmas may arise with Bill's research project?*
- *What are Annissa's ethical responsibilities in this situation?*
- *What is the responsibility of the primary care agency related to research conducted within the agency?*

Informed Consent

As noted previously, voluntary participation in a research study requires full disclosure. Informing potential participants of the research purpose, expected commitment, risks and benefits, any invasion of privacy, and ways that anonymity and confidentiality will be addressed are included in the process of **informed consent**. The researcher must ensure that the person who is agreeing to participate in the study understands the information included in the consent and has a chance to receive clarifications and additional information when needed. Printed consent forms should be written in common language without jargon. Since literacy level affects how people understand both written and verbal instructions and documents, researchers need to assess and document the literacy level of the person signing the informed consent. Additionally, the person agreeing to participate in the research must be mentally and emotionally competent to make the decision.

Munhall (2012) suggest that the process of informed consent provides a way of including the person as a collaborator in the research rather than as a mere "subject." We must, however, guard against the element of coercion. One review of nursing research protocols found more ethical concerns arising from the relationship between the researcher and study participant than from physical harm (Olsen & Mahrenholz, 2000). When the nurse who cares for the patient is on the research team and is the one obtaining the informed consent, determining whether the patient is giving consent to the "nurse" or to the "researcher" can be somewhat tricky. The nurse-researcher must determine whether the patient truly feels the freedom to refuse to participate.

The Code of Federal Regulations (2009) lists basic elements that need to be included in informed consent:

1. A statement that the study involves research, an explanation of the purpose of the research and the expected duration of the subject's participation, a description of the procedures to be followed, and identification of any procedures that are experimental.

2. A description of any reasonably foreseeable risks or discomforts to the participant.

3. A description of any benefits to the participant or to others that may reasonably be expected from the research.

4. A disclosure of appropriate alternative procedures or courses of treatment, if any, that might be advantageous to the subject.

5. A statement describing the extent, if any, to which confidentiality of records identifying the subject will be maintained.

6. For research involving more than minimal risk, an explanation as to whether any compensation and an explanation as to whether medical treatments are available if injury occurs and, if so, what they consist of, or where further information may be obtained.

7. An explanation of whom to contact for answers to pertinent questions about the research and research subjects' rights, and whom to contact in the event of a research-related injury to the subject.

8. A statement that participation is voluntary, that refusal to participate will involve no penalty or loss of benefits to which the subject is otherwise entitled, and that the subject may discontinue participation at any time without penalty or loss of benefits to which the subject is otherwise entitled.

Nurses who are assisting with research or who work on units where research is being conducted must be familiar with these elements of informed consent. If consent forms do not contain these elements, nurses should bring this to the attention of the investigators or the institution's ethics committee. Nurses also need to be familiar with the Health Insurance Portability and Accountability Act (HIPAA) policies and guidelines of the institutions in which they work. HIPAA requires institutions to establish procedures for handling individually identifiable patient health information (PHI) for all areas of patient contact. The goal of these procedures is to protect privacy and ensure confidentiality regarding PHI. HIPAA regulations may add additional privacy protection for patients regarding their participating in a research study and researcher access to protected health information necessary for a research study. The written, signed authorization from research participants to use PHI for research purposes must include the purpose for which the PHI will be used, what PHI will be disclosed, who will have access to the PHI, and the right of the participant to review the PHI that is recorded for research (Arford, 2004; Erlen, 2005).

Special Considerations: Vulnerable Populations

Nurses must be especially attentive to protection of human rights in research with vulnerable populations. These populations include persons with physical, mental, or emotional disabilities or challenges; children or elderly persons; those who are dying, sedated, or unconscious; persons who are institutionalized or incarcerated; pregnant women; and fetuses. Because people in these populations are vulnerable to deception and coercion, and may have decreased ability to give informed consent, advocates or guardians who have the person's best interest in mind must be involved in decisions regarding their participation in research. In both research and

Case Presentation

Nurses, Research, and Informed Consent

Juan, a registered nurse, works in a small rural hospital clinic that has a strong commitment to the under-served population in its area. The hospital has been struggling financially because of the large number of indigent patients and recent federal cutback of funding for health services. There has been talk of possibly eliminating some positions because of the financial crisis. In a recent staff meeting he learned that a pharmaceutical company has negotiated an agreement with the physicians to use a new medication with their hypertensive patients, and to gather data about side effects of this medication. A sizable financial reimbursement for the hospital is part of the agreement. As the RN, Juan will be responsible for checking patients' blood pressures and completing the side effect surveys. Juan asks about informed consent and is told that the pharmaceutical company said it is not needed because this medication has been through the clinical trials already. Juan does not feel comfortable about participating in the project, but recognizes that the money is needed by the hospital and, in fact, may make the difference in avoiding elimination of staff positions.

Think About It

Decisions About Participating in Research

- *What issues do you identify in this case situation?*
- *What ethical principles are being violated or potentially violated?*
- *What ethical dilemmas do you think Juan is experiencing?*
- *What do you think Juan should do, and why?*
- *How might potential consequences affect the decision-making process?*

clinical care, the less able the person is to give informed consent, the more important it is for nurses to advocate for the person, assuring that rights are protected. Guidelines for research involving children age 7 to 18 provide one example of special considerations regarding consent, which is obtaining the **assent** of the child to participate in a research study in addition to the consent of the parents or guardians. The principle of respect for persons acknowledges that persons, to the degree that they are capable, have the right to choose what will or will not happen to them. In accordance with this principle, U.S. federal guidelines direct researchers to inform children of any intended research activity, even if the parents or guardians have already agreed to the child's participation in a research study. This process of obtaining the child's *assent* includes describing, in language appropriate for the age and competence of the child, the purpose of the research and providing an explanation of the risks and benefits associated with the child's participation in the research. Younger children are asked to assent orally to participate in the proposed research, while older children may be asked to sign an assent form or the parent permission form indicating their willingness to participate in the study. Assent needs to be documented in the research protocol. Nurses who work with these populations need to be especially aware of their roles as advocates, particularly when research is proposed or being conducted in their settings.

More Than Protection of Human Rights

Although protection of human subjects is a very important consideration in nursing research, other issues deserve equal attention. Characteristics of ethical research that go beyond the protection of human rights, discussed by Wilson (1999), are still applicable. These include:

Scientific objectivity—reporting all data, both supportive and unsupportive of hypotheses, and not engaging in misconduct, fraud, or acts of bad faith;

Cooperation—submitting proposals to and following recommendations of those authorized to review the research for protection of human rights;

Nobility—working actively to ensure protection of participants from harm, deceit, coercion, and invasions of privacy, even when this may inconvenience the study;

Integrity and truthfulness—honestly describing the research process, including the purpose, procedures, methods, risks, discomforts, benefits, and findings;

Impeccability—ensuring anonymity and confidentiality of data and using discretion with information learned about people;

Illumination—publishing and presenting research findings in order to enhance nursing's body of scientific knowledge;

Equitability—noting contributions of others in publications and presentations;

Forthrightness—disclosing funding sources and sponsorship in publication and presentation of research findings; and

Courage—being willing to request public clarification of apparent distortions of research findings made by others.

When nurses are working in agencies or institutions where research is being conducted, whether or not they are directly involved in the research, they must be aware of standards for ethical research in order to guard against violations of these standards.

Nurses who participate in conducting research may at times experience role conflict. A nurse is held to standards of professional practice that delineate the nurse's concern as safeguarding the health and well-being of the patient. A researcher is focused on processes and outcomes of a study in which patients may be used as sources of data. Nurse researchers need to incorporate humanistic values in decisions regarding research participants. When questions arise regarding potential harm to a patient involved in a research study, the advocacy role of the nurse and the therapeutic imperative takes precedence over the integrity of the research protocol (Munhall, 2012). Ignorance of ethical and legal guidelines related to research is no excuse for a nurse failing to be a patient advocate in research situations. Although research is necessary for development of scientific and therapeutic knowledge, a balance between principles guiding scientific inquiry and those guiding nursing practice must be maintained.

When nurses are employed, particularly in institutions that are research focused, they need to clarify what is expected of them in regard to research. Nurses should know prior to accepting a position whether they will be required to gather data or administer treatments as part of research protocols, and whether such treatments may have potential risks to patients. Nurses in such settings need to know whether their positions will be jeopardized if they refuse participate as part of a research team. When participation in research is expected as part of a nurse's job, the nurse must know the protocol, whether it has been approved by the IRB, and whom to consult with any concerns about the research process and effect on patients.

ASK YOURSELF

What Takes Precedence—Research or Nursing Care?

Questions that Fowler (1988, p. 354) posed over 20 years ago continue to be worth pondering:

- Is the good of the patient ever subservient to the acquisition of nursing knowledge?
- Does the therapeutic imperative of clinical care and the good of the patient always preempt the mandate to enlarge the nursing profession's body of knowledge?
- At what point must a nurse stop a specific nursing research project?
- When must a nurse intervene to halt a specific medical research project?
- Are there conditions under which a nurse should not include a specific subject in a study, even though consent has been secured?

Ethical Treatment of Data

Scholarship issues regarding data include how the data is handled during the collection and analysis process and how the data is reported. **Ethical treatment of data** implies integrity of research protocols and honesty in reporting findings. The honesty and integrity of the researcher are of utmost importance in the ethical treatment of data. Taking care to ensure that only those who are involved in the research process have access to the data and to maintain confidentiality were mentioned previously. A critical ethical obligation of qualitative nursing researchers is to present and describe the experiences of others as authentically and faithfully as possible, even when it is contrary to our own aims (Munhall, 2012). The imperative to report the findings as accurately as possible is an ethical obligation in quantitative studies as well.

Nurses involved in research are accountable to professional standards for reporting findings. Principles that guide academic honesty apply as well to nurse researchers in reporting outcomes of studies. It is dishonest to exaggerate results, withhold negative findings, or adjust facts of a study in order to maximize or minimize particular outcomes or hypotheses. When information from someone else is included in a report without appropriate referencing, this is plagiarism. Scientific misconduct continues to be a concern within the scientific community. Articles have been published in professional journals reporting studies that were never conducted, findings that were fabricated, or findings that were intentionally distorted by researchers (Horner & Minifie, 2011; Karcz & Papadakos, 2011; Nylenna & Simonsen, 2006; Schnoor, 2006). Although these reports have related more to biomedical studies than to nursing research, such reports present problems to disciplines whose clinical practice may be changed based on research findings. They also serve as reminders to nurses to be vigilant regarding ethical reporting of research findings.

Case Presentation

Ethical Issues in Handling Research Data

A classmate and good friend is in the process of doing a research project required for graduation. You know she is frustrated because the surveys she sent out are not being returned, and the project needs to be completed soon if she is to graduate on time. She also needs to do well on this project in order to graduate with honors. In order to have a large enough sample, she tells you that she is going to fill in several forms herself and asks if you will do some for her too, noting that several other friends have already completed forms. She says that, after all, the object of the assignment is to see if one can collect and analyze the data. You are also aware that the best studies will be published in the student nursing newsletter.

Think About It

Honesty in Nursing Research

- *What is your reaction to her plan and request?*

- *Discuss the ethical issues involved in this scenario.*

- *Describe the appropriate ethical stance in this situation. What factors would enable or mitigate to prevent you from taking this stance?*

- *What would you do with this information, and what principles would guide your actions?*

ASK YOURSELF

Consequences of Reporting Fraudulent Research

Pause and think about the havoc rendered by publication of fraudulent research.

- How might this affect how others view the integrity of the profession?

- How might this affect a reader's response to other research published in the same journal?

- How would this affect your ability as a nurse to determine whether you should adjust your practice based on reported research?

- Imagine that you have just read the report of a research project for which you gathered data and discovered that the process described was quite a bit different from what you had done, making the results take on a different meaning. How would you react and what would you do?

SUMMARY

Nurses are expected to exhibit principled behavior in all situations. This chapter has focused on principles related to scholarship issues facing nurses. Decisions related to academic honesty face nursing students before they ever encounter a patient. Because personal values affect professional behavior, choices made in the academic arena concerning actions such as plagiarism, cheating, or forgery may foreshadow values used to guide future professional decisions. Nurses must be familiar with principles guiding ethical practices in research and reporting of research findings. These principles guide nursing decisions about research protocols, participation, and advocacy for patients related to research issues. Ethical practices regarding scholarship are essential to the integrity of both the professional and the profession.

CHAPTER HIGHLIGHTS

- Principles of veracity and integrity are core to academic honesty and to ethical treatment of research data.

- Nursing research and researchers must adhere to nursing standards regarding the ethical conduct of research that affirm a participant's right to freedom from intrinsic risk of injury, right to privacy, and right to anonymity.

- Protection of human rights, a prime focus of research ethics, is based on principles of beneficence, respect for human dignity, and justice. These principles imply protection from physical, emotional, spiritual, economic, and social harm; voluntary participation in research; and assurance of privacy and equitable treatment of all research participants.

- Informed consent for research studies, which helps to ensure that a participant's rights are protected, must include the elements contained in the Code of Federal Regulations.

- When there is a question of potential harm to a patient involved in a research study, the nurse's advocacy role and the therapeutic imperative take precedence over the integrity of the research protocol. Nurses need to be especially attentive to protection of the rights of vulnerable groups in clinical and research settings.

- When considering employment, nurses should clarify expectations regarding potential participation in research.

DISCUSSION QUESTIONS AND ACTIVITIES

1. Review your school's policy regarding academic honesty, and discuss ethical principles that are violated in cases of academic dishonesty. Explore issues and policies related to academic honesty at the following websites:

    http://ori.hhs.gov/avoiding-plagiarism-self-plagiarism-and-other-questionable-writing-practices-guide-ethical-writing

    http://library.camden.rutgers.edu/EducationalModule/Plagiarism

    http://www.ryerson.ca/academicintegrity

2. Describe factors that persons reviewing cases of academic dishonesty should consider.

3. How did protection of human rights come to be required for research involving human subjects? Explore the following websites

for information about the Belmont Report and the Declaration of Helsinki:

> Belmont Report—
> http://www.hhs.gov/ohrp/humansubjects/guidance/belmont.html
>
> Declaration of Helsinki—
> http://www.wma.net/en/30publications/10policies/b3/world medical association

4. What guidance do nursing standards offer nurses who are participating in or conducting research? What principles underlie the ethical conduct of research? Discuss nursing roles related to these principles and standards.

5. Interview a nurse-researcher regarding how human rights are protected in the study. Have all the required elements been included in the informed consent?

6. Give examples of situations in which the nursing role of patient advocate and the role of researcher might be in conflict. Which role takes precedence and why?

7. Discuss potential effects of fraud and deceit in medical or nursing research on patient care.

8. Compare and contrast what the ANA (www.ana.org), the Canadian Nurses Association (www.cna-nurses.ca), and the International Council of Nurses (www.icn.ch) say about human rights in research and in nursing practice.

9. Explore one or more of the following websites and report back to the class what you discovered about informed consent and protection of human rights in research.

> Regulations and Ethical Guidelines—
> http://www.hhs.gov/ohrp/humansubjects/guidance/belmont .html#xinform
>
> Office of Human Research Protection—
> http://www.hhs.gov/ohrp
>
> Code of Federal Regulations—
> http://www.hhs.gov/ohrp/humansubjects/guidance/45cfr46 .html#46.116
>
> U.S. Department of Education—
> http://www2.ed.gov/about/offices/list/ocfo/humansub.html
>
> Alliance for Human Research Protection—
> http://www.ahrp.org
>
> HIPAA regulations—
> http://privacyruleandresearch.nih.gov/pr_02.asp

REFERENCES

American Nurses Association. (1985). *Human rights guidelines for nurses in clinical and other research.* Kansas City, MO: Author.

Arford, P. H. (2004). Working with human research protections. *Journal of Nursing Scholarship, 36*(3), 265–271.

Burns, N., & Groves, S. K. (2009). *The practice of nursing research* (6th ed.). St. Louis, MO: WB Saunders.

Calloway, S. J. (2009). The effect of culture on beliefs related to autonomy and informed consent. *Journal of Cultural Diversity, 16*(2), 68–70.

Childress, J., Meslin, E., & Shapiro, H. (Eds.). (2005). *Belmont revisited: Ethical principles for research with human subjects.* Washington, DC: Georgetown University Press.

Code of Federal Regulations. (2009). Title 45, Part 46. Retrieved February 17, 2012, from http://www.hhs.gov/ohrp/humansubjects/guidance/45cfr46.html#46.116

Covey, S. R. (1992). *Principle-centered leadership.* New York: Fireside.

DuBois, J. M. (2004). Universal ethical principles in a diverse universe: A commentary on Monshi and Zieglmayer's case study. *Ethics & Behavior, 14*(4), 313–319.

Erlen, J. A. (2005). HIPAA—Implications for research. *Orthopaedic Nursing, 224*(2), 139–142.

Fowler, M. D. M. (1988). Ethical issues in nursing research: A call for an international code of ethics for nursing. *Western Journal of Nursing Research, 10,* 352–355.

Horner, J., & Minifie, F. D. (2011). Research ethics III: Publication practices and authorship, conflicts of interest, and research misconduct. *Journal of Speech, Language & Hearing Research, 54*(1), 346–362.

Husted, G. L., & Husted, J. H. (2007). *Ethical decision making in nursing and health care* (4th ed.). New York: Springer.

Karcz, M., & Papadakos, P. J. (2011). Consequences of fraud and deceit in medical research. *Canadian Journal of Respiratory Therapy, 47*(1), 18–27.

Lafleur, W. R., Bohme, G., & Shimazono, S. (2007). *Dark medicine: Rationalizing unethical medical research.* Bloomington: Indiana University Press.

Monshi, B., & Zieglmayer, V. (2004). The problem of privacy in transcultural research: Reflections on an ethnographic study in Sri Lanka. *Ethics & Behavior, 14*(4), 305–312.

Munhall, P. L. (2012). *Nursing research: A qualitative perspective* (5th ed.). Sudbury, MA: Jones & Bartlett Learning

Nylenna, M., & Simonsen, S. (2006). Scientific misconduct: A new approach to prevention. *Lancet, 367,* 1882–1884.

Olsen, D. P., & Mahrenholz, D. (2000). IRB-identified ethical issues in nursing research. *Journal of Professional Nursing, 16*(3), 140–148.

Schnoor, L. (2006). Fraud in science. *Environmental Science & Technology, 40*(5), 1375.

Shrader-Frechette, K. (2007). EPA's 2006 human-subject rule for pesticide experiments. *Accountability in Research, 14*(4), 211–254.

United States National Commission for the Protection of Human Subjects of Biomedical and Behavioral Research. (1979). *The Belmont Report: Ethical principles and guidelines for the protection of human subjects of research.* Retrieved from http://www.hhs.gov/ohrp/humansubjects/guidance/belmont.html

U.S. Department of Health and Human Services. (n.d.). Office for Human Research Protections (OHRP). Retrieved February 17, 2012, from http://www.hhs.gov/ohrp

Wilson, H. S. (1999). *Introducing research in nursing* (2nd ed.). Redwood City, CA: Addison-Wesley.

Wynia, M., & Boren, D. (2009). Better regulation of industry-sponsored clinical trials is long overdue. *Journal of Law, Medicine & Ethics, 37*(3), 410–419.

GLOBAL ISSUES THAT INTERFACE WITH NURSING PRACTICE

Part IV recognizes each person as part of an interrelated global population affected by many interacting forces. Focusing on nursing, this part begins by addressing twenty-first-century issues that require global consciousness. This section explores considerations related to the ethical and professional responsibility and accountability of nurses, individually and as a profession, in ever-changing local, national, and global health care systems. These chapters encourage nurses to be responsible professionals and citizens in acknowledging and participating in decisions and health policy related to issues that influence health care delivery and outcomes worldwide.

Chapter

13

GLOBAL CONSCIOUSNESS IN THE TWENTY-FIRST CENTURY

What we remember, we can change; what we forget we always are.

(Tafoya, 1996)

OBJECTIVES

After completing this chapter, the reader should be able to:

1. Discuss the relationship between Earth health and human health.

2. Describe the role and ethical responsibility of nursing in addressing local, national, and global environmental issues.

3. Discuss nursing role, responsibility, and ethical stance in responding to local, national, and global issues such as disaster, displaced persons, war and violence, epidemics, and toxic chemicals and other pollutants.

4. Discuss historical events and patterns of health care delivery that have helped to shape Western systems of health care delivery in the United States.

5. Describe trends and challenges of accessibility and financing facing health care delivery systems around the globe.

6. Discuss factors prompting a renewed interest in traditional healing systems worldwide.

7. Briefly describe factors affecting health care delivery for rural and urban aggregates.

INTRODUCTION

There are many global concerns that have a significant impact on the health and well-being of people and the planet. Ethical and other issues associated with these concerns call for both personal and professional responses from nurses at local, national, and international levels. Examples of these issues include Earth health, natural and other disasters, displaced persons, famine and malnutrition, child labor, human trafficking, use of torture, war and violence, genocide, unexploded bombs and land mines, pollution, global warming, epidemics and drug-resistant organisms, bioterrorism, and access to and financing of health care (both modern and traditional systems). Nurses need to be aware of both overt and covert human rights violations that are at the heart of, or result from, many of these global concerns. Discussion of nursing role, responsibility, and ethical considerations for several of these concerns is included in this chapter. Students are encouraged to explore and discuss appropriate nursing role and response related to global health issues not discussed here.

EARTH ETHICS AND HEALTH

Discussions of ethics, especially health care ethics, generally refer to principles and practices related to human experiences, values, and ways of being in the world. Rarely is there any consideration of ethical treatment of the other-than-human world—indeed, the Earth as a whole—the health of which is so intricately connected to human health. Our sense of relationship with the natural world is based in our worldview or cosmology. The Western scientific perspective flows from a worldview that holds that there is a radical distinction between humans as subjects and the natural world as object (Berry, 2009; Swimme & Tucker, 2011; Uhl, 2004). This sense of human experience being separate from and in opposition to nature has engendered and permitted a destructive attitude toward Earth, and has supported the belief that all species and resources of the Earth have been put here primarily for human use. One significant assumption of the Western worldview (that is now spreading globally) is that the more we try to control and "fix" nature, the more we are doing what is right and good. This idea is based in a view (that began emerging in the seventeenth century) of Earth and all her inhabitants (including the human body) as a complex machine with ordered, predictable laws. This shift—from an organic understanding of reality where everything is alive, to a mechanistic view of reality—engendered the belief that humans have a right to do anything they want with nature. Such an attitude results in little sense of ethical responsibility toward the other-than-human world. To the contrary, it has allowed us to turn a blind eye to our complicity in the exploitation of the planet. After several hundred years of demoting the natural world to a collection of material objects available for exploitation, we are now realizing that the complete disregard for the realities of ecological systems and the limited capacity of the natural world to sustain such exploitation and destruction are contributing to the ill health of humans and to the planet itself.

When we destroy the source of our life and sustenance, our health (physical, mental, emotional, and spiritual) suffers. Indigenous peoples continue to teach what many people in the West are only now beginning to remember: that all things are connected, and that we belong to a whole universe, not just to a city, culture, or nation. They remind us that, as part of the interconnected web of life, what we do to the Earth we do to ourselves. Indigenous peoples, mystics of many traditions, and contemporary scholars understand the world to be a seamless garment in which there is no separation between humans and nature, the sacred and the secular. They also recognize that we cannot have healthy minds or communities without healthy land and environment (Nelson, 2004). Understanding that we are all one single, sacred, Earth community, we recognize the interdependence and unity of all in the natural world, and appreciate that all species have an intrinsic right to exist. As we move beyond a human-centered focus, we begin to relate to the Earth community as having core value in itself, and incorporate Earth ethics into our nursing ethics. When we understand that, as humans, we are only one part of the interconnected Earth community, we recognize that our ethical principles must address the integrity and health of the entire community of life, and we understand the moral imperative to apply principles of beneficence, nonmaleficence, and justice to our treatment of the whole Earth community. This in no way diminishes human rights; rather, it augments human well-being by fostering the rights of humans to live within healthy ecosystems and receive the life-supporting benefits of the diversity, community, and beauty of the natural world.

Earth health is a critical global issue because, as noted, we cannot be healthy if the Earth is not healthy. The manipulation of nature through scientific and technological exploration has brought many benefits to human health, life, and general well-being. These benefits, however, have come with a high price—a disruption of the life systems of Earth, violence toward and degradation of much of the natural world, and disruption of both the human and bioregional communities. These disruptions have led to poisoning of the air we breathe, the water we drink, and the soil and seas that provide us food. Examples of health problems or potential problems related to disruptions of the natural balance in nature include asthma; birth defects; autism; deformed frogs; trees dying from acid rain; toxins in air, water, soil, and human tissues (including breast milk); drug-resistant organisms; and malnutrition. Recognizing that some health care practices and products (during manufacture, use, or disposal) can harm both humans and the environment, nurses are taking a leadership role in issues of environmental health (Alliance of Nurses for Healthy Environments, 2012; Sattler & Lipscomb, 2003).

Environmentally responsible health care requires awareness and action at many levels. One level involves seeking to move beyond the symptoms of an illness to address the source of the health concern. This may need to be done on an individual, community, or global level. The impact of smoking and second-hand smoke on asthma and pregnancy outcomes is one example of linking an environmental pollutant to a health concern and taking action to decrease the pollutant. Many health problems are related to toxic chemicals and other pollutants in the environment. These pollutants come from many sources, such as industrial production, everyday use in homes, heath care and other institutions, manufacturing, agribusiness, waste disposal, and military actions. We take these chemicals into our bodies through the food we eat, the water we drink, the air we breathe, and through our skin. It is alarming to realize the impact of these toxins on human health (Crinnion, 2010; Gaudry & Skiehar, 2007; Geller, 2009). Addressing the source of these toxins requires action at the personal level, such as responsible use and recycling of plastic; at the professional or local level, such as reducing the use of and providing for the responsible disposition of disposable plastic equipment in the hospital; and at the global level, such as working for legislation that mandates industry to provide a process for recycling components of disposable products that they manufacture in a way that does not create more pollution.

Nurses are positioned to be proactive in addressing the impact of the health care system on the health of the environment. This includes considerations such as attention to the health impact of chemicals found in products used in health care institutions; how the institution disposes of toxic and other waste; the proper disposal of unused or outdated medications; the impact of antibiotics, hormones, and chemotherapy that get into water and soil through human waste; and unnecessary water and electric consumption. Nurses can take leadership roles in instituting recycling programs; helping to develop institutional policies aimed at using energy-efficient, recycled, and environmentally friendly products wherever possible; and the like. The **precautionary principle** provides a useful guide for ethically addressing the potential risk or harm to human health or the environment of new products, processes, interventions, or technologies. This principle states "when an activity raises threats of harm to human health or the environment, precautionary measures should be taken even if some cause and effect relationships are not fully established scientifically" (Raffensperger, 2004, p. 44). The precautionary approach affirms that when there is reasonable suspicion of harm and scientific uncertainty regarding cause and effect, people have a duty to take action to prevent harm. With this approach, the developer or proponent of a product must provide sufficient information about and reasonable assurances of its safety before it can be marketed. (Currently the burden of proof of the harmfulness of a product lies with the public or government, generally after the product is already in use.) The precautionary approach suggests action steps that include setting goals; examining all reasonable alternatives for achieving the goal and choosing the least harmful way; monitoring results; heeding early warnings; making mid-course corrections as needed; and assuring that all decisions include the affected parties and be open, informed, and democratic (Chaudry, 2008; Myers & Raffensperger, 2006; Science & Environmental Health Network [SEHN], 2012). The ultimate goal of the precautionary approach is to determine how little harm is possible with a new product or development.

The Earth Charter and Nursing

The Earth Charter (http://www.earthcharter.org) can provide guidance to nurses and others for promoting ethically responsible relationships with Earth and the global community. This charter is a people's treaty resulting from a decade-long, worldwide, cross-cultural conversation about shared vision and goals for global interdependence and shared responsibility for the well-being of the human family and the larger living world. As a declaration of fundamental principles for building a just, peaceful, and sustainable global society, the Earth Charter recognizes that issues of human rights, environmental protection, equitable human development, and a culture of peace are interdependent and indivisible. The Charter provides a framework and ethical vision for addressing these issues. The following is a summary of the principles set forth in the Earth Charter—http://www.earthcharterinaction.org/content/pages/What-is-the-Earth-Charter%3F.html:

Respect and care for the community of life, which includes:

- Respecting Earth and life in all its diversity

- Caring for the community of life with understanding, compassion, and love

- Building democratic societies that are just, participatory, sustainable, and peaceful

- Securing Earth's bounty and beauty for present and future generations

Ecological integrity, which includes:

- Protecting and restoring the integrity of Earth's ecological systems with special concern for biological diversity and the natural processes that sustain life

- Preventing harm as the best method of environmental protection and, when knowledge is limited, applying a precautionary approach

- Adopting patterns of production, consumption, and reproduction that safeguard Earth's regenerative capacities, human rights, and community well-being

- Advancing the study of ecological sustainability and promoting open exchange and wide application of the knowledge acquired

Social and economic justice, which includes:

- Eradicating poverty as an ethical, social, and environmental imperative

- Ensuring that economic activities and institutions at all levels promote human development in an equitable and sustainable manner

- Affirming gender equality and equity as prerequisites to sustainable development and ensuring universal access to education, health care, and economic opportunity

- Upholding the right of all, without discrimination, to a natural and social environment supportive of human dignity, bodily health, and spiritual well-being, with special attention to the rights of indigenous peoples and minorities

Democracy, nonviolence, and peace, which includes:

- Strengthening democratic institutions at all levels and providing transparency and accountability in governance, inclusive participation in decision making, and access to justice

- Integrating into formal education and life-long learning the knowledge, values, and skills needed for a sustainable way of life

- Treating all living beings with respect and consideration

- Promoting a culture of tolerance, nonviolence, and peace

ASK YOURSELF

What Is an Ethic of Care for the Earth?

- What does your culture teach about your relationship with Earth and the other-than-human part of a global community of life?

- How do you see principles of beneficence, nonmaleficence, and justice reflected in the Earth Charter?

- What can you do, personally and professionally, to promote environmentally conscious practices in your local area and health care setting?

- What do you see as the role of nursing in developing and promoting an ethic of care for the Earth?

DISASTER—NURSING RESPONSE AND ETHICAL CONSIDERATIONS

Throughout the world nurses play an important role in providing emergency care and in meeting the ongoing humanitarian needs of people affected by disasters. Disasters are generally described as sudden events of massive proportion that result in large numbers of victims, displacement of people, material damage, disruption to society, or a combination of these (Brewer, 2010). Disastrous situations around the world, which may be linked to sudden events and require long-term as well as immediate interventions, include drought, famine, and epidemics (such as HIV/AIDS). Disasters may be termed natural (such as hurricanes, earthquakes, or tsunamis); technological (such as major chemical leaks); or accidental (such as a ship capsizing). The proportion of the disaster may be due to a combination of these factors. For example, the 2011 Japan tsunami and Haiti earthquake and the 2005 Hurricanes Katrina and Rita were natural disasters, while the nuclear power plant failure brought on by the tsunami was a technological disaster. Another example is human alteration of the land through activities such as massive logging and deforestation that contribute to the severity of some flood-related disasters. Scientists see a link between the increase in the number and severity of natural disasters over recent years and climate change, which is occurring in great part through human activity (Uhl, 2004).

Emergency and continuous health care are essential parts of any disaster response. Disasters, from the health professional's view, are situations in which there is an often sudden, unforeseen imbalance between the needs of people whose health and well-being are threatened and the resources and capacity of the health care system to meet these needs (Brewer, 2010;

World Medical Association, 2011). Many health-related problems arise in a disaster. Disasters require prompt action, yet responders must often deal with inadequate supplies and resources as well as the need to get to victims who are in places that may present health risks, be dangerous, or be difficult to reach. The World Medical Association offers guides for ethical practice for physicians in a disaster situation, which are summarized in the following discussion. These apply as well to nurses. In the emergency phase, prioritizing treatment and management, or triage, is the first ethical consideration. Triage must be done quickly and by an experienced person (often a nurse) who is aware of available resources. Based on medical needs and intervention capabilities, victims are separated into groups of those who can be saved and those whose condition exceeds the available therapeutic resources. Those who can be saved are separated into groups of those whose lives are in immediate danger and require urgent attention, those who are not in immediate danger and who need urgent but not immediate attention, those needing only minor treatment, and those with primarily psychological trauma. Because of the nature of trauma, regular reassessment of victims in each group must be done. Perhaps the most difficult ethical consideration of triage is the sense of abandoning a person whose injuries or care needs are beyond the available care. In the aftermath of Hurricanes Katrina and Rita, a number of nurses reported having to make very difficult decisions about which patients to save when electricity, medications, and other needed supplies and equipment were no longer available. Issues faced by those providing emergency care in disasters such as the earthquake in Haiti or the tsunami in Japan include difficulty reaching victims; lack of basic necessities such as food, water, shelter, and sanitation; large numbers of victims and very limited resources such as medical supplies; language barriers; and limited transportation. The ethical stance in these situations is to save the greatest number of persons who have a chance of recovery, restrict morbidity to a minimum, and do as much as possible to show compassion and respect for those who are dying.

Ethical care of victims in disasters requires nurses to provide impartial assistance to every victim without waiting to be asked, incorporating emotional as well as technical care. Nurses need to obtain a person's consent and address cultural differences as often as possible. Triage decisions should be based solely on a person's emergency status and not on any nonmedical criteria. Nurses need to respect cultural customs, religious practices, and other traditions, especially those associated with dying, mourning, and emotional and psychological response and needs. Other considerations are to assure confidentiality as much as possible, particularly when dealing with media and other third parties, and to be objective and respectful of the emotional and political climate associated with the disaster.

Nurses need to be aware of and prepared to intervene with health needs beyond the emergency response to a disaster. Principles of humanitarian action basic to this care include meeting critical human needs and restoring personal dignity. Critical human needs that may become serious problems during and following a disaster include nutrition (availability, quality, and special needs of children); economic security; environmental health (water, sewage, air quality, and vector control); communicable disease control; emotional and mental health (including attention to rape and other forms of violence); basic health care (both preventive and curative); and family and social support. Disaster preparedness is becoming a very important set of skills for nurses worldwide. Students are encouraged to explore the resources related to disaster preparedness at these websites:

American Nurses Association (ANA)—
http://www.nursingworld.org/MainMenuCategories/WorkplaceSafety/
DPR/Disaster-Preparedness.pdf

International Council of Nurses (ICN)—
http://www.icn.ch/Links/Disaster-Response-Network/Page-2.html

International Committee of the Red Cross (ICRC)—
http://icrc.org

DISPLACED PERSONS AND VICTIMS OF ARMED CONFLICT

In the past decades disasters, wars, political instability, and armed conflict have forced growing numbers of people worldwide to become refugees or displaced persons. Refugees are persons who have fled their countries and who cannot or do not want to return due to well-founded fears of death or persecution because of their religion, race, political opinion, nationality, or membership in a particular social or ethnic group. Internally displaced persons are those who, because of war, persecution, or other threats, have been forced to leave their homes, but who have not crossed an internationally recognized border (ICN, 2006b). Victims of major disasters and those in areas of famine or severe economic upheaval can become displaced persons either temporarily or long term. Victims of human trafficking (discussed in Chapter 16) are a less visible group of displaced persons. Displaced persons often have serious health and social problems related to deprivation (including basic human rights), physical hardship, stress, poor nutrition, and generally poor health status. Displacement often separates family members and cuts people off from community support, employment, educational opportunities, and cultural ties. Refugee settlements are often overcrowded and may lack sufficient resources, including food and sanitation, to meet basic necessities and health care needs. The majority of displaced persons around the world are women and children. The conditions in refugee settlements engender emotional cruelty and gender-specific violence such as rape, sexual abuse and harassment, spousal battering, and forced prostitution, and may also give rise to political unrest, particularly when internment in such camps becomes long term.

Although international humanitarian law provides for protection of civilians in times of war, large humanitarian groups such as the ICRC and United Nations organizations must have the permission of the ruling power in order to work in a country. Humanitarian aid often is unavailable to internally displaced persons, who may also be victims of repressive governments. These people may be left without basic necessities to suffer and die because the ruling government persecutes the group in various ways, provides no assistance, and denies permission for outside aid. The ongoing

Think About It

Nursing Response to the Plight of Displaced Persons

Baroness Cox of Queensbury (Interview, 2003), former co-editor of the International Journal of Nursing Studies, *is actively involved in international humanitarian work. She calls for nurses to address ethical, legal, and professional implications of the plight of displaced persons worldwide by posing the following questions:*

- *If nursing is concerned for all humanity, why are we silent when vast numbers of people are left to suffer and die unaided?*

- *Should nursing not be raising the issue of denial of access to those suffering under repressive regimes?*

- *Where is the nursing profession's voice urging governments to press repressive regimes to allow humanitarian and human rights organizations access to groups in need in their countries?*

- *How can nurses use professional conferences, journals, and media to try to find professional, legal, and ethical solutions to these problems?*

- *If nurses, who have a professional mandate to advocate for those who are suffering, remain silent, who else will speak? (p. 445)*

    How would you respond to Baroness Cox? How would principles of beneficence, justice, and respect for human dignity guide your response?

    How do her suggestions compare with the recommendations of the ICN?

    What action steps are needed individually and as a profession to address these issues?

situation and resulting genocide in Sudan is an example of such treatment of internally displaced persons.

Nursing involvement with refugees and displaced persons can occur at levels of emergency needs, care and maintenance, and seeking ongoing solutions. The ICN (2006b) suggests a number of action areas for nursing involvement with issues of displaced persons. These include raising public awareness and lobbying governments regarding the situation, identifying nursing and health needs of displaced persons and mobilizing resources to address these needs, assisting with emergency and resettlement programs, planning for provision and evaluation of health services for displaced persons, implementing educational programs for nursing personnel, and assisting nurse refugees. Recognizing that we live in a global community, principles of beneficence, justice, and respect for human dignity compel nurses to advocate for those who are suffering both close to home and globally.

WAR AND VIOLENCE

We live in a troubled world, perhaps made more so by ease of global travel and instant electronic communication. Conflict, violence in many forms, and war touch our lives in many ways, either directly if we live in an area experiencing the violence, or indirectly through the media or the presence of family or friends in war-torn areas. We cannot escape the impact of war and violence on our lives, nor can we escape the need, as nurses, for an appropriate ethical response to these realities. Inherent in national and international codes of nursing is respect for life and dignity of people, and adherence to principles of beneficence, nonmaleficence, and justice. In the face of modern warfare and increasing acts of violence worldwide (including torture and terrorism), we need to ask ourselves what the ethical stance of nursing needs to be.

As noted in earlier chapters, the principle of beneficence directs nurses to do good and prevent or remove harm. This includes defending and protecting another's rights, seeking ways to keep people out of harm's way, and intervening to assist if the person is in danger. Nonmaleficence directs nurses to do no harm, which includes the directives not to inflict suffering or to kill another. Justice refers to fair and equitable treatment of individuals regardless of their backgrounds. Fair, equitable, and appropriate distribution of resources in society is termed **distributive justice**. Applying these ethical principles to issues of war and violence raises many ethical considerations, which are discussed briefly here. Students are urged to pursue further reflection and discussion about these critical global issues.

Precepts of doing good, avoiding harm, and preventing or removing harm impels nurses to understand the effects of war and violence in order to know what and where the needs are and how to intervene. One tragic effect of modern warfare is that frequently civilian casualties, especially women and children, are more extensive than those of the soldiers (Tschudin & Schmitz, 2003). Even after a war is over, unexploded land mines and bombs left in the region continue to create casualties. The devastating effects of war and violence affect individuals and society and include physical, emotional, spiritual, and social components. Physical and emotional trauma sustained in war is compounded by poverty; destruction of societal infrastructure, such as roads, sanitation, and communication; spread of infectious diseases, sometimes in epidemic proportions; and strain on or destruction of resources necessary to meet basic health care needs. Traumas that have become common in armed conflict around the world, such as rape, torture, and maiming, and the stress of displacement and having to rely on charity for basic needs contribute to the increase of health concerns such as hypertension and post-traumatic stress disorder. Fear, depression, insomnia, flashbacks, and nightmares are part of the often life-long psychological fallout of war and violence. An example of this is a man who survived the Nazi Holocaust and moved to a small town in the United States after World War II. He became a successful businessman and was well respected in the community. He owned a nice house in a friendly and safe neighborhood, but rarely lived there because he felt insecure there. He lived instead (until his death at age 82) in a small apartment, with several locks on the door, above a store in the downtown area because of fear that someone would come for him in the night.

Environmental degradation resulting from war and armed conflict includes soil and water pollution; destruction of crops, trees, other vegetation, and animal habitat; and general ecological disturbances. This affects the ability of the land to support the needs of the people for even the basic requirements of food and water. A country's resources are strained and possibly depleted by warfare, limiting its ability to provide for the basic needs of its people. The lack of care and the physical and emotional traumas sustained during the war can cause the impact of war to affect a person's health throughout life. The cost of war includes not just the resources needed for the military action, but also the impact on the lives and health of individuals and communities, and the resources needed for cleaning up, rebuilding, and repairing the various levels of devastation caused by the war.

Nurses have an ethical responsibility to work to prevent war and conflict and the consequences of devastation that they cause. The response to war and violence must move beyond local and national considerations and embrace a global consciousness. This response requires taking leadership roles at the national and international levels "advocating the prevention of conflict, developing and teaching nonviolent ways to resolve conflict, being aware of international issues of professional concern, learning how to exercise the profession's political voice, and making politicians and governments aware of the devastation and misery caused by aggression and its drain on national and international economic, ecological, humanitarian, and emotional resources" (Tschudin & Schmitz, 2003, p. 358).

Understanding that world peace is a prerequisite for developing, fostering, and maintaining health, the ICN (2006a) affirms the ethical responsibility of nurses to eliminate threats to life and health caused by weapons of war and conflict. The ICN calls on national nurses' associations to work toward elimination of these weapons and land mines and to work to prevent the consequences of all types of weapons. Action steps that the ICN poses for nurses individually and collectively include educating the profession and the public about the social, economic, and environmental consequences of weapons that cause large-scale devastation; collaborating with human rights and health groups, disaster prevention agencies, the media, and other groups in lobbying manufacturers and governments against the production, distribution, and use of these weapons; developing strategies for taking action to reduce the threat of these weapons; and actively participating in disaster preparedness and response planning.

Along with working to prevent and avert war and armed conflict, nurses are called upon to deal with issues related to the immediate experience of war and violence. This includes working to alleviate the suffering of and providing equitable care for injured persons on all sides of the conflict. It is important as well to assure, to the best of our ability, that human rights and dignity are maintained for all in our care, and to assure that our practice

---

ASK YOURSELF

What Is My Personal Response to War and Armed Conflict?

Morally justify your responses to the following questions using ethical principles.

- Have I personally or professionally spoken out against the global devastation caused by war and armed conflict?

- How many people must be injured, killed, or displaced, and where must the violence occur in order for me to find my voice and take action?

- Are war and its multi-level costs ever justified?

- Who is most affected by war and armed conflict and its aftermath?

- Who should pay for the cost of war?

(Adapted from Silva & Ludwick, 2003.)

is aligned with the ethical standards of the profession. In areas of armed conflict, nurses may be called on to care for civilian as well as military casualties, provide basic health care for displaced persons, and work with both private and governmental agencies in procuring and providing basic necessities for those in need. Considerations discussed in the previous section on disasters apply as well in situations of war and armed violence. In times of war, nurses and other health care professionals may be asked or directed to participate in treatment of or practices related to patients or other persons that they consider ethically questionable. In such circumstances, the ethical stance for nurses is to follow the professional codes of ethics, seeking support and guidance from professional organizations and others as necessary. Professional codes mandate that nurses provide ethical and equitable care with respect for human dignity for all victims of war, including civilians, military, and even prisoners of war.

HEALTH CARE ACCESS AND FINANCING

Addressing global health issues at their source requires an awareness of the interconnectedness of the whole Earth community. The challenge to provide health care for people worldwide requires increasing effort, creativity, and global consciousness. Many variables play a part in this challenge, not the least of which is the health of the Earth itself. Other critical factors include economics, culture, politics, epidemics, disasters (natural and technological), war and violence, national crises, and global travel. The problems are further compounded by limited appreciation of what it means to live in a global community, national versus private health insurance, methods of health promotion contrasted with curative methods of treating illness, tenuous relationships between conventional medicine and traditional healing systems, and ignoring the health of the environment in health care policies and practices. These factors all affect the functioning of health systems and the care they provide around the world (Ausubel, 2004; Berry, 2009; Bodeker & Burford, 2007).

The fundamental principles upon which the health care delivery system is based and the way it is financed define the parameters within which nurses and other health care personnel function. Issues of health care delivery and the effectiveness of the health care delivery system are concerns worldwide. In the United States and most of the Western world, delivery of health care is much like a runaway train of high technology with its proliferation of markets for new medications and expensive treatments. Further, this system is challenged to provide for an ever-increasing global population with decreasing resources, both natural and monetary. Basic to this global concern is the state of the health of the planet itself and the ever-increasing cost of health care and the issue of its sustainability. Scientists are bringing our attention to the growing concerns of climate change and the issues of clean air, clean water, and environmental toxins. Developed and developing countries recognize that the current and future health care systems have at their foundation expensive technologies and medication, many of which have to be imported from other regions of the globe.

Health care systems must address global changes and challenges if they are to survive in the twenty-first century. Important questions arise about how best to meet the health care needs of people worldwide. Can countries address the needs of their people without relying on expensive medications and treatments? Can local, existing systems of health care be utilized to provide basic health services to rural and urban poor communities? In developing countries, can traditional methods and systems of health care be utilized to promote health and prevent disease, thus reducing the burden on the system? Has modern Western health care practice been lax in preserving and utilizing traditional healing methods in favor of technology, and at what cost? What ethical principles need to be considered when addressing issues of cost limits, access, rationing, justice, need and medical necessity, and quality of care? In order to gain an understanding of some of the major issues facing Western health care, it is useful to explore the history of various contemporary health care systems and their financing, including traditional systems.

ASK YOURSELF

What Cultural Influences Affect Your Health Care Practices?

All persons have roots in beliefs and cultural heritage from their family of origin and place of birth.

- What do you know about the health care practices of your cultural origins?
- Have you or anyone you know ever utilized any healing modalities that are not part of what would be deemed modern health care?

A BRIEF HISTORY OF HEALTH CARE DELIVERY: THE EURO-AMERICAN EXPERIENCE

From the earliest civilizations there is evidence of some type of health care. The methods of health care were often a mixture of religious, civil, and mythological belief that combined to keep away disease, prevent wars, and ensure survival of populations in order to keep the group strong. Traditional healing systems generally recognize the interconnection between human health and the health of the Earth and incorporate this understanding into their healing practices. In every culture there have been individuals designated to provide care to the sick. Some were formally trained as nurses and physicians, while others seemed to have a natural gift for the art of healing. Asian and Middle Eastern peoples, such as the Mesopotamians, Babylonians, Hebrews, Persians, Hindus, and Chinese, have recorded some type of system for the delivery of health care. In all of these cultures, religious or civil laws enforced systems of disease prevention in matters of hygiene and diet, some of which were connected to the various religious practices of the ancient civilizations.

Early Eras of Health Care Delivery

There is evidence to suggest that it is the Sumerians, rather than the ancient Greeks and Romans, who are the parents of Western healing systems. Archeological findings in the area of ancient Sumer, which is located in the vicinity of modern Iraq, include numerous prescriptions and two tablets that are considered to be the oldest medical text in existence (Achterberg, 1990). Sumerian knowledge of healing and theories of disease were dispersed to other areas through trade with the Phoenicians, Greeks, and Egyptians.

The ancient Greek civilization represents a major force in the systematic organization of education, both in secular and scientific fields. The most well-known name in ancient Greek medicine and health care is Hippocrates, known as the Father of Medicine. His approach of separating medicine and health care from religion, magic, and myth was considered purely scientific for his time. He diagnosed from observed symptoms, with emphasis on treating the whole patient, and he promoted continuous bedside care. His method of systematic record keeping of the patient's appearance, vital signs, and general bodily functioning became a standard for health care. Hippocrates approached medicine and health care from the highest ethical standard, believing medicine to be the noblest of arts. In addition, he believed that the physician's conduct should be of the highest quality and above reproach. Hippocrates gave the health care system organized writings of medical books that included detailed descriptive case histories, technical practices, and reports of research on various disease treatments, including treatments that worked and those that did not, in order to avoid repeating errors in care (Kennedy, 2004; Magner, 2005).

As nations and populations expanded, knowledge was disseminated from culture to culture, constantly redefining the approach to health care, research, and practice. Alexander the Great, who conquered Greece in about 339 BCE, spread what he learned in Greece throughout the entire known world. He established medical schools in Egypt that included clinics, laboratories, and libraries. Physicians were supported by the government, and could devote their time to practice and research. Gradually, through various wars and assimilation of culture, Greek medicine supplemented or replaced practices throughout the known Western world.

The empire of Rome replaced methods of health care that were based on folklore and magic with a knowledge base developed in Greece. Within this developing culture, medicine and health care soon became a part of the necessary education of upper-class men, and women's health issues and childbearing practices regained importance. Midwives became key figures in the care of women. Important contributions to health care delivery from the Roman Empire include public health sanitation and public health law. The Romans instituted city planning that provided for development of sewage systems, aqueducts, and baths. In addition, they can be credited for the development of hospitals with male and female attendants to care for the sick (Kennedy, 2004; Magner, 2005).

A new era in the care of the sick occurred after Christianity became the official religion of Rome. The Christian attitude of care for persons, based on a strong belief in the sanctity of human life, was derived from Hebrew tradition as well as the teachings of Christ. Bishops assigned individuals to care for widows, orphans, the sick, and the poor. Hospitals to care for the sick and institutions to care for the poor offered combinations of outpatient and welfare services. Monastic orders of monks and nuns, who were generally better educated than the ordinary person, controlled the health care institutions. Their writings documented the care given to the sick and techniques used, which provide us with early records of diseases, practices, and research for cure and care (Bullough & Bullough, 1978).

Changes from the Middle Ages to the Industrial Revolution

During the thirteenth and fourteenth centuries, the organization and founding of medical schools and universities and the advent of book binding all worked to promote a better-educated health care provider. Nurses, who were not as fully established as physicians, functioned as attendants who made beds and gave baths to the sick.

As noted in Chapter 1, amidst the religious revolution (known as the Reformation) that had taken place against the Church of Rome in the early sixteenth to seventeenth centuries, the disbanding of convents and monasteries led to severe impediments in the care of the sick. During this time, some progress was made in midwifery, medicine, and nursing. However, it was not until the mid-nineteenth century and the Industrial Revolution, when the demand for intellectual freedom brought about expansion of educational institutions for both men and women, that the health care system as we know it began to emerge. During the nineteenth century, Florence Nightingale's leadership influenced not only nursing education and nursing care, but also the health care of the world (Dossey, 2000; Dossey, Selanders, Beck, & Atwell, 2005; McDonald, 2010; Nightingale, 1859/1992; Selanders, 2010a, 2010b).

ASK YOURSELF

How Have Things Changed?

- Consider the discussion of the early era of the health care delivery system and identify problems in early civilization that might still be seen in today's world.

- Consider how Florence Nightingale's profound influence on health care systems worldwide continues to affect health care today. How can nurses continue this legacy in the twenty-first century?

Nightingale is perhaps best known for crafting the standards of Western secular nursing education and practice. Her leadership was also felt in the area of public policy and social reform. She spearheaded improvements in British military medicine, and greatly influenced public health reform in Great Britain and India. She promoted what we now call holistic health, recognizing the role of body, mind, spirit, and the environment in health and healing. Appreciating the importance of environmental factors in healing, Nightingale directed her nurses to assure that patients had clean water, sanitation, clean air and good ventilation, and limited noise. She was a pioneer in using evaluative statistics to monitor the various factors influencing health and the effectiveness of the health care system.

Changes Influencing Development of Modern Health Care in the United States

Health services in the United States developed from health care models in European countries. These systems share the products of medical innovations that took place from the late nineteenth century to the time of World War I, a time when major nations were changing from agricultural to industrial economies. Such innovations as the use of anesthesia in surgery and the recognition of bacteria as a causative factor in many widespread diseases provided the impetus that led to the development of the modern hospital as it exists today. The dissemination and incorporation of this knowledge among the large number of practicing physicians took at least a generation to accomplish. Consequently, the importance of the place of the modern hospital in society was not felt until the late nineteenth century and into the early twentieth century. At the time of this revolution of knowledge, physicians, who were the primary health care practitioners, engaged primarily in a private, fee-for-service practice that included office and home visits.

Physicians and Hospitals

In the United States, hospitals were generally privately funded, while European nations had both tax-supported charity hospitals and private hospitals for those patients who had the ability to pay for their own health care (Kennedy, 2004; Rutkow, 2010). The primary purpose for hospitals built in Europe was ministry to the low-income or charity patient, while in the United States, hospitals that were built by private funding were open to charity patients as well as private-pay patients.

The development of hospitals affected European physicians by creating a class of specialists who operated in the general hospital and also had the option of treating private-pay patients. These specialists often created their own cottage hospitals, where they could treat their private-pay patients. All other physicians in that system were excluded from practicing in a hospital. In the United States, on the other hand, practitioners sought out appointments to the hospital system in order to be able to admit patients, while at the same time maintaining private offices in which to see their patients. This began a new approach to the use of the hospital system, in which resources were used more extravagantly and the system was more democratic in its care of patients than the European system. The U.S. health care system became immersed in greater use of technology, industrial and management skills, and scientific methods, creating by some estimates the best health care system in the world, and the most expensive (Rutkow, 2010).

As an outgrowth of the development of hospitals, a greater awareness of public health problems arose. Prevention programs for the public, such as sanitation, environmental issues, control of communicable diseases, and maternity and infant care, developed. Curative programs, which were generally hospital-based, were supported by private and public funding. Hospital clinics that provided outpatient services became the primary site of health care for low-income and indigent patients. During that period, physicians provided these outpatient services free of charge and, in return, were able to participate in the hospital system, where the latest in knowledge and technologies was being introduced. This information could then be applied to the care of large numbers of both private and charity patients. Hospitals provided physicians an opportunity to develop their skills and to provide service to the public, thus fulfilling the physician's commitment to the public interest (Rutkow, 2010).

Twentieth- and Twenty-First-Century Changes and Challenges

The U.S. health care delivery system in the later nineteenth century was affected by sources of funding (private or public), the ability of the patient to pay, and the type of control exercised by independent practitioners, which now included physicians, pharmacists, and dentists. The development of an industrialized society in the United States, the growth of the economy, and the increased capability of a growing health care system produced a healthier and more aware population. However, twentieth-century changes created new challenges for the health care system. Figure 13–1 presents some of the significant events that have influenced health care in the United States in the nineteenth and twentieth centuries.

Date	Event
1862	William Rathbone opened a nurse training school, the Liverpool Royal Infirmary, in consultation with Florence Nightingale.
1869	The first Board of Health was established in Massachusetts.
1872	The American Public Health Association was established.
1886	The Visiting Nurse Society of Philadelphia was established.
1893	The Henry Street Settlement, under the direction of Lillian Wald, was founded to provide health promotion, disease prevention, case finding, and follow-up care. Out of this system came the first school nurse, Lina Rogers, who was assigned to the public school system.
1896	The Nurses Associated Alumnae of the United States was established, later to become the American Nurses Association.
1901	The Army Nurse Corp was established by an act of Congress.
1903	North Carolina was the first state to legislate the licensing of nursing.
1910	The Flexner Report exposed abuses in medical education and proposed reforms.
1916	The Pure Food and Drug Act was enacted.
1918	An influenza epidemic produced 500,000 deaths in the United States.
1918	The Chamberlain-Kahn Act established the Venereal Disease Division of the United States Public Health Service.
1921	The Sheppard-Towner Act was passed, providing grants-in-aid to enable states to create their own bureaus of maternal and child health.
1923	The Goldmark Report was published, entitled *Nursing and Nursing Education in the United States*.

FIGURE 13–1 **Selected Significant Events in Health Care History— Nineteenth and Twentieth Centuries (*continued*)**

Date	Event
1925	Mary Breckinridge developed rural health care programs that become the Frontier Nursing Service.
1935	The Social Security Act authorized grants to aid public health programs.
1940	Sister Elizabeth Kenny brought her method for treating poliomyelitis to the United States.
1946	The Hospital Survey and Construction Act, known as the Hill-Burton Act, provided for matching funds to states and local communities for the building of hospitals.
1948	The Brown Report, *Nursing for the Future*, was published by Esther Lucille Brown, emphasizing higher education for nurses.
1948	Eli Ginzberg's report, *A Program for the Nursing Profession*, recommended two levels of nursing: professional and practical.
1956	The Health Amendments Act was passed to provide traineeships for public health personnel. It gave nurses an opportunity for advanced preparation for positions in teaching, administration, and supervision.
1962	State nurses' associations eliminated discriminatory membership barriers.
1965	The American Nurses Association published its "Position Paper."
1965	The Social Security Act was amended to provide funds for the health care of the elderly (Medicare—Title XVIII) and the health care of the medically indigent (Medicaid—Title XIX).
1972	Revision of the New York State Practice Act acknowledged nursing as an autonomous profession.
1977	Nurse practitioners providing rural health care were authorized to receive Medicare payment.
1978	Louise Brown, the first test tube baby, was born in England.
1981	AIDS was identified in the United States.
1982	Maryland was the first state to grant direct third-party reimbursement for nurse practitioner services without physician supervision.
1983	A prospective payment system based on Diagnosis Related Groups (DRGs) was created under Medicare.
1986	The National Institute of Nursing Research (NINR) was established at the National Institutes of Health (NIH).
1989	The Omnibus Budget Reconciliation Act (OBRA '89) phased in new Medicare payment scales for physicians. It mandated direct Medicaid reimbursement for pediatric and family nurse practitioners.

FIGURE 13–1   *(continued)*

Date	Event
1990	The Patient Self-Determination Act and the Americans with Disabilities Act were enacted.
1992	Congressional mandate created to establish the Office of Alternative Medicine at the NIH.
1993	The Omnibus Budget Reconciliation Act (OBRA '93) established an all-time record cut in Medicare funding and contained the Comprehensive Childhood Immunization Act to provide vaccines for Medicaid-eligible and Native American children.
1994	President Clinton's health reform proposal, the American Health Security Act, failed.
1997	Medicare reimbursement for nurse practitioners and clinical specialists authorized by federal legislation.
	Children's Health Insurance Program (CHIP) established.
1998	The NIH Office of Alternative Medicine was elevated to status of the National Center for Complementary and Alternative Medicine, and was mandated to facilitate research on and provide public information about alternative medical treatments.
1999	The National Institute of Nursing Research (NINR) became the lead institute dealing with palliative care and end-of-life issues.
2000	Landmark legal decisions against tobacco companies related to the health hazards of tobacco use.
2000	Needlestick Safety and Prevention Act signed into law.
2000	Several states included on their ballots health care reform measures calling for universal health care.

FIGURE 13–1

In the early part of the twentieth century, a growing nation experienced population increases and a greater influx of immigrants, with over one million immigrants from southern and eastern Europe in 1905 alone. The need for health care and related services warranted attention. Medical schools and nursing schools expanded to provide personnel to meet the demand. Science, technology, public health services, and medicine progressed at an increased rate. Physicians and scientists began to use such diagnostic tools as x-rays. They made strides toward reduction of infectious organisms through the use of rubber gloves. They began to research the causes and cures of diseases such as yellow fever and typhoid, and began to use radiation to treat breast cancer. Amid such major advances as the discovery of penicillin, the proliferation of science and technology, the advancement of the professions of nursing and medicine, and the changing conceptualization about disease,

ASK YOURSELF

How Do Nineteenth-Century Concepts Affect Twenty-First-Century Health Care?

- What concepts or practices regarding health care from the late 1800s and early 1900s still affect a patient's access to health care today?

- How is the health care delivery system that we know different from the system at the turn of the nineteenth and twentieth centuries?

- What is your vision for health care for the twenty-first century?

a phenomenon unique to the United States emerged: the American hospital system. This phenomenon has shaped the health care system in the twentieth century and into the twenty-first century as well.

The later part of the nineteenth century and the first two decades of the twentieth century saw the transformation of hospitals from asylums for the poor to modern institutions, dedicated to science and improved patient care. Physicians expanded surgical interventions such as tonsillectomies, removal of tumors, and many gynecological operations. Nurses began to take a more active role in managing the hospital environment to control infection, and began to have more responsibility for technical management of patient care through duties such as taking the patient's pulse, temperature, and blood pressure (Judd, Sitzman, & Davis, 2009). Patterns that developed in the health care delivery system in the early part of the twentieth century can still be seen today. Physicians gained a new and strong identity and prestige, and the American Medical Association (AMA) became a powerful force. Physicians gained increased authority in the routine workings of hospital systems, shifting the balance of power from boards of trustees to the medical decision makers (Stevens, 1989).

As a result of battlefield experiences in World War I, nurses, physicians, and other health care workers designed and set up streamlined, technically proficient, and very efficient specialized hospitals for the acutely ill or injured patient. On the home front, in response to ever-increasing numbers of immigrants, models of health care with emphasis on prevention and community interaction were developed. Prior to the war, the elite area of nursing was public health, with nurses at the forefront of campaigns for infant care and welfare, tuberculosis, and infectious disease. The war, however, emphasized the glamour of hospitals, and by 1920, more than half of the general hospitals in this country had schools of nursing attached to them. Student nurses staffed hospitals and were socialized into the hospital system. Because of this socialization, nurses tended to work more in the acute health care hospital environment than in public health and the social aspect of health care.

After World War I, the idea of group practices for physicians began to take hold, and the movement for health insurance began to develop. With the encouragement of President Theodore Roosevelt, workers' compensation was the first form of social insurance to become prominent in this country. By 1919, 37 states had passed laws that sanctioned workers' compensation. Through this movement, the cost of injury and damage to workers because of job-related hazards was passed on to industry. The health insurance movement entered a fast track, supported by the AMA and various physicians' groups around the country. During this time, the struggle for access to care and control of fees and services escalated (Rutkow, 2010).

The 1920s were years of growth and expansion of the health care industry. Consumerism flowered in direct relationship to the growth of the health care industry. As the public became aware of the availability of modern techniques, they wanted the best available. The health care delivery system developed into a middle-class entity in which many advances were taking place in private care, while the poor were increasingly underserved. By the end of this decade, there was increasing criticism of the cost and financing of the health care system, and the question of equal care for all income levels was raised. The rich and middle class were accused of having the best care available primarily to them, while the poor were viewed as manipulative of the very system that wanted to provide *charity* care to them.

During the Great Depression, government and charity hospitals were overrun with patients unable to afford health care, causing health care institutions to lose income and question their survival. The various health care professions pulled together to care for the sick, and a renewed sense of dedication kept a strained system afloat. Continually rising costs of health care led to development of plans for health insurance for everyone in the 1930s. The original Blue Cross plans were an outgrowth of the need for payment for continued growth of hospital and health care technologies. Thus, a prepayment insurance plan was born, and the health care delivery system grew by leaps and bounds. During the ensuing years, major federal grant programs such as the Hill-Burton Act of 1946 funded the construction of health care facilities, and the science of medicine expanded through laboratory and clinical research. World War II prompted advances in health services that included therapy for prevention and treatment of shock, better blood replacement techniques, and research on gamma globulin, steroids, and other drugs, all of which increased the possibilities for successful

Think About It

How Do World Events Affect Health Care Delivery?

In reviewing history it is evident that seemingly nonrelated events can steer the course of other events, as has been noted in the development of the health care delivery system.

- *How have major world events of your lifetime affected the course of health care delivery?*
- *Identify ethical issues that have arisen in association with these events.*

treatment in surgery and internal medicine (Magner, 2005; Murray, 2007). Expansion in the health care industry continued in the postwar years.

Between the passing of the Hill-Burton Act in 1946 and the enactment of Medicare legislation in 1966, the U.S. health care delivery system hit a new wave of expansion. The most widely known image of expansion in hospitals was the intensive care unit, with the greatest expansion between 1950 and 1965. In the early 1960s, coronary care units began to flourish, and by the mid-1960s premature nurseries, respiratory units, physical therapy units, and units dealing specifically with postoperative surgeries and neurosurgery were functioning in every fully operational hospital. Because of technological expansion, the cost of health care increased rapidly.

Expanding Health Insurance Coverage

Seeing a need and opportunity, the insurance industry began to compete with Blue Cross plans to provide third-party coverage for health care. These insurance plans removed the anxiety related to paying large hospital and health care bills, and also removed incentives from health care institutions to keep their costs down. Hospitals passed down increased costs to insurance companies, who in turn passed the cost on to the individual insurance subscriber. Because individual citizens had insurance, they demanded more and better service, and the system drove itself through the supply and demand cycle (Morrisey, 2008; Murray, 2007).

Medicare Parts A and B, which were passed in 1965 and enacted in 1966, essentially gave hospitals and other health care institutions a license to spend, and "bigger and better" were the watchwords. The health care delivery system was caught up in a whirlwind that has escalated to the point where the system is facing the need for serious change and the possibility of rationing at the beginning of the twenty-first century. Spiraling costs have prompted development of cost-containment mechanisms such as Diagnostic Related Grouping, case management, and managed care systems, which affect current health care delivery. Standardization and the constraints of health insurance plans are more and more defining the care that patients receive in the present health care delivery system. The Medicare Part D drug benefit program, developed in response to the increasing cost of medications for the elderly on fixed incomes, has had loopholes that limit its ability to meet the needs of many Medicare recipients. The future of the system is uncertain, and continues to be influenced by political structures, economic constraints, and worldwide societal needs and demands.

According to the 2010 census, 13 million more people in the United States were uninsured in 2010 than in 2000 (DeNavas-Walt, Proctor, & Smith, 2011). In addition, nearly 25 million Americans are underinsured, meaning they have very high deductibles or spend 10% or more of their income on medical expenses. Caring for people with limited or no health insurance results in health care institutions having to provide charity care similar to that which existed in the first part of the twentieth century. Limited access to health care by so many people due to lack of health insurance prompted the passage by the U.S. Congress in 2010 of the Patient Protection and Affordable Health Care Act. This law puts in place over several years comprehensive insurance reforms focused on closing existing gaps in health care coverage. Several key provisions of this law include prohibiting insurance companies from placing lifetime limits on the dollar value of essential benefits, retroactively cancelling health insurance policies, charging higher premiums based on health status or gender, or denying coverage for people with pre-existing conditions; closing (by 2020) the Medicare Part D "donut hole"; requiring new group and individual health plans to provide free preventive care for recommended preventive services; tax credits for small businesses that offer health insurance to employees; student loan programs for those in nursing, primary care, and pediatric programs; increased funding to community health centers for serving more people with limited health insurance coverage; establishing grants for developing primary care "medical home" teams and school-based health clinics; allowing parents to keep children on their health policies to age 26; and increasing Medicare reimbursement for primary care services. Students are encouraged to further explore provisions of the Affordable Care Act and its implications for nurses and patients. Several resources for this exploration are listed at the end of this chapter.

GLOBAL NEEDS AND FINITE RESOURCES

Health care resources worldwide are limited, and making choices regarding who receives these resources is difficult at all levels of care. Although ethical principles direct us to distribute health care resources justly and equitably, there are powerful local and global social, political, and economic forces that urge both for and against the rationing of health care (Povar et al., 2004). In developing countries, access to modern health care may be very limited for much of the population because of limited governmental resources for health care, distance from facilities, and limited ability to pay. Basic health care services that we take for granted in the West, such as immunizations, antibiotics and other medications, and common surgical and other treatments, are unavailable or too expensive. Health care needs may be addressed by traditional healing practices, local outreach workers who do their best with limited resources, periodic visits from health care teams from the government or abroad, or not at all. Difficulty accessing health care is often compounded by political unrest, economic instability, and social, cultural, and other factors that contribute to a large gap between the rich and the poor. Ultimately, a large portion of the population in many of these countries suffers from poor health.

On the other hand, all industrialized nations, with the exception of the United States and South Africa, have some form of universal health coverage that covers basic health care needs. However, all of these programs are not equal and most function less smoothly than one would hope. These systems vary in regard to the amount of government and private involvement in health care delivery and contributions for health insurance. Some countries have a combination of several methods. Germany, France, and Japan, for example, mandate benefits coverage, the cost of which is shared by employers, employees, and government tax revenues. These health care delivery systems share three traits with the system in the United States: Medical care is offered through private physicians and through private and public hospitals, patients may choose their providers, and most people in these countries have health insurance coverage through their place of employment. Health insurance is offered to the citizens of these countries through multiple third-party insurance agencies. Similar problems to those in the United States exist, such as high costs and increased spending for technology. However, every citizen has some type of health care coverage. In an attempt to hold down rising health care spending, all have instituted direct controls on the price of health care. Canada and Great Britain have developed national health care systems that provide health care for their citizens. The government-run plans provide cradle-to-grave services that are financed through taxes. These plans enable patients to receive free services, and to choose their own hospitals and physicians. The plans pay salaries to physicians and operate their own hospitals.

There are both champions and critics of the national health insurance systems in Canada and Britain. Some say the systems are sound, while others say they are flawed. In Canada, for example, citizens can go to physicians or hospitals of their choice when they need care. Physicians bill the province for patient care. Patients do not pay for services, nor are they required to fill out endless forms. Negotiations for fees, cost-containment measures, and salaries take place between the provinces and the health care system.

The national health insurance systems in these countries have their critics. Some say the systems are flawed, and that being insured in this way sets up a system of rationing because of insufficient funds for specialized health care. It has been said that waiting for care in these systems sometimes means death. Access to certain procedures and technologies is limited. Waiting lists are getting longer. Critics say that there is an unequal access to health care from province to province, depending on the affluence of the province. Some Canadian citizens who can afford to pay out-of-pocket come to the United States for specialized care and surgeries. In all instances, the increase in health care spending due to the high cost of technologies and research is having an impact on these systems in much the same ways as it is across the globe (Canadian Health Care, n.d.; Health Canada, 2012).

Information about national health care systems worldwide is available at http://www.allianzworldwidecare.com/national-healthcare-systems. Students are encouraged to visit this website to compare and contrast what is offered by health care systems in various countries.

In the United States, the burden of dealing with issues of health care access, limited resources, justice, rationing, and quality involves many players, including insurance companies, governmental agencies, managed care organizations, individual clinicians, and patients. A workgroup convened by the American College of Physicians and the Harvard Pilgrim Health Care Ethics Program developed a statement of ethics of managed care (Povar et al., 2004). The interdisciplinary group consisted of patients, nurses, physicians, social workers, medical ethicists, and managed care representatives. The four principles set forth in this statement are summarized as follows:

1. *Relationships are critical in the delivery of health services. They should be characterized by respect, truthfulness, consistency, fairness, and compassion.* This implies truthfulness and openness among patients, clinicians, and health plan purchasers; maintaining accurate and honest records; supporting the importance, intimacy, and ethical obligations of the patient-clinician relationship; and honesty on the part of patients regarding their health conditions and needs.

2. *Health plan purchasers, clinicians, and the public share responsibility for the appropriate stewardship for health care resources.* This implies including all parties in public dialogue to shape policies on access to and quality of care, and on resource allocation decisions, recognizing that a clinician's duty is to promote the good of patients, practice effective and efficient care, use resources responsibly, and advocate as vigorously for vulnerable and disadvantaged patients as for any other patient. Included in this principle is the understanding that all

involved parties (patients, clinicians, and insurers) are in discussion about what health care needs can reasonably be met with available resources, that all parties understand and honor the rules and coverage of their contracts, and that all commit to effective, quality health care with consistency and fairness.

3. *All parties should foster an ethical environment for the delivery of effective and efficient quality health care.* Implicit in this principle is the understanding that agreements between clinicians, health plans, and health care organizations are congruent with professional ethical standards, and that all parties share the ethical obligation to protect the confidentiality of patient health information.

4. *Patients should be well informed about care and treatment options and all financial and benefit issues that affect the provision of care.* This implies that patients receive sufficient and appropriate information to support informed consent or refusal of treatment, that clinicians disclose any potential conflict of interest to patients, and that purchasers and health plans inform patients of any arrangements that may influence care.

These principles do not solve the socioeconomic and political problems contributing to the rising cost and limited resources faced by the health care system. While nurses need to work to address these issues individually and as a profession, they must continue to deal with the ethical and moral dilemmas associated with these difficult issues in the changing health care environment. The purpose of these principles is to provide some guidance for ethical practice in a health care system where resources do not always meet the need, regardless of the setting.

ASK YOURSELF

Access to Health Care—Rights and Responsibilities

Much of the discussion regarding the health care delivery systems of the United States, as well as those of many countries in the world, is a commentary on access to what is termed *modern medical care.*

- How does access to health care affect an individual's participation in the health care system?

- What is our individual responsibility in the big picture of these vast health care systems?

- Do you consider health care a basic right? If it is a right, what are our individual responsibilities in ensuring this right for all citizens?

- What ethical issues arise when access to care is limited for some people and available to others?

ALTERNATIVE TRADITIONS OF HEALTH CARE

Indigenous populations in cultures throughout the world have traditional forms of health care that view humanity as connected to the wider dimensions of the Earth and nature. In developing countries, these forms of traditional healing systems provide comprehensive approaches to prevention of illness and promotion of health that go beyond the scope of modern medical care. The World Health Organization (WHO) refers to these systems as holistic—that is, viewing a person in totality within a vast ecological spectrum, and emphasizing the notion that illness or disease occurs as a result of an imbalance between the person and his or her ecological systems (WHO, 2012).

An important component of traditional systems of health care is their basis in models that take into account mental, spiritual, physical, and ecological factors in assessing health and well-being. A basic concept of all traditional health care systems is that of balance between mind and body, function and need, and individual, community, and environment. Illness or disease is thought to be a breakdown in the balance in one or more of these areas. Treatments are designed to restore health and balance between the individual and his or her internal and external environments. While these models of traditional health care systems have been considered primitive and unsophisticated by modern practitioners, increasing numbers of developing countries are showing a new interest in program development toward revitalizing these traditional systems. There are several factors at work in promoting this resurgence of interest.

The majority of rural populations of developing countries cannot afford Western types of medical health care. Rural people have to travel many days to reach the larger health care centers, resulting in loss of wages in addition to money spent for travel and medicines. For example, 80 percent of the population in some Asian and African countries depends on traditional medicine for primary health care (WHO, 2012). In Asia, the traditional systems are being incorporated into other, more formal health care systems to provide for care and to ease the burden of cost. India has over 200,000 traditional practitioners. In Thailand, the Ministry of Health promotes the use of traditional medicinal plants in primary health care, state-run hospitals, and health service centers. In Korea, 20 percent of the national health care budget is directed to traditional health care services. Health insurance coverage is available for both Oriental medical treatments and traditional health care methods (Bodeker & Burford, 2007).

In Africa, the governments are facing huge bills for the exploding AIDS crisis. These governments are exploring their traditional indigenous medicinal treatments for inexpensive and effective ways to relieve the suffering of AIDS patients. Health care providers in Uganda have been active in promoting research into traditional medicine for treating people with AIDS.

China has had a policy of integrating traditional health care into the national health care policy for over 40 years. The Chinese are trying to combine the modern and the traditional as formal components of health care provision. In China, the traditional health care providers perform the majority of care in the poor and rural communities. The country physicians are educated in a 3-year program that includes a combination of traditional medicine and modern medicine. Modern Western medicine is being strongly pursued at great financial cost to the government, but at the same time hospitals and health care systems offer a choice to patients. Persons who take advantage of these choices are often the older and the less affluent. As the country is opening up to capitalist beliefs and free enterprise, some Chinese citizens who now have the financial means to make different choices are choosing Western methods of treatments, and often ignore the tried-and-true Oriental methods for status reasons. The younger generation of Chinese seem to believe that what is Western is always better. In observing some of the health care delivery in China, there is evidence that the government, while allowing the practice of the ancient Oriental medicine, is putting a strong emphasis on the belief that technology is the answer to health care in this heavily populated country. This is especially disconcerting, in view of the fact that Oriental medicine and the tradition of health care with alternative choices have been functioning well for two thousand years, and Western health care providers are beginning to research and utilize these traditional systems of care in order to offer them to their patients.

ASK YOURSELF

What Do You Know About Traditional Healing?

Traditional methods of healing and health care have kept indigenous populations healthy and functioning for thousands of years. Many countries are trying to reinstate these practices to promote health and reduce the cost of health care and health care delivery.

- How do you think traditional and modern healing systems should relate to each other?
- What traditional methods of health care are available in your community or nearby area?
- With what traditional or folk health practices are you familiar? Have you or persons you know utilized these practices?

CHALLENGES FOR RURAL AND URBAN AGGREGATES

Problems in the delivery of health care to populations around the world occur not only because of expensive technology or lack of money to pay for insurance, but also because of geographic barriers. Rural populations in the United States and abroad often have to do without services because of lack of providers and facilities within a reasonable distance from their homes. Health care for persons in these populations requires a day off of work for travel and waiting in crowded waiting rooms. Many rural areas lack health care personnel, and emergency care is often nonexistent. In one mid-Atlantic state, all counties boast of an access to a 911 emergency number, but for some, the switchboard and EMT vehicle are three counties away and travel is over narrow mountain roads. Patients often delay treatment or do not become involved with prevention or health education plans because they require so much effort to accomplish. In addition, many rural citizens tend to be older persons for whom travel and finances are a great consideration in health care services.

The urban poor face similar access problems, not because care is geographically distant, but because access requires trips to places they cannot afford or free clinics, where lines are long and workers are few. Individuals are often required to take time from work, like their rural counterparts, in order to see a provider. Medications may be unaffordable. Large immigrant populations live in overcrowded situations in the urban setting. In addition to financial constraints, there may be language and cultural barriers and lack of knowledge about how to access the system.

Think About It

Health Care Changes and Challenges

The challenges and changes in health care can seem insurmountable and overwhelming. It can seem as though only the very wealthy will be able to have health care services. Some sociologists say that the middle class is disappearing and that this country, as well as other countries, will have only the rich and the poor. Health care costs are rising, and there seems to be no end to it.

- *How should these issues be addressed? What are appropriate nursing responses to these issues?*

- *What issues have you encountered in accessing health care providers for you and your family?*

- *Are you able to afford a comprehensive health plan? If not, what do you do when you become ill?*

- *How does the Affordable Health Care Act address some of these issues and concerns?*

SUMMARY

Global consciousness is needed to address twenty-first-century health care needs and issues. Nurses must be aware of and prepared to address the global concerns that have a significant impact on health and well-being of people and the planet. Nurses need to apply principles of beneficence, non-maleficence, and justice to their relationship with Earth as well as to humans. Recognizing that human health depends on the health of Earth, nurses must engage in and promote environmentally responsible health care locally and internationally. Examples of issues that need to be addressed include natural and other disasters, displaced persons, famine and malnutrition, child labor, human trafficking, use of torture, war and violence, genocide, unexploded bombs and land mines, pollution, global warming, epidemics and drug-resistant organisms, bioterrorism, and access to and financing of health care.

Historical awareness enables us to have a more informed view of circumstances in the present. Contemporary issues and concerns regarding health care delivery and financing are related to the historical interplay of advances in scientific and medical knowledge, social and political climate, and waxing and waning of economic and other resources. Current parameters within which health care providers function are changing. Acute-care hospitals are changing the focus of, and in some cases limiting, services, and many people are looking to the traditional healing systems of various cultures to provide needed health care services. Although some countries ensure access to basic health care services for their citizens, many individuals throughout the world have limited or no access to basic health care. Questions regarding access to and availability of resources are not new, but they must be addressed anew in light of the various currents within contemporary society. The future of the system is uncertain, and we must consider whether issues of the past are destined to repeat themselves. Perhaps we can take what is positive from the past, and blend this with both traditional and modern healing approaches in order to rescue a flawed health care system in this country and around the world.

CHAPTER HIGHLIGHTS

- Earth health and human health are intricately interconnected, and nurses need to include ethical considerations of our relationship with Earth into nursing practice. Twenty-first-century health care needs and issues require global consciousness. Nurses need to work individually and collectively both to meet the needs of those affected by global issues such as war, violence, disaster, famine, epidemics, and displaced persons, and to work as well to prevent the devastation these issues cause.

- Systems of health care, which have existed to address societal needs for healing from early civilization to the present, have been influenced by cultural, political, economic, religious, and scientific factors throughout history.

- Scientific and medical innovations, coinciding with the shift in Western nations from agricultural to industrial economies in the later nineteenth and early twentieth centuries, provided a basis for modern-day health care. Societal changes such as wars, women working more outside the home, and the influx of immigrants have raised new issues and concerns for health care delivery at various times in U.S. history.

- Skyrocketing health care costs can be traced to the advent of health insurance (1930s and later) and the enactment of Medicare and Medicaid (1960s), which removed incentives from health care institutions and physicians to keep costs down, and to public awareness of the availability of medical interventions, which prompted consumers to demand the best care and services available. Difficult decisions emerge with issues of access, cost, and justice.

- Expansion of hospital and other health care services has reached a point of crisis in which out-of-control health care costs have prompted imposition of external controls on institutions and health care providers. Many people have no means of paying for expensive services. Provisions of the Affordable Health Care Act of 2010 address issues related to limited health insurance coverage.

- Some nations provide basic health care services for their citizens, while people in many areas suffer from limited access to or availability of such services. People in both developing and industrialized countries are exploring ways to incorporate traditional and modern healing practices into contemporary health care systems, in an effort to utilize the benefits of both systems in meeting the health care needs of society.

- Problems of access to and payment for health care services are of special concern among rural populations and the urban poor.

DISCUSSION QUESTIONS AND ACTIVITIES

1. Read the Earth Charter at http://www.earthcharter.org and compare the principles it sets forth with those found in nursing codes and position statements such as those found at http://www.nursingworld.org, http://www.cna-nurses.ca, and http://www.icn.ch. How can the Earth Charter help us to integrate Earth ethics into nursing practice?

2. At the nursing websites just noted, explore, compare, and contrast position statements and policies related to disaster preparedness, displaced persons, war, violence, and other global health issues. Discuss with classmates.

3. Investigate disaster preparedness plans and policies in your town or city and health care agency.

4. Interview or read a biography of a person who worked as a nurse during or within the decade following World War II or the Vietnam War, and discuss nursing roles and duties, types of health concerns for which patients were hospitalized, and what were considered new therapies at the time. Compare the information you obtain to your experience of health care today.

5. Review nursing and medical journal articles and texts from the mid-twentieth century regarding issues of concern in practice and to the profession. Compare and contrast these issues to issues of current concern.

6. Imagine that it is the year 2040, and you are being interviewed by a nursing student about factors that affected health care delivery and financing in your early days in nursing. What would you say?

7. Discuss global issues related to health care delivery. Which of these issues would have the greatest impact on your nursing practice and why? Investigate health care issues in a non-industrialized country. Share with classmates how these issues might affect your nursing practice.

8. Describe the impact of health delivery and financing on patient care and outcomes. Identify potential ethical dilemmas related to current systems of delivery or financing. Study provisions of the Affordable Care Act at the following websites and discuss the impact of this law on patients, nurses, and the health care system.

    http://www.aarp.org/health/health-care-reform/info-01-2011/health_law_benefits_2011_and_to_come.html

    http://www.aarp.org/health/health-care-reform/

    http://nursingworld.org/MainMenuCategories/Policy-Advocacy/HealthSystemReform

    http://www.commonwealthfund.org/

    http://healthreform.kff.org

9. How would you suggest that traditional and modern healing practices and practitioners relate to each other?

REFERENCES

Achterberg, J. (1990). *Woman as healer*. Boston: Shambhala.

Alliance of Nurses for Healthy Environments. (2012). Retrieved from http://envirn.org

Ausubel, K. (Ed.). (2004). *Ecological medicine: Healing the Earth, healing ourselves*. San Francisco: Sierra Club Books.

Berry, T. (2009). *The sacred universe: Earth, spirituality, and religion in the 21st century*. Mary Evelyn Tucker (Ed.). New York: Columbia University Press.

Bodeker, G. C., & Burford, G. (2007). *Traditional, complementary, and alternative medicine: Policy and public health perspectives*. London, England: Imperial College Press.

Brewer, K. (2010). Who will be there? Ethics, the law, and a nurse's duty to respond in a disaster. *ANA Issues Brief*. Retrieved from http://www.nursingworld.org/MainMenuCategories/WorkplaceSafety/DPR/Disaster-Preparedness.pdf

Bullough, B., & Bullough, V. (1978). *The care of the sick: The emergence of modern nursing*. New York: Prodist.

Canadian Health Care. (n.d.) Canada's healthcare system. Retrieved February 28, 2012, from http://www.hc-sc.gc.ca/hcs-sss/index-eng.php

Chaudry, R. V. (2008). The precautionary principle, public health, and public health nursing. *Public Health Nursing, 25*(3), 261–268.

Crinnion, W. J. (2010). The CDC Fourth National Report of Human Exposure to Environmental Chemicals: What it tells us about our toxic burden and how it assists environmental medicine physicians. *Alternative Medicine Review, 15*(2), 101–108.

DeNavas-Walt, C., Proctor, B. D., & Smith, J. C. (2011). Income, poverty, and health insurance coverage in the United States: 2010. Washington, DC: U.S. Census Bureau. Retrieved from http://www.census.gov/prod/2011pubs/p60-239.pdf

Dossey, B. M. (2000). *Florence Nightingale: Mystic, visionary, healer*. Springhouse, PA: Springhouse.

Dossey, B., Selanders, L., Beck, D. M., & Atwell, A. (2005). *Florence Nightingale today: Healing, leadership, global action*. Kansas City, MO: American Nurses Association.

Gaudry, J., & Skiehar, K. (2007). Promoting environmentally responsible health care. *Canadian Nurse, 103*(1), 22–26.

Geller, A. M. (2009). The susceptibility of older adults to environmental hazards. *Generations: Journal of the American Society on Aging, 33*(4), 10–18.

Health Canada. (2012). Health care system. Retrieved February 28, 2012, from http://www.hc-sc.gc.ca/hcs-sss/index_e.html

International Council of Nurses. (2006a). Codes and declarations: Towards elimination of weapons of war and conflict—ICN position. Retrieved from http://www.icn.ch/images/stories/documents/publications/position_statements/E14_Elimination_Weapons_War_Conflict.pdf

International Council of Nurses. (2006b). Resources for disaster. Retrieved February 28, 2012, from http://www.icn.ch/disas_relatedpubs.htm

Interview. (2003). Baroness Cox of Queensbury. *Nursing Ethics, 10*(4), 441–445.

Judd, D., Sitzman, K., & Davis, G. M. (2009). *A history of American nursing: Trends and eras.* Sudbury, MA: Jones and Bartlett.

Kennedy, M. T. (2004). *A brief history of disease, science, and medicine.* Mission Viejo, CA: Asklepiad Press.

Magner, L. N. (2005). *A history of medicine.* Boca Raton, FL: Taylor & Francis Group.

McDonald, L. (2010). Florence Nightingale: Passionate statistician. *Journal of Holistic Nursing, 28*(1), 92–98.

Morrisey, M. A. (2008). *Health insurance.* Chicago, IL: Health Administration Press.

Murray, J. E. (2007). *Origins of American health insurance: A history of industrial sickness funds.* New Haven, CT: Yale University Press.

Myers, N. J., & Raffensperger, C. (Eds.). (2006). *Precautionary tools for reshaping environmental policy.* Cambridge, MA: MIT Press.

Nelson, M. (2004). Stopping the war on Mother Earth. In K. Ausubel (Ed.), *Ecological medicine: Healing the Earth, healing ourselves* (pp. 228–230). San Francisco: Sierra Club Books.

Nightingale, F. (1859/1992). *Notes on nursing: What it is and what it is not* (Commemorative ed.). Philadelphia: Lippincott.

Povar, G. J., Blumen, H., Daniel, J., Daub, S., Evans, L., Holm, R. P., ... Campbell, J. D. (2004). Ethics in practice: Managed care and the changing health care environment. *Annals of Internal Medicine, 141*(2), 131–137.

Raffensperger, C. (2004). The precautionary principle. In K. Ausubel (Ed.), *Ecological medicine: healing the earth, healing ourselves* (pp. 41–52). San Francisco: Sierra Club Books.

Rutkow, I. (2010). *Seeking the cure: A history of medicine in America.* New York: Scribner.

Sattler, B., & Lipscomb, J. (2003). *Environmental health and nursing practice.* New York: Springer.

Science & Environmental Health Network (SEHN). (2012). Precautionary principle. Retrieved from http://www.sehn.org/precaution.html

Selanders, L. C. (2010a). Florence Nightingale: The evolution and social impact of feminist values in nursing. *Journals of Holistic Nursing, 28*(1), 70–78.

Selanders, L. C. (2010b). The power of environmental adaptation: Florence Nightingale's original theory for nursing practice. *Journal of Holistic Nursing, 28*(1), 81–88.

Silva, M. C., & Ludwick, R. (2003). Ethics and terrorism: September 11, 2001 and its aftermath. *Online Journal of Issues in Nursing.* Retrieved July 24, 2006, from http://www.nursingworld.org/ojin/ethicol/ethics_11.htm

Stevens, R. (1989). *In sickness and in wealth.* New York: Basic Books.

Swimme, B., & Tucker, M. E. (2011). *Journey of the universe.* New Haven, CT: Yale University Press.

Tafoya, T. (1996, May). Embracing the shadow: Mending the sacred hoop. Paper presented at the South Texas AIDS Training (STAT) for Mental Health Providers: The Human, Transcultural, and Spiritual Dimensions of HIV/AIDS, San Antonio, TX.

Tschudin, V., & Schmitz, C. (2003). The impact of conflict and war on international nursing and ethics. *Nursing Ethics, 10*(4), 354–366.

Uhl, C. (2004). *Developing ecological consciousness: Path to a sustainable world.* Lanham, MD: Rowman & Littlefield.

World Health Organization. (2012). Traditional and complementary medicine. Retrieved February 28, 2012, from http://www.who.int/medicines/areas/traditional/en/

World Medical Association. (2011). *WMA Declaration of Montevideo on disaster preparedness and medical response.* Retrieved from http://www.wma.net/en/30publications/10policies/d3/index.html

C h a p t e r

14

HEALTH POLICY ISSUES

". . . every community is established for the sake of some good (for everyone performs every action for the sake of what he takes to be good)."

(Aristotle, Trans. 1931)

OBJECTIVES

After completing this chapter, the reader should be able to:

1. Describe the process by which issues become "political issues."

2. Distinguish between the terms *political* and *partisan*.

3. Give examples of specific political issues related to health care.

4. Discuss your personal stand on various political issues in relation to ethics.

5. Describe the health policy process.

6. Discuss the role of ethics in policy making.

7. Explain the role of nurses in the policy-making process.

8. Describe various methods of influencing public policy.

INTRODUCTION

We can view health policy in a number of different ways. In the current political climate, some perceive health policy as a political process, strongly influenced by ideology and party politics. Others view the health-policy-making process as a thoughtful one, by which decisions are made based on data and the rational analysis of needs, outcomes, and costs. In reality, the health policy process is a combination of both informed rational judgments and ideological partisan politics.

Nurses have become more involved in the political process, particularly in the realm of health policy. Nurses view health, at least in part, as dependent upon various environmental factors that can be altered by health policy decisions. Recognizing the role of patient advocate, and acknowledging the importance of being involved in regulatory processes, nurses are assuming more responsibility in the political arena. This chapter features examples of selected political issues as related to health policy, and describes specific methods that nurses can utilize to influence policy.

POLITICAL ISSUES

The term **political** relates to the complex process of policy making within the government. Government is an essential element of society, and politics is inherent in government. **Political issues** are those that are created, affected, or regulated by decisions within either the executive, judicial, or legislative branches of government. **Political parties** are organized groups with distinct ideologies that seek to control government. When political parties take opposing positions on an issue, the different opinions and subsequent decisions are said to be **partisan**. Though individuals may genuinely and independently agree with the position of a particular party, partisanism is sometimes portrayed in a negative light—that is, consisting of blind, prejudiced, and unreasoning allegiance to one political party. Because many people think that every problem in society can be solved by passing a law, legislatures make more and more laws to satisfy demands. Depending upon the existence of legitimate need or the interest or whims of society at large, special-interest groups, individuals, or government, any issue can become a political one.

An issue can become "political" in a number of ways. As discussed in Chapters 6 and 8, the administrative branch of government is involved in the operation of government agencies. State boards of nursing and medicine, for example, are administrative agencies charged with regulating the activity of specific groups of professionals or particular aspects of health care. Rules and regulations promulgated by these groups can have a profound effect upon health care delivery. Because positions on these boards are often granted through the process of political appointment, decisions are occasionally viewed as partisan. Examples of political issues influenced by the administrative branch include prescriptive authority for nurses in advanced practice and implementation of mandatory standards of care.

Think About It

Abortion—A Moral and Political Issue

Abortion, a moral issue, raises questions about basic beliefs regarding life and death, sanctity of life, the beginning of life, and a woman's individual rights. Over time, abortion has become a political issue. Examples of this change include legal arguments over women's choice versus the right to life, as in Roe v. Wade (1973); congressional discussions regarding public funding of abortions, including debate related to the level of coverage; and the definition of acceptable circumstances surrounding conception and abortion. Within the last two decades, the two major American political parties have polarized on the issue. One party supports the freedom of a woman to make her own decision, while the opposing party advocates the fetus's right to life. As a result, abortion has become a partisan issue.

- *What is your moral stand on abortion?*
- *How did you develop this stand?*
- *How is your opinion about abortion related to the position of the political party to which you belong?*
- *Would you support a particular party based solely upon one issue?*
- *What is the government's role related to moral issues? Explain your position.*
- *How does your opinion influence your ability to give quality care?*

The judicial branch of government influences health care professions and health care delivery through the common law system. As was noted in Chapter 8, judicial precedents take on the force of the law. Consider, for example, the profound effect on the American health care system of the landmark Supreme Court decision in *Roe v. Wade* (1973). Although the Supreme Court is considered a nonpartisan entity, partisan politics plays a tremendous role in judicial appointments. Supreme Court appointments are particularly important to political parties because of the potential to apply party ideology through the unusual power granted the Court in the United States, the small number of justices, the durability of Supreme

ASK YOURSELF

Is the Supreme Court Partisan?

Supreme Court justices are appointed by the president of the United States, with the advice and consent of the Senate. The Senate Judiciary Committee holds a series of hearings, during which the appointee is questioned on judicial and legal matters. The committee makes a recommendation on the suitability of the appointee; the entire Senate then votes to confirm or reject the president's appointment. Try to recall the confirmation process of nominees for the Supreme Court within the past 10 years.

• Were the prospective justices questioned about issues with moral/ethical implications?

• Were they questioned about their position on specific partisan issues?

• Why do you think it is important to political parties that judges with certain beliefs are appointed to the Supreme Court?

• What role does the Supreme Court have in shaping the country's health policy?

Court decisions, the Court's relative freedom from special-interest groups, and the fact that Supreme Court justices are appointed for their lifetime.

Nurses are most familiar with political issues in the legislative arena. These issues are the ones decided through the passage of federal or state laws. Within the legislative forum, nurses can influence the outcome of various political issues. Examples of well-publicized legislative issues with health care implications include: Medicare and Medicaid revisions; health insurance reform; and issues related to advanced practice nursing, such as prescriptive authority, scope of practice, and third-party reimbursement.

Nurses function in a variety of roles. They are citizens, knowledgeable consumers of health care, professionals whose practice is regulated by government, and advocates for patients. Responsible political involvement is an important function of each of these roles. Because nurses are individuals with a variety of backgrounds, experiences, beliefs, and values, their opinions about political issues are diverse. This diversity, when coupled with sensitivity to moral and ethical implications, provides a foundation for productive and fair policy discussions.

Political issues of particular interest to nurses fall into four distinct categories involving moral values, professional regulation, the health of individuals in society, and distributive justice. Nurses' opinions on these issues are based upon personal experience, ethical orientation, religion, cultural bias, and a number of other factors. Naturally, there is a healthy diversity of opinion among nurses on most issues—particularly those involving moral values. Figure 14–1 shows examples of selected political issues of interest to many nurses.

Issues Involving Moral Values
Beginning-of-Life Issues

- Abortion
- Use of Fetal Stem Cells
- Genetic Testing
- Contraception and Sterilization
- Human Cloning

Health Care Issues

- Medicare and Medicaid funding
- Medically Assisted Pregnancy
- Deciding for Infants and Children
- Procurement and Distribution of Harvested Organs
- Use of Animal Organs for Research and Treatment
- Informed Consent
- Patient's Bill of Rights
- Electronic Health Records and Health Records Privacy
- Prescription and Diversion of Controlled Substances

End-of-Life Issues

- Support for Home Care at the End of Life
- Active and Passive Euthanasia
- Physician-Assisted Suicide
- Patient Self-Determination

Issues Involving Professional Regulation
Nursing Education

- Entry into Practice
- Funding for Nursing Education and Research

Workplace Issues

- Mandatory Overtime
- Nurse-Patient Ratios

Advanced Practice Issues

- Third-Party Reimbursement
- Prescriptive Authority
- Scope of Practice

Issues Involving the Health of Individuals in Society
Environmental Health

- Clean Indoor Air

FIGURE 14–1   **Selected Examples of Political Issues**

- Clean Groundwater
- Air Pollution Control

Public Health

- Emerging Pandemic/Epidemic Diseases
- Bioterrorism
- Treatment and Reporting of STDs
- Family Planning Programs and Regulations
- Tobacco Legislation
- Childhood Immunizations
- Gun Control
- Seatbelt and Helmet Laws

Issues Involving Access to Care

- Social Security
- Medicare and Medicaid
- Regulation of Private Insurance
- Managed Care Legislation

FIGURE 14–1   (continued)

HEALTH POLICY

Because health plays a critical role in the physical, psychological, and economic condition of individuals, it affects society in general. The central purpose of health policy, therefore, is the improvement of the overall health of the population. Health policy is far reaching; it influences the behavior and decisions of people in relation to their environment and living conditions; it affects lifestyle and personal behavior; and it affects availability, accessibility, and quality of health care services. Health-related issues receive considerable attention in the policy-making forum.

Different people define health in different ways. The culture's prevailing definition of health affects the investment society is willing to make in specific health care programs. For example, if society defines health narrowly in terms of absence of illness, policy makers might choose to fund programs that focus on treatment of illness, but neglect programs that support health-promoting behaviors. In contrast, a society that defines health positively, in terms of wellness, would place more emphasis on funding programs to prevent illness or maximize health potential.

Health policies are formal and authoritative decisions focusing on health. Health policies are made in the legislative, executive, or judicial branches of government, and are intended to direct or influence the actions, behaviors, or decisions of others. Policy is comprised of a very large set of decisions. Examples of health policy include legislation, rules and regulations established for the purpose of implementing legislation, rules and regulations established to operate the government and its various programs, and judicial decisions related to health. **Statutes** or **laws** are pieces of legislation that have been enacted by legislative bodies and approved by the executive branch of government. **Rules** or **regulations** are policies that are established to guide the implementation of laws and programs. **Judicial decisions** are authoritative court decisions that direct or influence the actions, behaviors, or decisions of others. In addition to these different types of policies, there are also two broad categories of health policies—allocative and regulatory.

Allocative policies determine what programs are funded—that is, where the resources are allocated. This is the area in which we see distributive justice in practice. Allocative policies are essentially economic in nature. In most countries, these policies are geared toward guaranteeing access to goods and services for the disadvantaged. Allocative policies are based upon fundamental beliefs about which distinct group or class of individuals or organizations should receive the benefits. Policy makers realize that some will receive benefits, some will not, and others will bear the expense. Ideally, these decisions are based upon public objectives (Longest, 2010). The most well-known examples of allocative health policies are those of Medicare and Medicaid. All of the major nurses associations actively promote various allocative policies. For example, the Canadian Nurses Association (CNA) actively pursues legislation focused on human resources in the workforce; the International Council of Nurses (ICN) pursues international policies on health services for migrants, refugees, and displaced persons; and the American Nurses Association (ANA) promotes equitable third-party reimbursement for advanced practice registered nurses.

Regulatory policies are those designed to direct the actions, behavior, and decisions of individuals or groups. These policies place rules on health care delivery. There are five basic classes of regulatory policies:

1. Market-entry restrictions;

2. Rate or price-setting controls on providers;

3. Provider quality controls;

4. Market-preserving controls; and

5. Social regulation (geared toward such socially desired ends as safe workplaces and nondiscriminatory provision of health care). (Longest, 2010)

As with all policies, the purpose of regulatory policy is to ensure that public objectives are met. Many nurses do not realize the impact regulatory policies have on nursing practice. Following are selected examples of recently debated regulatory policies: policies that would allow people their choice of providers, including advanced practice nurses; policies to require health records privacy; policies to protect workers from accidental needlestick; policies to restrict mandatory overtime; policies to set nurse-patient ratios; and policies to require employers who provide health insurance to include contraception coverage.

The Health Policy Process

The process of health policy includes three distinct phases. These phases are both consecutive and circular. The first phase is that of **policy formulation**. This phase includes such actions as agenda setting and the subsequent development of legislation. The second phase is that of **policy implementation**. This phase follows enactment of legislation, and includes taking actions and making additional decisions necessary to implement legislation, such as rule making and policy operation. The final stage is **policy modification**. The purpose of this stage is to improve or perfect legislation previously enacted. This might entail only minor adjustments made in the implementation phase, or it may involve major changes or the elimination of particular statutes (Longest, 2010).

Policy Formulation

The first phase of policy making is policy formulation. This phase is divided into two distinct sequentially related sets of activities: agenda setting and legislation development (Longest, 2010). At any point in time, there is a complex mix of three variables: health-related problems, possible solutions and alternatives, and diverse political interests. As agenda setting progresses, the emerging issues can proceed to the development of legislation.

Problems. The existence of real or perceived problems is the impetus for the policy-formulation phase of policy making. Problems may become evident in a number of ways. Some problems occur as the result of the interaction of certain variables related to previous policy. For example, it is likely that the predicted shortfall of Social Security is related to a policy that did not take into account inequities between promised benefits and escalating costs. Other problems may gain attention as they reach unacceptable levels. Growth in the numbers of people with AIDS is an example of this type of problem. Other problems emerge as a result of some specific event that forces public attention. Examples of this type of problem include the discovery of medical waste products washing up on beaches and the development of a new drug for treating AIDS that is so expensive few people can afford to purchase it (Longest, 2010). Nevertheless, the mere existence of problems is not always sufficient to ensure the formulation of legislation. There must also be feasible solutions to the problems and the political will to enact legislation.

Solutions. Someone must come up with an idea to solve a problem before legislation is initiated. The process of offering solutions to problems involves generating ideas for solving the problems, refining the ideas, and selecting from among the options (Longest, 2010). *Nursing's Agenda for Health Care Reform* (ANA, 1991) is an important example of the profession's early attempt to participate in the formulation of specific solutions to problems of health care access.

Political Circumstances

Even if nurses identify a serious problem and offer feasible solutions, they may not be able to influence legislation. Legislation can only progress through the process with the sponsorship of influential policy makers who believe in the issue and invest time and energy. Potential sponsors are sensitive to the political will of their party, constituents, and colleagues. Factors that influence political will include public attitudes, concerns, and opinions surrounding an issue; the preferences and relative ability to influence political decisions; the positions of key political leaders on the issue; and the other competing items on the policy agenda. Creating a political thrust forceful enough to cause policy makers to formulate and implement new policy is often the most difficult problem (Longest, 2010). Nurses are a significant percentage of the voting population. They are in a good position to collectively influence political decisions and enhance the political will essential to formulate health policy.

Policy Implementation

Policy implementation immediately follows the enactment of legislation. Because legislation seldom contains explicit language on how it is to be implemented, details are left to the process of rule making. For example, the various states' boards of nursing are responsible for promulgating rules related to nursing practice. Generally, these organizations accept input from affected groups during the rule-making process. Interest groups routinely seek to influence rule making, because they are so often the targets of rules established to implement health policies. **Lobbying** is one of the major means by which interest groups attempt to influence policy makers. Lobbying is especially intense when various interest groups disagree upon the formulation of a particular policy.

Think About It

Health Care Reform Initiatives

Health care access has been a critical social issue since the 1980s and has become one of the most divisive political issues of the past three decades. On September 22, 1993, President Bill Clinton introduced the American Health Security Act. Following months of high-level negotiation and planning, this reform package included many of the ideas presented in at least 11 separate proposals made within the preceding 5 years. Administration officials thought the public and many special-interest groups were demanding a radical reform of the health care system. Leah Curtin (1996), nursing leader and ethicist, predicted in May of 1991 that there would be a universal access system within 3 to 8 years. Yet Clinton's proposal, along with all of its predecessors, failed. Universal access did not become a reality. In 2010, President Barack Obama signed into law the Patient Protection and Affordable Care Act, a law that phases in reforms of some aspects of private and public insurance programs by prohibiting exclusion of pre-existing conditions and expanding insurance access to millions of Americans (H.R. 3590—111th Congress: Patient Protection and Affordable Care Act, 2009). This law had an extreme polarizing effect on the political parties, with many political leaders praising the law as landmark legislation and others vowing repeal it.

- *A great deal of time and energy was invested in the policy-formulation phase of health care reform. How effective do you believe leaders were in this phase of each bill?*

- *What was the problem being addressed? How clear was the problem?*

- *Do you think the influence of special-interest groups affected the eventual outcome of the two proposed bills? Explain your thinking.*

- *At what point in the policy-making process do you think the proposals succeeded or failed?*

Policy Modification

Policy modification occurs when outcomes, perceptions, and consequences of existing policies indicate either that the original problems still exist or that new problems have arisen from unforeseen circumstances or from the policy itself. The policy-modification phase is intended to spiral backward, with feedback, into the agenda-setting and legislation-development stages of the formulation phase—potentially creating new legislation—and spiral forward into the rule-making and policy-operation stages of the implementation phase, stimulating changes in rules or operations. Many programs are routinely amended, some of them repeatedly, over a period of many years. These modifications may reflect, among other things, the development of new technologies, changing economic conditions, and public demand (Longest, 2010). The change in Medicare that added prescription drug coverage is an example of the policy-modification process.

Ethics in Policy Making

Policy making is an inherently ethical endeavor because it affects people's lives, their relationships, and the distributive justice process. The outcomes and consequences of most health policy affect large groups of people. There are two equally important functions of ethics in public policy making. In the policy-formulation phase, ethics can guide the original development of new policies. Ethics is also useful in the policy-modification phase as a means to examine the immediate and far-reaching effects of policies that are already implemented. There is, however, some practical difficulty in adhering strictly to specific ethical principles during the policy-making process. Policy formulation and criticism involve more complex data and forms of reasoning than ethical principles can handle. Disagreements about public policy can turn on differences in basic beliefs and interpretations, as well as uncertainties. Ethical principles provide the moral background for policy decisions, but participants must take into account complex empirical data and specialized disciplinary knowledge such as that of nursing and medicine (Beauchamp & Childress, 2008). Thus, health policy is so complex that it prohibits the strict and exclusive use of specific rules or principles in guiding policy formulation; rather, the authors suggest that ethical considerations must be accompanied by the rational use of empirical data.

Think About It

Ethics and Politics of Tobacco Sales

The sale and distribution of tobacco products has become a highly publicized political issue. The tobacco industry is increasingly affected by legislative and judicial decisions regarding the health effects of tobacco.

- *What are the ethical issues of which the policy makers should be aware?*
- *Can you think of ethical arguments in favor of regulating the production and sale of tobacco products?*
- *Can you think of ethical arguments in favor of allowing the industry to operate on the free market, unrestricted?*
- *There are judicial precedents that assign at least some responsibility for the health problems of smokers to the tobacco companies. Is this a legal, ethical, or political issue, or some combination of these?*
- *Is this an issue in which nurses should be interested? What factors determine whether nurses should be interested in this issue?*

Research Data in Policy Making

To influence policy we must furnish officials with important and reliable information. If they have reliable facts and research findings, policy makers are able to identify problems, make comparisons, confirm trends, and establish policy based on evidence. Because time is a precious commodity, officials are often more interested in research findings than unsubstantiated personal opinion. When preparing to discuss policy with officials, nurses should carefully review objective data, pertinent research findings, and a few particularly attention-getting personal stories. Cost savings often gets attention when other facts elicit little response.

The federal government recognizes the importance of health care research in the development of policy. Established by Congress as part of the 1989 Omnibus Budget Reconciliation Act, the Agency for Healthcare Research and Quality (AHRQ) was created to improve the quality, safety, efficiency, and effectiveness of health care for all Americans. The agency supports and disseminates health services research to improve the quality of health care and promote evidence-based decision making. The AHRQ is a bridge between clinicians, consumers, policy makers, payers, and other health officials.

NURSING, POLICY, AND POLITICS

Not since the days of Lavinia Lloyd Dock have nurses been so actively involved with health policy. It is through the perspective of knowledge, experience, and intimacy with the health care needs of people that nurses are in the unique position to bring insight and balance to the policy-making process. Moreover, professional codes of ethics identify the goals and values of the profession, and explicitly call for nurses to be involved in policy formulation. For example, the ICN *Code of Ethics for Nurses* (2006) calls for nurses to share with society the "responsibility for initiating and supporting action to meet the health and social needs of the public, in particular those of vulnerable populations." The ANA *Code of Ethics for Nurses* (2001) clearly describes nurses' responsibility for health policy participation as follows:

> The nurse collaborates with other health professionals and the public in promoting community, national, and international efforts to meet health needs. The nurse has a responsibility to be aware of ... broader health concerns such as world hunger, environmental pollution, lack of access to health care, violation of human rights, and inequitable distribution of nursing and health care resources. [The nurse] participates in legislative and institutional efforts to promote

health. In addition, the nurse supports initiatives to address barriers to health, such as homelessness, unsafe living conditions, and lack of access to health services. Nurses can work individually as citizens or collectively through political action to bring about social change. It is the responsibility of a professional nursing association to speak for nurses collectively in shaping and reshaping health care within our nation, specifically in areas of health care policy and legislation that affect accessibility, quality, and the cost of health care. Here the professional association maintains vigilance and takes action to influence legislators, reimbursement agencies, nursing organizations, and other health professions. In these activities, health is understood as being broader than delivery and reimbursement systems, but extending to health-related sociocultural issues such as homelessness, hunger, violence, and the stigma of illness.

The formulation of health policy requires strong nursing leadership and an understanding of the crucial role of local and national policy making. To do this, nurses must develop the ability to think, teach, research, and act in ways that are relative to policy. They must be aware of the impact that policies have on health and on clinical practice. They must conduct research on health policy issues and find strategic ways to influence state and national policy agendas. Recognizing health problems as policy issues is the first step toward policy formulation.

Nursing's Political Strengths

Nursing enters the political arena with notable strengths. First, because it is the most sizable group of health care providers, the nursing profession boasts an extremely large number of political constituents. Acting together, nurses have the potential to be a formidable political force. Second, nurses have traditionally been perceived favorably by the public. Research has repeatedly shown that the public views nurses with respect, trust, and admiration. They view nurses as being honest and having ethical integrity. Third, once nurses become involved in health policy, they usually continue to be active (Gebbie, Wakefield, & Kerfoot, 2000).

Nursing's Political Weaknesses

The profession also has a number of political weaknesses. First, being relatively new to the political arena, many nurses are not astute or comfortable in policy-making or lobbyist roles. Second, there has historically been a lack of ideological and political unity within the profession, a weakness Hadley (1996) believes stems from the lack of uniform educational requirements and titles. Third, though nurses comprise the largest number of professionals, they have fewer funds specifically earmarked for intense lobbying than many other special-interest groups.

Policy Goals for Nursing

How do nurses become aware of the issues that are important and require energy and focus? Each of us has the responsibility to reflect upon problems and potential solutions. In addition, one of the major functions of professional organizations is to provide leadership and assistance to members in political and other matters. Congruent with nursing codes of ethics, each of the major nursing associations provides specific issues and strategies for nurses interested in policy making. Each organization clearly highlights its legislative and policy agendas on its website. Organizations such as the ANA, the CNA, the ICN, and the American Academy of Nurse Practitioners share the goals of maintaining nursing control of nursing practice, making a positive impact on health care policy, advocating on behalf of the vulnerable, and instituting workplace reforms.

Think About It

Nurses Take Positions on Political Issues

The American Nurses Association (ANA) has been a powerful lobbying force for many years. Issues of interest to members of the organization are freely accessible through the ANA's website at http://www .nursingworld.org/. This site includes ANA legislative position statements, fact sheets, and transcripts of congressional testimony. It also includes transcripts of some pertinent legislation. The ANA has been active in advocating policy for many issues, including the following: campaign finance reform, child and elder care, civil rights, collective bargaining, domestic violence, drug control policy, family and medical leave, gun control, homelessness, malpractice/liability reform, migrant and seasonal farm worker health issues, pay equity, rural health care, and sexual harassment. These are but a few of the issues the ANA has been involved in over the past decade.

- *Why do you think the professional organization published these position statements?*
- *Why are nurses concerned with issues such as campaign finance reform and gun control?*
- *What impact do you think the profession could make if each nurse became familiar with all of the issues and promoted them to policy makers?*
- *Can you identify any issues within your state that affect the health of your patients or your practice?*
- *How could you begin the process of health policy formulation for this issue?*

LOBBYING

Sometimes nurses are privileged to be legitimate members of governmental or institutional policy-making bodies. More often, the nurse's role in policy formulation, implementation, and modification is that of informal lobbyist. Lobbying involves advocating for an issue that is affected by the decisions of policy makers. Lobbyists cultivate relationships and employ the art of persuasion as they attempt to influence officials toward their point of view. Lobbying is essential to the proper functioning of the U.S. government and is specifically protected by the First Amendment to the Constitution: "Congress shall make no law ... abridging ... the right of the people peaceably ... to petition the Government for a redress of grievances." Lobbying provides a forum in which to resolve conflicts among diverse and competing points of view. It also provides information, analysis, and opinion to policy makers, which promotes informed and balanced decision making.

Lobbyists have a powerful voice in determining the policy-making process, from agenda setting to policy modification. In fact, some nurses believe it is a nurse's duty to participate in political **activism**. There are others who believe that constrained, subtle, and persistent political activity is more effective in the long term than overt activism.

To be effective in the political domain, nurses need to become politically astute. Nurses who are politically active must be aware of trends in the political climate, must access powerful political leaders, and must learn how to play the game. Knowing the power players in the political arena is one of the most important steps in the lobbying process.

Methods of Lobbying

The most familiar type of lobbying is the face-to-face approach. This process involves either meeting directly with a policy maker to request a desired action or testifying at a hearing. When possible, both paid and volunteer lobbyists should utilize the face-to-face method of lobbying. A second form of lobbying is **grassroots lobbying**. Grassroots lobbying involves mobilizing a committed constituency to influence the opinions of policy makers. Different types of grassroots lobbying include organized letter writing and implementing campaigns designed to mobilize public opinion.

One of the most important facets of lobbying is knowing whom to lobby. In seeking help to promote a particular legislative agenda, nurses want to begin by enlisting policy makers who have the following characteristics: (1) legitimate power, (2) an interest in the problem, (3) an affinity for nursing or for health care issues in general, (4) time and energy to invest in the process, (5) the respect of colleagues, and (6) committee or other positions that are appropriate to the particular legislation. Finding an official with all of these characteristics will greatly improve the probability of legislative success. New lobbyists waste time and energy lobbying officials who are uninterested, have conflicting loyalties, are powerless, or are not respected by their colleagues. The first step in lobbying is to connect with the appropriate policy makers.

The Lobbying Campaign

Once nurses have identified the appropriate policy-making officials and are familiar with the issues and the legislative and regulatory process, the lobbying campaign can begin. There are two basic types of lobbying: direct and indirect. Indirect lobbying strategies are geared toward influencing public opinion, which in turn will influence policy makers. Methods of indirect lobbying include media broadcasts, newspapers and other written materials, dissemination of the results of opinion polls, paid advertisements, educational campaigns, and organizations' agendas. Direct methods include party platforms, political elections, membership on committees, participation in agency regulation development, face-to-face lobbying, letter writing, and contact with policy makers during social events (deVries & Vanderbilt, 1992).

Letter Writing. Handwritten, personal, mass letter and e-mail writing is a powerful grassroots lobbying technique. Certain letter-writing techniques have been found to be more effective. Here are some practical tips for letter writing:

- Whenever possible, individualize and legibly handwrite or type letters on personal stationery or send e-mails. Though more effective than no letters at all, form letters are much less likely to be read by officials than personal correspondence.

- Write the letter or e-mail in your own words, using your own thoughts and logic and drawing pertinent inferences.

- Identify yourself as a nurse and state your reason for writing in the first paragraph, including the title and number of the legislation in which you are interested.

- Be specific and include key information and examples supporting your position.

- Be explicit. Tell the official exactly what you want. If you are writing to ask for co-sponsorship or a vote for or against a bill, say so.

- Be brief but informative.

- Include only one topic.
- Never threaten or use hostility. This immediately destroys your chances of developing a cooperative relationship.
- Offer your assistance as a resource.
- Promptly thank the official for favorable votes.

Personal Visits. A personal visit is usually a more powerful lobbying tool than letter writing. Whenever possible, nurses should seize the opportunity to meet with policy makers face to face. Following are a few suggestions for personal visits with policy-making officials:

- Be prepared. Develop your plan of action and know what you intend to say.
- Be on time for your appointment and be patient if the official is late.
- Be courteous and greet the official with a firm handshake, introduce yourself, and present your business card.
- Identify the subject of the meeting and present your facts in an orderly, succinct, calm, and direct fashion.
- Support your position with personal experiences and anecdotes; use valid research and statistics when appropriate.
- Keep your presentation simple. Avoid technical language and professional jargon. Your goal is to inform and influence, not to impress.
- Close the meeting strongly and effectively, asking for the official's support.
- Leave a short fact sheet summarizing the issue and your position. Include the names and telephone numbers of contact people.
- Send a letter within a few days thanking the official for the meeting, restating your position, and including any information requested during the meeting.

Political Campaigns

One very effective direct lobbying technique is for nurses to become involved by either supporting candidates or running for elective office themselves. To begin, nurses can become involved in campaigns and elections. This can be done in any number of ways. First, nurses can become involved in political party organizations. Political party activity serves as a vehicle for developing important relationships with elected officials. Involvement in a political party is essential to building a political network. Second, nurses can become involved through district and state nurses' associations. These organizations

Think About It

Be Careful of Your Wording

Nurses must be careful in choosing words to use when lobbying. One nurse relates a story of her first experience testifying before a state legislative committee. Feeling that her presentation was well prepared and would be effective, the nurse decided at the last minute to substitute the words nurse voters *for the word* nurses. *There were many people giving testimony that day. Following the completion of the testimony phase, the legislators were given an opportunity to make comments or ask questions. There were no questions. Every comment was directed toward the nurse, who was surprised to learn that the legislators perceived the term* nurse voters *as a veiled threat. They did not hear the substance of the presentation, but rather the perceived threat, "If you do not support our position, we will vote you out of office." By unintentionally giving this impression, the nurse ruined a productive relationship with these legislators. The legislation that the nurses were supporting failed.*

- *Why do you think the nurse changed the wording of her presentation in the first place?*

- *What words would you have used?*

- *Describe similar circumstances in which you were speaking and the reaction of the listeners was based upon their inferences from your choice of words rather than their intended meaning.*

- *How can nurses avoid mistakes of this sort?*

provide an opportunity to meet candidates, form relationships, and offer candidates forums. Forums remind a candidate that nurses are an organized group interested in politics and public policy and acquaint nurses with the candidate's position on important issues. Third, nurses can become actively involved in campaigning for candidates who support their positions on various health care issues. This may take the form of campaigning door-to-door, stuffing envelopes, or publicly endorsing candidates. Actively supporting candidates for public office helps to forge relationships with officials and elect candidates to public office who will sympathize with issues important to nurses. Involvement with political parties and the consequent relationships with public officials can also lead either to nurses' candidacies and election to public office or nurses' appointments to important policy-making positions.

SUMMARY

Many political issues are important to nurses. Most issues for which nurses are actively concerned relate to health policy: issues of a moral nature, issues related to professional regulation, issues related to public health, and issues related to distributive justice. Fulfilling the role of advocate, nurses are challenged to become politically active: to know and become involved with important issues, to learn the political process, to form relationships with public officials, and to become astute in methods of influencing health policy.

CHAPTER HIGHLIGHTS

- The term *political* relates to the policy-making process within the government.
- Political issues are those that are created, affected, or regulated by any of the government branches.
- Political parties are organized groups with distinct ideologies that seek to control government.
- Partisan issues are those issues for which the political parties have distinct ideology.
- Health policies influence the actions, decisions, and behaviors of people in the domain of health.
- Society's definition of health reflects the extent to which society is willing to move toward maximizing the health of citizens.
- Allocative health policies are designed to provide benefits to a distinct group.
- Regulatory policies are designed to influence others through directive techniques.
- The process of health policy includes the phases of policy formulation, policy implementation, and policy modification.
- There are two important functions of ethics in public policy making— guiding the original development of policy and criticizing previously implemented policy.
- Nurses are able to affect health policy through various political means.

DISCUSSION QUESTIONS AND ACTIVITIES

1. Explore the following websites, paying close attention to health policy issues and strategies:

   a. American Nurses Association: http://www.nursingworld.org

   b. Canadian Nurses Association: http://www.cna-nurses.ca/CNA/default_e.aspx

   c. International Council of Nurses: http://icn.ch/index.html

2. Discuss the issues on the organization sites listed previously. How do the issues fit with the organizations' codes of ethics? How would you prioritize the issues?

3. Visit the Kaiser Family Foundation website at http://www.kff.org/. Which of the issues highlighted on the website are health care policy issues? Discuss how nurses could impact the policy makers on these issues.

4. Discuss the issues listed in Figure 14–1 in class. How do classmates' positions compare to those of the major political parties? Are each student's opinions politically consistent from issue to issue?

5. Discuss the following question in class: What purpose do political parties serve?

6. Compile a list of political issues and classify them as to the branch of government with which the issue is most closely aligned—administrative, judicial, or legislative.

7. Discuss methods for influencing health policy in the administrative and judicial domains.

8. Compile a list of at least five political issues related to health that have been decided within the judicial domain. How have the judicial decisions affected health care delivery?

9. Compile a list of political issues related to moral values. Discuss the role of the professional organization in guiding members' actions related to these moral issues.

10. Discuss popular definitions of health and determine how each definition, if adopted by government, would affect health care delivery.

References

American Nurses Association. (1991). *Nursing's agenda for health care reform.* Kansas City, MO: Author.

American Nurses Association. (2001). *Code of ethics for nurses.* Washington, DC: Author.

Aristotle. (trans, 1931). *Politics* (C. D. C. Reeve, Trans.). Indianapolis, IN: Hackett.

Beauchamp, T. L., & Childress, J. F. (2008). *Principles of biomedical ethics* (6th ed.). New York: Oxford University Press.

Curtin, L. (1996). *Nursing into the 21st century: Health care reform, restructuring, practice, leadership.* Springhouse, PA: Springhouse.

deVries, C. M., & Vanderbilt, M. W. (1992). *The grassroots lobbying handbook: Empowering nurses through legislative and political action*. Washington, DC: American Nurses Association.

Gebbie, K. M., Wakefield, M., & Kerfoot, K. (2000). Nursing and health policy. *Journal of Nursing Scholarship, 32*(3), 307–315.

Hadley, E. (1996). Nursing in the political and economic marketplace: Challenges for the 21st century. *Nursing Outlook, 44*(1), 6–10.

H.R. 3590—111th Congress: Patient Protection and Affordable Care Act. (2009). In *GovTrack.us* (database of federal legislation). Retrieved from http://www.govtrack.us/congress/bill.xpd?bill=h111-3590

International Council of Nurses. (2006). *The ICN code of ethics for nurses*. Geneva, Switzerland: Author. Retrieved July 12, 2006, from http://icn.ch/icncode.pdf

Longest, B. B., Jr. (2010). *Health policymaking in the United States* (5th ed.). Ann Arbor, MI: AUPHA Press/Health Administration Press.

Roe v. Wade, 410 U.S. 113 (1973).

C h a p t e r

15

ECONOMIC ISSUES

I begin with the assumption that suffering and death from lack of food, shelter, and medical care are bad. I think most people will agree about this. . . .

(Singer, 1972, p. 229)

OBJECTIVES

After completing this chapter, the reader should be able to:

1. Describe the role of economics in health care.

2. Explain the concept of distributive justice.

3. Discuss utilitarian, libertarian, communitarian, and egalitarian theories.

4. Discuss basic questions related to the distribution of health care resources.

5. Describe recent trends in health care economics and the relationship of economic trends to the delivery of health care.

6. Discuss ethics in relation to managed care systems of health care delivery.

INTRODUCTION

Nursing, other health care professions, and the overall health care delivery system exist to deliver health care to society. Over the past several decades, dynamic forces have worked together to create a complex system that has been called the best in the world. From advances in knowledge and technology to changes in health care financing, the system has experienced rapid and drastic changes. It is not unusual to hear the term "crisis" used to describe the state of the current health care system. This crisis relates to problems with cost, quality, and access to health care services. Current debates about social justice are fueled by inequalities in access to health care and health insurance, combined with dramatic increases in the costs of care. Thoughtful, systematic consideration of ethics is necessary for the process of devising solutions to the current problems. This chapter discusses particular aspects of health care economics, distributive justice, and emerging trends.

OVERVIEW OF TODAY'S HEALTH CARE ECONOMICS

Though given its own twists, the history of economic thought is closely associated with the utilitarian movement in the last century (Honderich, 2005). One of the main assumptions in traditional economics is that we should judge the institutions of a society by the preferences of the people whom those institutions affect. There are different ways to judge the total preference of society. One method claims that one arrangement is better than another only if it satisfies the preferences of some people and does not frustrate the preferences of any others. This idea is at the center of what is known as welfare economics. Another method suggests that one arrangement is better than another only if it is preferred by people allowed to make a collective choice. Given that institutions are only properly judged according to the preferences of the people they affect, the institution of health care should be judged by the people it serves. Discussion and debate about the current state of health care economics is integral to the process of evaluating the present system and formulating one that is more just.

Today's problems in the health care system have a long history, with many intervening factors. Partially as a result of lawsuits, we have produced a system with progressively higher standards that require the most and best care for a large segment of the population, regardless of cost. This spiraling pattern is combined with irresponsibility caused by a third-party reimbursement system that (in the past, at least) did not require the providers or patients to be careful of cost. This has led to a skewed model that focuses heavily on technology and personal autonomy, and ignores basic principles of social responsibility and distributive justice. Except for newer managed care programs, this system features an odd split between the patients and physicians who make the spending decisions and the third-party payers who must actually pay for those decisions (Morreim, 1995). Moreover, there are staggering contrasts within this system. In an age when millions of dollars are spent on futile care, much of the population has no access to even basic health care services.

Before the advent of managed care, most health care was "fee-for-service" in which ethics was predominately driven by codes of ethical behavior and patients' rights statements, with a strong focus on the principle of autonomy. The fee-for-service model focuses on the individual patient, protects physician autonomy, promotes treatment that offers potential benefit or prolonged life, and assumes unlimited resources. Much of health care continues to be financed in this way. Analysts have recognized that there are ethical problems associated with this model, including the paradoxical extremes of overutilization and rationing of care.

ASK YOURSELF

Paying for Futile Care

One hears stories about elderly patients with terminal illness—and even "no code" status—who remain in intensive care settings for extended periods of time, often because family members insist that everything be done for their loved ones.

- Is the expenditure of expensive health care resources appropriate for these types of situations? Explain your position.
- Who should bear the financial burden for futile care?
- What are the ethical principles that conflict in situations of this sort?

Though most people agree that modern health care in America is highly sophisticated and technologically advanced, they also recognize that there are many deficiencies in the system. First, health care services and resources have been inaccessible to a large segment of the population. Second, health care costs are accelerating at an unsustainable annual rate, consuming a huge portion of the gross domestic product. Third, the high cost of health care threatens the competitiveness and profitability of business and industry. Fourth, the benefits to the individual and corporate providers within the system are often pursued at the expense (and sometimes harm) of persons who are in need of health care. DeBlois, Norris, and O'Rourke (1994) propose that the real problems with the current system are related to its priorities and the values and commitments that support them, the most significant of which are:

1. An extreme form of individualism that routinely prefers individual interests over concerns about the community of persons;

2. An endorsement of profit making as a primary motive for providing health care services; and

3. An uncritical acceptance of technology as morally neutral and as un-ambiguous in the service of human goods and goals. (deBlois et al., 1994, p. 55)

DeBlois et al. charge that the health and well-being of people subjected to a system under the influence of these values are often threatened by the kinds of services offered, the manner in which they are provided, and the priorities that determine both. Further, if improvements in the system are intended to promote health and well-being of people, efforts need to be ethically grounded and challenge the values that drive the present system.

DISTRIBUTIVE JUSTICE

The ethics of **justice** relates to fair, equitable, and appropriate treatment in light of what is due or owed to persons, recognizing that giving to some will deny receipt to others who might otherwise have received these things (Beauchamp & Childress, 2008; Honderich, 2005). The "others" may be those living in a person's community, those in other communities, or even those yet to live. For example, if Social Security becomes bankrupt through excessive expenditures in the present, others who would have received benefits in the future (even if they are not yet born) will be denied these benefits. As mentioned in Chapter 3, the relevant application of the ethical principle of justice within the health care system focuses on the fair distri-bution of goods and services. This application is called **distributive justice**. Beauchamp and Childress (2008) define distributive justice as the fair, eq-uitable, and appropriate distribution of diverse benefits and burdens such as property, resources, taxation, privileges, and opportunities. Because there is a scarcity of resources and competition for resources and services, it is impossible for all people to have everything they might want or need. One of the primary purposes of government is to formulate and enforce policies that deal with distribution of scarce resources.

Three areas of health care are relevant to questions of distributive justice: Which population groups should be the recipients of health care resources? What percentage of society's resources is it reasonable to spend on health care? Recognizing that health care resources are limited, which aspects of health care should receive the most resources? These are important questions that are both practical and ethical in nature.

Entitlement

In deciding questions of distributive justice, we must ask, "Who is entitled to these services?" As with all of ethics, there is no universally accepted answer. Distribution of limited resources is the function of various levels of governing bodies. In attempting to distribute limited resources fairly, leaders will seek systematic means of deciding. Historically, these questions have been answered by **material rules** such as the following: to each person an equal share, to each person according to need, to each person according to merit, to each person according to social contribution, to each according to the person's rights, to each person according to effort, to each person according to ability to pay, or to each person according to the greatest good to the greatest number. Most societies will utilize several of these principles in establishing public policies. We find many of these principles in effect in the United States, where, for example, welfare payments and many health care programs are distributed on the basis of need; jobs and promotions in many sectors are awarded on the basis of demonstrated achievement and merit; comparably high incomes of some are awarded on the basis of superior effort, merit, or potential social contribution; and the opportunity for basic education is distributed equally to all citizens (Beauchamp & Childress, 2008).

ASK YOURSELF

Is Health Care a Right or a Privilege?

- Discuss whether you think health care is a right or a privilege. Explain your thinking.
- Should all people have access to the same health care services regardless of ability to pay? How should ability to pay influence access to health care services?
- If you believe health care is a right, to how much health care is each person entitled?

Right to Health Care

In examining who should receive care, we ask questions about the basic right to health care. Is health care a right, or a privilege? This is a question that is debated fiercely in the media, in the professional and political arenas, and around the dinner table. Is society responsible for providing health care for all citizens, and if so, to what degree? Should each person be eligible for minimum basic health care, or should everyone be allowed to have everything there is to offer, from organ transplants to tummy tucks? Would the public benefit from a strict free-market system that would provide health care services only to those who can pay, or should the government be responsible for the health care needs of all citizens? If health care is a right and health care resources are scarce, what resources are allocated to which group of people? These and other questions fuel the debate about the right to health care.

Discussion of health care as a right is not new. On December 10, 1948, the General Assembly of the United Nations adopted the Universal Declaration of Human Rights, which identifies medical care as a necessary social service. Article 25 of the document states that "Everyone has the right to a standard of living adequate for the health and well-being of himself and of his family, including food, clothing, housing and medical care and necessary social services, and the right to security in the event of unemployment, sickness, disability, widowhood, old age or other lack of livelihood in circumstances beyond his control" (United Nations, 1948). In 1983, the President's Commission for the Study of Ethical Problems in Medicine and Biomedical and Behavioral Research (1983) concluded that society has a moral obligation to ensure that everyone has access to adequate care without being subject to excessive burdens. The commission made a clear distinction between society and government, recognizing that a collective or societal obligation does not imply that government should be the primary institution involved in making health care available but, rather, that government should participate with the private sector.

The issue of health care as a right has some basis in constitutional law. Some argue that the "general welfare" clause in the Preamble of the U.S. Constitution implies the protection of basic needs, including a right to the protection of health. The President's Commission for the Study of Ethical Problems in Medicine and Biomedical and Behavioral Research (1983) reported that neither the Supreme Court nor any appellate court has found a constitutional right to health care, but many federal and state statutes have been interpreted to provide statutory rights in the form of entitlements to some vulnerable groups. As a consequence, these groups have benefited from many legal decisions.

The concept of health care as a right is not universally accepted. There are those who believe that health care is a privilege to be enjoyed by some, but beyond the common advantage of all citizens. The entrepreneurial model of libertarianism declares that health care is not a right, but rather a commodity that must be purchased on the open market like any other service. This model compares the health care professional's right to conduct a practice and charge fees with other business's right to do likewise. It can be argued that this model provides health care only for those who can pay, or for those who are given health care services as a gift. It is hypothesized that, as a result of a free-market system of health care delivery, supply-and-demand and pricing competition would result in lower health care costs. This in turn would result in health care services becoming more accessible to a larger portion of the population. Except for the fact that professionals can choose to provide services free of charge, this model makes little allowance for children and the very poor (Beauchamp & Childress, 2008).

How Much and to Whom?

If one accepts that health care is a right or that society has an ethical obligation to provide health care services to vulnerable populations, then one is required to examine the question of how much health care is to be provided, and to whom. There are two broad views about the right to access to health care: some believe all should have equal access to health care, while others believe the right extends only to a decent minimum of health care. Consider the following case.

Case Presentation

Should Public Funds Pay for Extraordinary Procedures?

There was a recent court case in which a middle-aged indigent woman who suffered from insulin-dependent diabetes mellitus demanded that Medicaid pay for a pancreas transplant. This patient was reported to be uncooperative in her previous diabetic regimen and disliked giving herself insulin injections. Even though Medicaid in that state has a fiscal policy that denies payment for this surgery to all program recipients, the state supreme court ruled that this woman had a right to the surgery because other people with insurance or adequate funds have access to the surgery. The decision was based on the principle of nondiscrimination.

Think About It

Decisions About Entitlements

- *Do you think the patient had a "right" to this surgery? Why or why not?*
- *Should society (through taxes) pay for the surgery, even though the patient was known to be nonparticipative in her previous regimen? Why or why not?*

(continued)

- *Should the government make arbitrary decisions permitting or prohibiting certain therapies? Explain.*
- *Do you think there were others who might have received benefits but were subsequently denied them because extraordinary funds were used for this patient?*
- *What are the ethical implications of the court decision?*
- *What are ethical arguments for and against the court decision?*

Fair Distribution

The court's decision to require public payment for the pancreas transplant in the previous case study raises questions about restricting health care services. Few people would argue that there are enough resources to pay for all services. Think about your household budget. If you have only $300 to spend on Christmas gifts for your three sisters and you also need to purchase groceries for the week and antibiotics for yourself, it would be foolish to spend $200 on one gift. By doing that, you would ensure that your sisters would not be treated equitably, that you probably would not be eating very well for the next week, and that you would not feel well anyway, since you could not afford your prescription medication. The same principle applies to health care dollars. The limited public budget must be divided among many interests. In order to maintain a functioning infrastructure, the government must ensure that public schools, highways, police, national defense, Social Security, and other services in the public domain have a proportionate share of the total budget. Policy makers are charged with the difficult task of making equitable decisions about distribution of resources. These decisions must balance health care spending with other programs, and must carefully avoid both extravagant excess spending and frugality that threaten the health of citizens.

Distribution of Resources

Limited health care dollars must be spent wisely. There are several different criteria that have been proposed to make distributive justice decisions. One method involves making judgments about cost in relation to predicted benefit. For example, we could question the practice of allowing patients in the last stages of terminal illness to monopolize limited and expensive intensive care beds, thus utilizing the most expensive kind of health care for the least benefit. Some propose that the best way to avoid making arbitrary decisions in these kinds of situations is to set mandatory guidelines. For example, some suggest that expensive therapies, such as dialysis or organ transplant, be reserved only for those below a certain age. A second method involves making judgments about the usefulness of given therapies. Immunizations, for example, are cost effective and benefit a large percentage of the population. Some would suggest that less costly therapies that are nearly guaranteed to help a large number of people are the ones that should have priority.

Theories of Justice

Distributive justice is based upon common morals and ethics. Several theories have been proposed to determine how resources and services should be distributed. Utilitarian, libertarian, communitarian, and egalitarian theories are examples of popular theories of justice. Because of society's fragmented beliefs about social justice, no single theory can be expected to bring coherence to the situation. Many countries seek the best possible health care for all citizens, while at the same time instituting cost-containment programs. The U.S. health care system promotes the ideal of equal access to health care while maintaining some aspects of free-market competition. The goals of superior, accessible, and affordable health care are very difficult to reach simultaneously. Pursuing one goal may cripple another (Beauchamp & Childress, 2008). Recognizing that no single theory will satisfy society by fulfilling all principles, we suggest that several theories of justice be used to understand competing social goals.

Utilitarian Theories

Based, in general, upon the rule that it is good to maximize the "greatest good for the greatest number," **utilitarian theories** favor social programs that protect public health and distribute basic health care in a manner that maximizes the overall benefit. This is based on the belief that the outcome of these programs maximizes utility. Although these theories are the basis of many social programs, there are problems in their application. For example, because utilitarianism places aggregate social good before individual rights, social utility might be maximized by denying access to health care for some of society's sickest and most vulnerable populations (Beauchamp & Childress, 2008).

Libertarian Theories

Libertarian theories propose that the just society protects the rights of property and liberty of each person, allowing citizens to improve their circumstances by their own effort. Libertarian theories support a private citizen's or group's right to own and manage a health care business. Libertarian theory does not classify health care as a right, but rather as a commodity that operates on the material principle of ability to pay either directly or indirectly through insurance. Strict libertarians view taxation as an unjust redistribution of private property, but do not oppose other methods of distribution if they are freely chosen. Market strategies and managed competition are proposals in the United States that are influenced by libertarianism (Beauchamp & Childress, 2008).

Communitarian Theories

Communitarian theories place the community, rather than the individual, the state, the nation, or any other entity, at the center of the value system. Less fully developed than utilitarianism or libertarianism, communitarianism emphasizes the value of public good and maintains that values are rooted in communal practices. Communitarians believe that human life will be better if collective and public values guide people's lives. They have a commitment to facilities and practices designed to help members of the community develop their common lives and hence their personal lives (Honderich, 2005). Modern communitarian writers disagree on the application of these theories to health care access. Some propose a federation of interlinking community health programs that are democratically administered by citizen-members. In this model, each individual program would determine which benefits to provide, which care is most important, and whether expensive services will be included or excluded. Another communitarian theory holds that community tradition includes commitments of equal access to health care, and suggests that as long as communal funds are spent, services must be equally available (Beauchamp & Childress, 2008).

Egalitarian Theories

Egalitarian theories are related to the concept of equality, in which people who are similarly situated should be treated similarly, though much depends on what kinds of similarity count as relevant and what constitutes similar treatment (Honderich, 2005). Promoting ideals of equal distribution of social benefits and burdens, egalitarian theories recognize the social obligation to eliminate or reduce barriers that prevent fair equality of opportunity. These theories are cautiously formulated to avoid requiring equal sharing of all possible social benefits. A leading proponent of egalitarianism, John Rawls, suggests that in making decisions of justice, one should examine the situation behind a veil of ignorance. In this hypothetical situation, "no one knows his place in society, his class position or social status, nor does anyone know his fortune in the distribution of natural assets and abilities, his intelligence, strength, and the like" (1996, p. 567). This veil of ignorance ensures that no one is able to design principles to favor his or her particular condition. Supporters of Rawls's theory recognize a positive social obligation to eliminate or reduce barriers that prevent fair equality of opportunity, and suggest that health policy formulated according to egalitarian principles would guarantee a safety net or minimum floor below which citizens would not be allowed to fall (Beauchamp & Childress, 2008).

ASK YOURSELF

Making Fair Decisions

- Which theory of distribution appeals to you as the most fair and equitable? Why?

- Do you think the theory you chose would be fair to all people in all circumstances? Discuss your thinking.

- Could you combine two or more theories to make a system that is fair and equitable?

RECENT TRENDS AND HEALTH ECONOMIC ISSUES

Questions of ethics and distributive justice began to be discussed well before the 1980s. Claims that the United States was experiencing a crisis in health care economics have escalated in the last three decades. Skyrocketing expenditures and a general tightening of health care dollars resulted in fiscal scarcity. Both government and business responded by attempting to gain control over expenditures. This tightening assumed a variety of forms, including managed care systems, prospective payment, Medicare and Medicaid, and utilization review. Sacrificing, in part, the traditional focus on the welfare of patients, health care corporations devised ways to cut costs, improve profits, increase efficiency, and branch out into more profitable ventures such as landscaping, catering, and laundry service.

Government was the prime mover of cost containment during the early 1980s. Having experienced virtually no incentives for cost controls up to this point, hospitals were unprepared in the 1980s when the government instituted the payment system based on Diagnosis Related Groups (DRGs). This shift represented the first major change in the way hospitals were paid for Medicare patients, and placed the responsibility for efficiency and cost savings on hospitals and physicians. Certificate of Need programs were established to restrain the building or purchasing of unnecessary and expensive technologies and capital construction. Organizations such as Professional Standards Review Organizations (PSROs) and Peer Review Organizations (PROs) were established to require physicians to develop more efficient practice standards (Sherrill, 1995). By the early 1990s, the system was in a state of disequilibrium. Large hospital corporations were finding ways to cut costs by utilizing such methods as eliminating support services and reducing nursing staff, and many small rural hospitals were closing as a result of the financial strain. Inherent problems were unsolved. Care remained excellent though expensive for some, but inaccessible to many.

Economic influences also arose from outside the health care system. Two of the major outside influences were increased malpractice litigation and employment-negotiated health insurance plans. Malpractice litigation resulting in huge awards and the subsequent birth of defensive medicine added to the expense of the system. Califano (1986) attributes this to dynamic forces that included elements from many distinct programs and entities. The system moved from one that traditionally called for community standards to one in which scientific invention; medical technology; specialization; Medicare and Medicaid; and regional heart, cancer, and stroke centers required nationalized standards of care for physicians. This resulted in the routine practice of ordering batteries of diagnostic tests to meet new, stricter standards. Fearing malpractice litigation, physicians began to lose a measure of the autonomy that would have allowed them to choose only the diagnostic tests they thought were appropriate.

Employment-negotiated insurance plans fueled the practice of overspending and added to these pressures. Negotiated as part of employment contracts, many health insurance plans featured 100 percent coverage of health care costs with a zero deductible. As a result, a large percentage of patients did not pay directly for any health care services; thus, the cost of the doctor or hospital was rendered irrelevant (Califano, 1986). Everyone expected the most and best. Being indifferent to the costs of the medical services, patients were much more likely to buy more of them, even those that were of marginal utility or duplicative. Hospitals and physicians were more than happy to participate. For hospitals and doctors alike, maximizing services resulted in increased cash flow and consequent lessening of financial problems. This trend contributed to even higher standards of care that required very aggressive diagnosis and treatment, resulted in greater costs, and opened the door for more malpractice litigation.

Health Care Reform

The President's Commission on the Health Needs of the Nation (1952) concluded that access to health care is a basic human right, and the President's Commission for the Study of Ethical Problems in Medicine and Biomedical and Behavioral Research in 1983 concluded that "society has an ethical obligation to ensure equitable access to health care for all" (p. 4). Even so, the U.S. federal government has experienced political controversy over its attempts to implement comprehensive health care legislation. Recognizing problems in the health care delivery system and sensing a groundswell of public support, the Clinton administration devised a health care reform proposal. Unveiled in the fall of 1993, this proposal called for universal access to health care through managed competition. It also described a system of financing that would be accomplished primarily through mandated coverage at places of employment, with employers required to pay a large percentage of the premiums. Subsidies were planned for small businesses, and the federal government assumed the employer responsibility for persons who were not covered by employer-based plans.

After months of highly publicized debate, the Clinton health care reform proposal was defeated. Examining the defeat in terms of ethics, Jean deBlois (1995) attributes the failure to four fundamental factors: a lack of social consensus on the question of a right to basic health care for all persons; the strength and energy of those who argued on behalf of individual rights and liberties over the needs of the community or the nation; unconstrained powerful interest groups; and little or no recognition that substantive reform required a significant challenge to the values that inform and drive health care.

Having lost features intended to ensure integrity within the new system, managed care was the only piece that emerged unscathed from Clinton's health care reform proposal. Existing as a small part of the U.S. health care system for several decades, managed care gained prominence as a preferred method of delivery and financing of health care services (deBlois, 1995).

As we move toward the second decade of the twenty-first century, there continues to be a global crisis of health care access. Millions of people in the United States and billions of people worldwide have limited access to health care services, often because of a lack of health insurance coverage. The uninsured population in the United States is growing rapidly. In 1982, there were an estimated 32 million uninsured citizens. Although the percent of uninsured peaked at 16.3 percent in 1998, the total number continues to increase. In 2000, the number was 38.7 million (U.S. Census Bureau, 2001). By 2010 the number of uninsured had risen to 49.9 million, which constituted 16.3 percent of the population (DeNavas-Walt, Proctor, & Smith, 2011).

As a result of the failure of Clinton's 1993 health care reform, piecemeal and incremental efforts by disparate public and private groups moved toward relieving the problem of health care access. A network of free clinics was established to serve the indigent in all 50 states. The National Association of Free and Charitable Clinics (2012) reports that over 1,200 free clinics serve the uninsured and underinsured patients, generating billions of dollars in health care services. The Children's Health Insurance Program (CHIP) provides health insurance in all states for uninsured indigent children who do not meet the Medicaid guidelines (U.S. Department of Health and Human Services, 2012). Various states have enacted or attempted legislation to improve health care access. Oregon enacted legislation to provide all citizens universal access to a basic level of care. The program was initiated in 1987 and continues to undergo policy modifications (Oregon Department of Human Services, 2004). Massachusetts enacted legislation in 2006 that requires all residents to purchase health insurance or face legal penalties. President Barack Obama sponsored a new plan for health reform in the United States. The bill passed the U.S. House and Senate, and on March 23, 2010, President Obama signed into law the Patient Protection and Affordable Care Act (PPACA). This law was the major health care reform legislation of the 111th U.S. Congress. The newly enacted law reforms some aspects of public and private health insurance, increases coverage for pre-existing conditions, and expands access to insurance to more than 30 million Americans. Although the previously listed strategies are based on different economic and ethical foundations, they are a few among many attempting to reach the same goal—improving health care access.

Managed Care

Managed care is a health care system that attempts clinically and financially to control primary health care services in a medical group practice through elimination of redundant facilities and services, for the purpose of reducing costs. It is an integrated form of health care delivery and financing that represents attempts to control costs by modifying the behavior of providers and patients. Managed care moves away from a system based on patient and provider autonomy. According to supporters, managed care lowers costs through the elimination of waste and excess. The lower costs result in benefits to each patient and the membership as a whole. Aiming toward lower premiums and preventive care benefits, managed care organizations claim that members receive appropriate, quality care. In this regard, managed care is attentive to the needs of the membership as a group, as well as the needs of individual patients. As a result of the goal of lower costs, some propose that patients in managed care plans can be saved from unnecessary tests and treatments, which are viewed as a risk inherent in the traditional system.

Raising questions about the ethics of managed care, Fiesta (1996) discusses four notable legal cases that have resulted in significant financial losses for managed care organizations. These cases involved patients who experienced unfavorable outcomes as a result of managed care providers' efforts to follow program policy in cutting costs. One case involves an infant who was febrile, moaning, panting, and flaccid when the parents consulted the managed care emergency line. (See Chapter 8, where this case was discussed in detail.) Even though there were closer hospitals, the parents were instructed to take the child to a hospital that was nearly an hour away because it offered reduced cost to the managed care plan. The infant suffered a cardiac arrest en route. After resuscitation, both of the child's hands were amputated as a result of extraordinary complications. The family was awarded a $45 million verdict in a malpractice suit against the health maintenance organization.

In another case, the court concluded that by limiting enrollees' choice of provider to those on a specified panel, there is an unreasonable risk of harm to members if the selected clinicians are incompetent or unqualified. Another case involved the refusal of a physician assigned to a particular patient to admit the patient to the hospital. Although assigned by the managed care organization as the primary care provider for the patient filing suit, the physician argued that a physician-patient relationship did not exist because he had never seen the patient. Refused admission to the hospital as a result of this disagreement, the patient experienced a stroke in the hospital's parking lot. The court held that the plan's designated physician owed the patient a duty of care as a result of an implied physician-patient relationship inherent in the plan's enrollment agreement. In another case, the court rendered a $90 million verdict based upon a managed care organization's refusal to cover a bone marrow transplant. The court held that the managed care organization's internal utilization review decisions were unduly influenced by financial incentives to minimize care. Each of these cases illustrates ethical problems associated with balancing utilitarian views of cost-effective care with a respect for persons and the traditional view of a duty to care.

ASK YOURSELF

Ethical Problems in Managed Care

- What ethical problems can you foresee with managed care economics?
- How do you think nurses will be affected by managed care?
- How do you think nurses can influence the resolution of ethical problems in managed care?

Ethics in Managed Care

We must pay particular attention to the potential for ethical abuses that occur as a result of managed care organizations' unique role of both payer and provider of health care services. Like American society as a whole, the ethics community was slow to recognize the profound ethical implications of managed care. Based upon the assumption that the basic ethical criterion for the planned allocation of resources in a managed care setting at the policy level is the well-being of the entire group for whom the decisions are being made, balanced by the requirement of respect for individual health care needs, the following list of considerations is suggested for managed care organizations:

1. Relationships are critical in the delivery of health services. They should be characterized by respect, truthfulness, consistency, fairness, and compassion.

2. Health plans, purchasers, clinicians, and the public share responsibility for the appropriate stewardship of health care resources.

3. All parties should foster an ethical environment for the delivery of effective and efficient quality health care.

4. Patients should be well informed about care and treatment options and all financial benefit issues that affect the provision of care. (Povar et al., 2004)

SUMMARY

Because health care is a scarce resource, citizens rely upon social institutions to make fair and equitable distributive justice decisions. There is little consensus on basic ethical questions such as: Who should receive health care resources? Is there a right to basic health care? How much should be spent on particular health care services? What percentage of the society's overall resources should be invested in health care? Utilitarianism, libertarianism, communitarianism, and egalitarianism are theories that attempt to describe fair means of distributing resources. Recent focus on problems related to the economic aspects of the health care delivery system of the United States has prompted debate on practical issues of distributive justice. Emerging from the struggle to reform the health care system, managed care is becoming a major component of the health care system. While moving from a traditional system that valued patient and provider autonomy to a system that values the economic delivery of health care to a particular population, close attention must be paid to ethical standards in health care.

CHAPTER HIGHLIGHTS

- The history of economic thought is closely associated with the utilitarian movement in the last century.
- The traditional health care system in the United States is fee-for-service.

- Within a fee-for-service system, there is a strong focus on the principle of autonomy.

- Justice relates to fair, equitable, and appropriate treatment in light of what is due or owed to persons, and recognizes that giving to some will deny receipt to others who might otherwise have received these things.

- Distributive justice is the fair, equitable, and appropriate distribution of benefits and burdens. Theories of distributive justice seek to render diverse principles coherent.

- Utilitarian theories are based upon the rule that it is good to maximize the greatest good for the greatest number.

- Libertarian theories propose that the just society protects the rights of property and liberty of each person, allowing citizens to improve their circumstances by their own effort.

- Communitarian theories place the community—rather than the individual, the state, the nation, or any other entity—at the center of the value system.

- Egalitarian theories are related to the concept of equality in which people who are similarly situated should be treated similarly.

- Scarcity of health care resources has led to a rethinking of the structure of health care economics.

- Managed care gives rise to ethical problems associated with balancing utilitarian views of cost-effective care with a respect for persons and the traditional view of a duty to care.

DISCUSSION QUESTIONS AND ACTIVITIES

1. Read the Summary of Conclusions of the 1983 President's Commission for the Study of Ethical Problems in Medicine and Biomedical and Behavioral Research on the following website: http://bioethics .georgetown.edu/pcbe/reports/past_commissions/securing_access.pdf. Discuss ways that the federal government has attempted to respond to the report.

2. Read Article 25 of the United Nations 1948 Declaration of Human Rights at http://www.un.org/rights/. List current private national and international efforts toward assuring this right.

3. Visit America's Health Insurance Plans online at http://www.ahip.org/ to find out the managed care perspective on various economic and policy issues.

4. Discuss current problems in health care economics with classmates. Is there a consensus regarding root causes, the right to health care, or the role of the government as a payer for health care services?

5. Go to the library and find a basic economics text. How does the health care system differ from other free-market systems?

6. Discuss the influence of utilitarian theory on the economics of the current health care system.

7. Why do patient and provider autonomy affect health care delivery and financing?

8. Define *distributive justice*. In class, discuss the material rules of distributive justice. Which material rule is most popular among classmates?

9. What method of distributing goods and services do you think is fair and equitable? Do your classmates agree with your theories?

10. Discuss health care ethics as related to managed care.

11. Discuss opinions about the Patient Protection and Affordable Care Act.

REFERENCES

Beauchamp, T., & Childress, J. (2008). *Principles of biomedical ethics* (6th ed.). New York: Oxford University Press.

Califano, J. A., Jr. (1986). *America's health care revolution: Who lives? Who dies? Who pays?* New York: Random House.

deBlois, J. (1995, Autumn). Ethical issues and managed care: Asking the right questions. *Health Care Ethics, USA*, 3(4), 6–7.

deBlois, J., Norris, P., & O'Rourke, K. (1994, Autumn). *A primer for health care ethics: Essays for a pluralistic society* (pp. 5–6). Washington, DC: Georgetown University Press.

DeNavas-Walt, C., Proctor, B. D., & Smith, J. C. (2011). *Income, poverty, and health insurance coverage in the United States: 2010.* U.S. Census Bureau, Current Population Reports (pp. 60–239). Washington, DC: U.S. Government Printing Office.

Fiesta, J. (1996). Legal update, 1995: Part 2. *Nursing Management*, 27(6), 24–25.

Honderich, T. (Ed.). (2005). *The Oxford companion to philosophy* (2nd ed.). New York: Oxford University Press.

Morreim, E. H. (1995). *Balancing act: The new medical ethics of medicine's new economics.* Washington, DC: Georgetown University Press.

National Association of Free and Charitable Clinics. (2012). About us. Retrieved from http://www.nafcclinics.org/about-us

Oregon Department of Human Services. (2004). Oregon health plan: A historical overview. Retrieved July 19, 2006, from http://www.oregon.gov/oha/healthplan/data_pubs/ohpoverview0706.pdf

Povar, G. J., Blumen, H., Daniel, J., Daub, S., Evans, L., Holm, R. P., . . . Campbell, A. (2004). Ethics in practice: Managed care and the changing health care environment: Medicine as a profession managed care ethics working group statement. *Annals of Internal Medicine, 141*(2), 131–136. doi: 141/2/131 [pii]

President's Commission on the Health Needs of the Nation. (1952). *The contribution of health education in meeting the health needs of the nation.* Washington, DC: U.S. Superintendent of Documents.

President's Commission for the Study of Ethical Problems in Medicine and Biomedical and Behavioral Research. (1983). Securing access to health care: A report of the ethical implications of differences in the availability of health services. Retrieved from http://bioethics.georgetown.edu/pcbe/reports/past_commissions/securing_access.pdf

Rawls, J. (1996). A theory of justice. In J. Feinberg (Ed.), *Reason and responsibility: Some readings in basic problems of philosophy* (pp. 567–572). Belmont, CA: Wadsworth. (Reprinted from *A theory of justice* by J. Rawls, 1971, Cambridge, MA: Harvard University Press.)

Sherrill, R. (1995, January 9–16). Medicine and the madness of the market. *The Nation,* 45–72.

Singer, P. (1972). Famine, affluence, and morality. *Philosophy & Public Affairs, 1,* 229–243.

United Nations. (1948). Declaration of human rights. Retrieved July 18, 2006, from http://www.un.org/rights/

U.S. Census Bureau. (2001). Health insurance coverage: 2000. Retrieved July 18, 2006, from http://www.census.gov/prod/2001pubs/p60-215.pdf

U.S. Department of Health and Human Services. (2012). Children's Health Insurance Program. *Medicaid.gov.* Retrieved from http://www.medicaid.gov/Medicaid-CHIP-Program-Information/By-Topics/Childrens-Health-Insurance-Program-CHIP/Childrens-Health-Insurance-Program-CHIP.html

16

SOCIAL ISSUES

What we are doing is just a drop in the ocean, but if that drop was not in the ocean . . . the ocean would be less because of that missing drop.

(Mother Teresa)

OBJECTIVES

After completing this chapter, the reader should be able to:

1. Explain how social conditions such as poverty, homelessness, intimate partner violence, human trafficking, an increasing elderly population, and racism affect health.

2. Apply the concept of justice to vulnerable populations, elaborating on the implications for society and the health care system.

3. Discuss the application of beneficence and nonmaleficence to vulnerable groups in light of today's health care system.

4. Identify the pros and cons of promoting autonomy for health care decision making among vulnerable populations.

5. Analyze evidence of victim blaming within the health care system.

6. Illustrate application of the concepts of advocacy and nonviolence to care of vulnerable populations.

7. Examine current research for application to culturally diverse groups.

INTRODUCTION

Health is unquestionably a product of the person and environment interchange. Thus, social conditions that alter the person and environment interchange process are critical concerns for nurses and nursing students. Nurses confront social issues that shape the health and health care management of individuals on a daily basis. These social issues may create conflicts in values and ethical dilemmas that must be addressed in order to determine appropriate health care interventions for involved individuals. The purpose of this chapter is to help elucidate the principles inherent in decision making when social issues create ethical dilemmas for the nurse.

SOCIAL ISSUES

Many pervasive social issues are of special concern to health care providers. Poverty, homelessness, intimate partner violence, human trafficking, an increasing elderly population, and racism are examples of some of these very important concerns. Each of these issues is reviewed briefly in this chapter, along with the dominant guiding principles for related ethical decision making.

Poverty

Poverty and homelessness continue to be prevalent in the United States as a consequence of the overall economy and changes in government assistance programs and taxes. Health care is influenced more and more by poverty, as increasing numbers of people lack health insurance due to lack of employment and limitations in employment-based health insurance. Due to shifts in governmental budget priorities and changes in federal and state guidelines, a publicly financed health care system for medically indigent adults has become available to fewer people, and meets only a fraction of the needs of enrolled individuals. Without health care coverage, the poor often postpone needed health care, or cope with public clinics that are often degrading and impersonal.

Except for children covered under the Medicaid Children's Health Insurance Program, federal programs for the indigent cover only about half of all individuals living on incomes below the poverty level. Individuals without coverage must find health care systems that will provide free care, or do without. For this reason, many people living below the poverty level do not participate in basic preventive care programs.

Poverty, growing worldwide, is known to have a negative impact on both the health of individuals and the receipt of health care services (Chaufan, Davis, & Constantino, 2011; Dashiff, DiMicco, Myers, & Sheppard, 2009; Kushell, Gupta, Gee, & Haas, 2006; Romeo, 2005; Sapolsky, 2005). Poorer people are sicker than people with adequate financial resources. While poverty is detrimental to the health of all individuals living with inadequate resources, it produces a next generation of citizens with more health problems than usual. Children living in poverty have a higher incidence of conditions associated with trauma, poor nutrition, drugs, burns, mental illness, and HIV infection (Child Trends Data Bank, 2012). Children living in poverty are more likely to experience poor nutrition, inadequate exercise, and diseases from environmental factors such as vermin or lead. They are more likely to grow up with chronic illnesses that require extensive health care resources. Overall, poverty and health are inextricably enmeshed.

Case Presentation

Socioeconomic Influences on Health

Martha D. is a 69-year-old African American woman who lives in a substandard, cold-water, third-floor walk-up apartment in a housing project with a high crime rate. She draws a small Social Security check that does not cover living expenses. Her income is supplemented by food stamps, housing assistance, and by working as a nanny for three small children for 20 hours a week. Ms. D. earns minimum wage for her job as a nanny, and accepts cash for her work to avoid any interference with her Social Security check. She uses public transportation to go to and from her job, spending $3.00 each working day on bus fare.

Ms. D. helps her alcoholic single daughter, age 47, with two teenage children, especially when the daughter is experiencing a drinking binge. The children frequently stay with Ms. D. and rely on her for food, shelter, and love. Mr. D. is an alcoholic and has not been home for 2 years; however, he does occasionally call from a homeless shelter or treatment facility. Neither the daughter nor Mr. D. contribute to household expenses, but Ms. D. is very devoted to her family, especially her two grandchildren.

Martha D. is 5'8" tall and weighs 285 pounds. She has hypertension, with her blood pressure ranging from 200/90 to 250/110. She is on medication for her blood pressure, and the physician has linked her with a county home health nurse to encourage a diet and simple exercise regime for her obesity and hypertension. Ms. D. is beginning to show signs of type II diabetes and has been encouraged to lose weight and adhere to a diabetic diet. In addition, Ms. D. has some small ulcerations on her left ankle.

The home health nurse visits Ms. D. and instructs her in the care of her ulcers, advising her to keep her left foot elevated as much as possible. The nurse spends considerable time explaining a 1,200-calorie diabetic diet with moderate sodium restriction to Ms. D., and talks with Ms. D. about the need to begin walking as soon as the ulcers on her foot heal. Ms. D. lets the nurse know she used to attend a weight control group and understands low-fat and diabetic diets. However, she says coming home to a nice pot of beans, fried chicken, and biscuits is her only daily pleasure. "I've lived 69 years on this diet, don't wish to change, and have nothing to lose if I remain on it the rest of my life." She also points out that it is not safe to walk in her neighborhood, so she stays inside. In addition, she indicates that she is too tired to exercise after working all day.

Think About It

Who Decides What Is Best for a Patient?

- *Consider Ms. D.'s decision to ignore recommendations regarding diet, exercise, and, perhaps, care of her ankle ulcerations in relation to autonomy, beneficence, and nonmaleficence.*

- *Since the principle of beneficence requires actively doing good for Ms. D., who decides what is good?*

- *Discuss implications of justice and health care for Ms. D.*

- *How would you approach Ms. D. about her health issues?*

Homelessness

Homeless individuals, although not a homogenous group, are increasing in society. While good census data are hard to obtain, estimates suggest that approximately 3.5 million people are homeless in the United States, 1.35 million of whom are children (National Coalition for the Homeless, 2012a). The homeless are not all mentally ill or substance abusers. The new homeless are often families, single women with children, veterans, and the elderly. Like those living in poverty, homeless people suffer from acute and chronic health problems. Their health problems include those resulting from limited access to care, those coincident with homelessness, and those associated with the psychosocial burden of homelessness (John & Law, 2011; Kushell et al., 2006; National Coalition for the Homeless, 2012a; Romeo, 2005). Health problems resulting from limited access to care include exacerbated or advanced conditions that would have responded to early and thorough intervention. Health problems coincident with homelessness include illnesses resulting from living with inadequate nutrition, warmth, hygiene, safety, and other basic needs. Health problems associated with the psychosocial burden of homelessness are primarily mental illnesses, suicide, assault, and substance abuse, which can dull the anxiety of homelessness. The percentage of homeless children who have a chronic health problem is well above the rate for children who are not homeless. The homeless, like those living in poverty, have few options for health care, limited access to care, and difficulty with follow-up treatment or compliance. This is due, in part, to the typical model of health care delivery in the United States.

The health promotion model generally views health as the absence of disease and associates common diseases with controllable risk factors. In this model, the key to improved health is deemed to be the provision of knowledge and skills to individuals. An assumption of the model is that people will use self-determination, individualism, and responsibility to secure adequate housing, employment, and proper nutrition. While this model may benefit people with good education, a continuum of options, and resources to elicit change, it is less applicable to those with limited choices and resources regarding their own destinies. As long as the dominant models for health care delivery inhibit patients' participation in their own care, poverty and homelessness will contribute to the poor health of American citizens.

Case Presentation

No Home to Go To

Ms. Brown, a 34-year-old Caucasian woman, comes into the emergency room to secure treatment for a head injury, plus minor bruises and abrasions that she reportedly received during an assault that happened about 20 hours ago. Ms. Brown is accompanied by her boyfriend, Roy. She indicates they were sleeping in a protected entrance to an elevator in the city parking garage when two young men began beating and kicking them. The two men took Ms. Brown's purse, a sack of food she and Roy had accumulated, and Roy's wallet, which contained $5.00. Ms. Brown indicates she has been homeless for over a year. She occasionally stays in city shelters but spends most of her time roaming the city and walking to secure meals at the various programs that feed the poor. She is tall and thin, with a variety of skin lesions. She came to the hospital due to dizziness that prevented her from walking to the church where she could eat. She and Roy occasionally work odd jobs, but use the bulk of their income to support Roy's drug habit. She is trying to get Roy to quit using.

The physician has the nurse clean Ms. Brown's scalp and apply a dressing to the traumatic lesion. A contusion is expected, and the physician suggests that Ms. Brown rest for a few days and go to the neurological clinic if the dizziness worsens. The nurse points out that Ms. Brown has no place to rest and cannot get to the clinic without access to public transportation. The physician realizes this but indicates it is beyond her control.

Think About It

When Resources Are Lacking

- *Apply the concepts of justice, nonmaleficence, and beneficence to Ms. Brown's care.*

- *Does society have any responsibility for Ms. Brown? If so, what?*

- *Can thorough treatment be denied if a client has no resources? If not, who pays for the treatment?*

Intimate Partner Violence

A third common social condition affecting health and health care delivery is intimate partner violence (IPV), the most common but least reported crime in the United States. Estimated numbers of battered women range from 2 to 12 million per year. Women comprise the vast majority of victims of IPV, although a small percentage of men also report IPV. Nearly one-third of women worldwide, including in the United States, report being physically or sexually abused at some point in their lives (Futures Without Violence, 2012; Office on Women's Health, 2012). Intimate partner violence flows from a historical position of sexism. Eisler (1987) describes how select tenets of Judaism, Christianity, and Islam support patriarchy, the inferiority of women, and women as the property of men. In the United States it was legal until 1899 for a husband to beat his wife to maintain his authority (Barner & Carney, 2011). Remnants of these beliefs are still threaded through society, affecting the way families socialize their children and the way communities tolerate gender inequity. Women have long been defined in American society by their roles as mothers and caretakers, with an implied dependence on men. While these role definitions are changing, daily events in society continue to perpetuate gender inequity. As long as gender inequity exists, domestic violence will remain a social problem.

The vast majority of abused women eventually leave their abusive partners. However, leaving is a process that takes time, energy, and resources. Many abused women will leave and return to their abusive partners several times before permanently terminating the relationship. Factors contributing to this include the inability to find housing or suitable jobs; the fear, loneliness, or poverty that results from being out on their own; concern for children who are experiencing relocation and other difficulties; relentless pressure from family and friends to try harder to make the relationship work; and poor support from the criminal justice system (Barner & Carney, 2011; Duffy & Hardacre, 2005; Lutz, 2005). It is sometimes easier to return to a familiar though unpleasant situation than to start over and deal with numerous unknowns.

Since sex is the risk factor, domestic violence affects women of all socioeconomic, racial, and ethnic groups (Futures Without Violence, 2012; Office on Women's Health, 2012; World Report on Violence and Health, 2012). All persons living in violent relationships will experience poorer health. Women living in abusive situations experience acute traumatic injuries and chronic physical and emotional problems (Macy, Ferron, & Crosby, 2009; Tweddale, 2006). They are especially vulnerable to battery during pregnancy and are at a higher risk than nonbattered women for poor pregnancy outcomes (Lutz, 2005; Melhado, 2005; National Coalition Against Domestic Violence, 2012; World Health Organization [WHO], 2012b). The health care system may add insult to abused women's injuries. Women may feel humiliated by and blamed for the abuse by a health care system that minimizes the abuse, makes insufficient referrals, and fails to acknowledge abuse as the culprit (Barner & Carney, 2011). Women who leave health care settings without having the domestic violence addressed often remain isolated and uninformed about their options. However, women who have domestic violence issues addressed by a health care provider may be more likely to use an intervention and subsequently exit the abusive relationship (McCloskey et al., 2006).

Case Presentation

Suspicions of Abuse

Maria P. is a 25-year-old woman who made an initial visit to the clinic for prenatal care when she was 18 weeks pregnant. She has returned for a second prenatal visit at 22 weeks of gestation. Maria has a 4-year-old son and a 2-year-old daughter. Her record indicates she had several bruises, lacerations, and a black eye during her last pregnancy that she attributed to clumsiness. Her 2-year-old weighed 4 pounds, 8 ounces at birth and was 17 inches long.

As part of routine prenatal care for the most recent pregnancy, Maria was tested for HIV antibodies. The test was positive, and the physician and nurse conveyed this information to Maria during her second prenatal visit. Maria, of course, was quite upset. She admits that her spouse has been physically abusing her for some time and that both have used intravenous drugs in the past. She has had no sexual partners other than her spouse.

The nurse encourages Maria to tell her spouse that she is HIV positive so that he can be tested for antibodies. She also encourages use of condoms during sexual intercourse to help avoid transmission to her spouse should he not be infected. Maria insists that her husband refuses to use condoms as they interfere with his pleasure. In addition, she says he would kill her if he knew she was HIV positive.

The nurse encourages Maria to go to a shelter for abused women and links her to both a counselor and a social worker who help her devise a safety plan. However, Maria ultimately decides to go home because she cannot abandon her children, and she does not want them in a shelter. She knows she cannot make it on her own, as she has neither income nor job skills. She requests that the clinic not interfere and that the clinic workers allow her to decide if, when, and how she will notify her spouse about her HIV status.

Think About It

When Patient Choices Place Them at Risk for Harm

- *Consider the principle of autonomy when determining the appropriate decision in this situation. Remember that confidentiality is an inherent part of autonomy.*

- *Who is the patient in this situation?*

- *If Maria's husband is notified by the clinic of her HIV status and he does significant harm to Maria, would liability become an issue?*

- *If Maria's husband discovers he is HIV positive in the future, blames Maria, and discovers the clinic has known she was HIV positive for some time, is there any liability? Explain.*

Human Trafficking

Human trafficking, also known as modern-day slavery, is another form of violence that is often unrecognized. Human trafficking involves the acquisition, harboring, and trade of persons through force, threats, deception, or other forms of coercion with the aim of exploiting them (United Nations Office on Drugs and Crime [UNODC], 2012). For example, people may be abducted by traffickers, threatened with harm to themselves or their families if they do not comply, or lured by such things as promises of jobs. Victims of trafficking may be exploited for forced labor, for their organs, and for sexual services. Trafficking victims have many faces, ranging from the poor in developing countries to the adolescent girl next door. Young women and children are the largest group of those who are trafficked, and most of them are trafficked for sexual exploitation. Human trafficking occurs both nationally and internationally. Although there are estimates of 2.5 million people in forced labor worldwide, the full extent of this global issue is hard to determine due to the covert nature of trafficking (Global Initiative to Fight Human Trafficking, 2012). The U.S. Department of State estimates that there are over 17,500 persons trafficked into the country annually (U.S. Department of State, 2011). Nurses may encounter victims of human trafficking when they are brought to health care facilities with acute physical, emotional, or sexual health concerns. Their overall health may be poor. They often present in ways similar to victims of domestic violence in that they seldom self-identify and are often accompanied by a person who is controlling, speaks for them, and does not leave the room. They may appear fearful and depressed, not have control of personal identification documents, not know their own address, have inconsistencies in their presenting story, and may not speak English. Nursing responsibility related to victims of trafficking includes recognizing signs and providing appropriate interventions and support, as well as working toward prevention of this form of violence. Students are encouraged to explore the online resources related to human trafficking listed at the end of this chapter and to complete the free human trafficking awareness training available at http://www.dhs.gov/xlibrary/training/dhs_awareness_training_fy12/launchPage.htm.

Increasing Elderly Population

In addition to poverty, homelessness, and domestic violence, the problems of the growing worldwide elderly population are another major health concern. The World Health Organization (WHO) notes that there will be 2 billion people age 60 and over worldwide by 2050, 80 percent of whom will live in the developing world (WHO, 2012a). In developed countries, such as the United States, those age 80 and older are the fastest growing population. People are living longer due to many factors, such as healthier diets, vaccines, medical advances, and improvements in the environment. Certainly advances in health care knowledge have contributed to greater longevity. However, health disparities exist. For example, in the United States, those in higher socioeconomic groups are expected to live up to 20 years longer than those in lower socioeconomic groups. In addition, many elderly, especially from minority populations, live without pensions and on incomes below the poverty level (Wright, 2005). The incidence of elder abuse is also increasing worldwide as the population ages, with estimates of 4–6 percent of older persons suffering some form of abuse (WHO, 2012a). Vast numbers of the elderly are socially isolated, in need of work to survive, and susceptible to economic hardship. Chronic illnesses, pain (especially from arthritic processes), frailties, cognitive problems, and disabilities occur with increasing frequency as people age. Health problems contribute significantly to the social isolation, financial burden, and general discomfort that may accompany aging.

The assumption in current prevailing health care models is that the frail elderly will be cared for at home by friends and family to alleviate strain on the health care system. In reality, family members may be unable to provide needed support due to geographical distance from the frail elderly family member or personal responsibilities. Caring for the elderly, particularly those with dementia, often causes emotional, relational, and financial strain for the caregivers. The caregivers often have to help with the finances of the elderly, since their fixed incomes cannot cover the basic cost of living as well as health care expenses. Reliance on friends and family for health care of the frail elderly is especially problematic for the elderly without the necessary social or financial resources.

Case Presentation

Aging, Poverty, and Illness

Mr. Chang is a 65-year-old widower who is diabetic with chronic kidney disease. He is supposed to receive dialysis three times a week but frequently misses his appointments due to not having transportation or not feeling well. His only hope for a cure is a kidney transplant, which Mr. Chang really wants. Mr. Chang is very frail with many health problems. He lives alone in a small garage apartment. The landlord is threatening to evict Mr. Chang because he is behind in his rent payments. Mr. Chang lives on a small pension and Medicare. His prescription costs are excessive and his Medicare Part D prescription plan requires large co-payments on the brand-name medications needed for his care

A home health nurse used to transport Mr. Chang to dialysis occasionally, as Mr. Chang lives outside the township limits and is unable to access public transportation services. The clinic, which does not believe Mr. Chang is a candidate for a transplant, has revised its policies regarding home visits due to changes in reimbursement mechanisms. The home health nurse can no longer visit Mr. Chang unless there is a reimbursable need such as a dressing change; and for liability reasons, she can no longer transport Mr. Chang to dialysis.

Think About It

What Health Care Should Society Provide for Its Citizens?

- *Consider the principle of justice in deciding if health care is a right or a privilege that comes with the ability to pay. If health care must be rationed, who decides what services an individual will receive?*

- *Is society prepared to pay health care costs for all citizens?*

- *Is there a level of care that society should provide to all citizens, with private financing providing all care beyond the set level? Explain.*

- *What is fair for Mr. Chang?*

Racism

Racism is another social concern that affects health. The term *race* generally refers to biological traits related to a person's genetic heritage, such as skin color, hair type and color, and facial features, that allow classifications of human beings on the basis of these characteristics. Ethnicity, on the other hand, refers to a shared cultural background such as nationality, language, practices, and beliefs. Although people within a racial group ascribe to many different cultural beliefs and practices, it is often race that stereotypes a group of people or engenders ethnocentric beliefs and moral conflicts in values. Racism is an ethical problem that violates the principle of respect for persons and contributes to human rights abuses.

Racial and ethnic minorities continue to experience disparities in health status and health care (Clark, 2009; Davitt & Kaye, 2010; Egede, 2006; Lillie-Blanton, Maleque, & Miller, 2008). According to all public health indicators, African Americans, Hispanics, and Native Americans have the worst health status of all American groups. In addition, they have the highest rates of risk behaviors for disease. Hunger has increased among these three racial groups. They have poorer cancer survival rates and higher incidences of stroke, hypertension, diabetes, and other problems. In addition, African Americans and Hispanics have the lowest levels of health insurance and the most inappropriate use of expensive emergency rooms. While socioeconomic conditions contribute to these health conditions, it is easy to discern possible racial influences on health.

Problems of access to care and inequity of treatment for racial and ethnic minorities are frequently cited as evidence of racial bias within the health care system. In addition, traditional solutions to health problems, such as health education and health promotion programs, are often not programmed for minority groups (Breton, 2000). More important, minority groups tend to demonstrate poorer health outcomes in some areas, revealing inadequate health care—for example, mortality from breast cancer is disproportionately high among women from racial and other ethnic minorities (Blackman & Masi, 2006).

There is significant interface of poverty, homelessness, IPV, an increasing elderly population, and racism. Poverty underpins homelessness. In addition, racial and ethnic minorities living in poverty are more likely to face homelessness (National Coalition for the Homeless, 2012a; WHO, 2012a). African Americans, Native Americans, and Hispanics are overrepresented among the homeless. Women experiencing intimate partner violence move frequently and often deal with homelessness and poverty as they try to improve their situations (Futures Without Violence, 2012; National Coalition for the Homeless, 2012b). Poverty and homelessness are linked to a high abuse rate, and there is a link between violence and poverty. The elderly are often made homeless as they face mounting health care and living costs on a fixed income. Persons experiencing poverty, homelessness, aging, domestic violence, and racism are vulnerable to poor health and inadequate health care delivery. Often these vulnerable groups are the least powerful and vocal persons in society, yet they are the groups most affected by ethical decisions regarding health care (Clark, 2009; Davitt & Kaye, 2010; Egede, 2006).

These social situations represent examples of classism, sexism, and racism. Each indicates prejudice or discrimination against a particular class, gender, or racial group. The implication is that one group of people is held to standards espoused by another group. Statistical data on these social situations, and the health of persons experiencing these social situations, explain why a feeling of helplessness may emerge when social situations are so intrinsically intertwined with health. Yet treating a person's symptoms without attending to the root causes of the problem may be viewed as inadequate health care.

ETHICAL PRINCIPLES APPLIED TO SOCIAL ISSUES

Ethical dilemmas involving classism, sexism, and racism are difficult to resolve. The common principles most essential in unraveling ethical dilemmas encompassing social issues include justice, nonmaleficence, beneficence, and autonomy. A brief discussion of each principle follows.

Justice

Justice is the duty to treat all people fairly without regard to age, socioeconomic status, race, or gender. This implies a fair distribution of the benefits and burdens among members of a society, with equal treatment to all or to those most in need. This could mean extending necessary treatment to those in need, even though they may not have the requisite means to pay for the treatment. For example, a frail elderly gentleman, beloved by his family, might receive an expensive but desired transplant procedure based on justice, even though there is only a moderate chance that the extensive surgery will prolong life or improve the quality of life.

ASK YOURSELF

Who Should Receive Limited Health Care Resources?

• In this day of declining health care resources, should those with the greatest need or those who have contributed more to society receive expensive restorative procedures? Or should these procedures be available to all? Support your position.

Nonmaleficence

Nonmaleficence is the duty to prevent or avoid doing harm, whether intentional or unintentional. This could mean refusing to discharge an abused woman to her home if there is a possibility of further injury. It might also entail ensuring a safe, hygienic environment before hospital release of a newborn infant and mother suffering from poverty or homelessness.

Beneficence

Beneficence is the duty to actively do good for patients. This requires us to act in ways that benefit others with attention to the psychological, social, and spiritual dimensions of disease or injury as well as the physical problems. This principle directs the nurse to make an effort to ensure that the homeless lady—with leg ulcers and diabetes, who walks all day in poor shoes to secure free meals and safe sleeping quarters—will receive treatment for the leg ulcers that includes adequate diet and rest, elevation of the legs, and proper hygiene. Treatment would have to go beyond the usual prescriptions for drugs and address the social conditions contributing to the physical problems.

Autonomy

Autonomy is the patient's right to self-determination without outside control. Related to this principle are the principles of veracity, privacy, confidentiality, and respect for all persons. Little (2000) reminds us that people must develop a sense of autonomy. She suggests that autonomy involves a set of skills that people possess to greater or lesser degrees. These skills often require someone to help us cultivate them, a context that sustains them, and help in exercising them when we are in a vulnerable position. One of these skills is the capacity to think through different options and imagine possibilities. Our social context, however, can get in the way of seeing our options. Autonomy would direct us to work with the abused woman to develop a stronger sense of herself and to help her to see various options

Think About It

The Impact of Social Conditions on Vulnerable Groups

Consider how social conditions affect other vulnerable groups, such as children, people who are mentally or physically disabled or challenged, undocumented immigrants, and people who are institutionalized or incarcerated.

- *Discuss the factors that make these populations vulnerable.*
- *Describe the issues related to these populations that give you concern as a nurse.*
- *Discuss the ethical concerns related to the needs and care of people in these groups.*
- *How would you apply the principles of justice, nonmaleficence, beneficence, and autonomy to health care concerns with people in each of these groups?*

and available support. We also recognize that limitations on autonomy that occur within an abusive relationship affect a person's ability to act autonomously. Thus, autonomy would direct us to honor her choice to return home—even if her safety is a concern—while continuing to offer support as she struggles with difficult decisions.

PERSONAL IMPEDIMENTS TO INTERVENING WITH VULNERABLE GROUPS

Victim Blaming

Working with people who are poor, homeless, experiencing intimate partner violence, victims of human trafficking, aged, or of a different race requires exploration of personal values to ensure that negative attitudes do not interfere with health care. Victim blaming is a real phenomenon that can affect attitudes and interactions (Adler & Stewart, 2009; Idisis, Ben-David, & Ben-Nachum, 2007). **Victim blaming** tends to hold the people burdened by social conditions accountable for their own situations and responsible for needed solutions. Victim blaming is often evident in language such as "she was asking for it," "he should have quit smoking," or "they're not willing to work; they just want to live off the state." When there is evidence of personal or systemwide victim blaming, the ethical stance is to treat each person with dignity and fairness while working to change attitudes toward the victim. To respect others by allowing them to make choices and decisions, when they are capable of doing so, requires an attitude of caring with a focus on advocacy. This implies facilitating patient empowerment, acknowledging their values and guarding their rights, and promoting social justice in health care. Reeducating nurses and other providers to be aware of situations of victim blaming and enhancing the advocate role may improve care within a health care agency.

Language of Violence

Another possible impediment to intervention, specifically with the social situation of violence, is the violence mode that colors speech and actions. Consider metaphors of violence commonly used in the health care system such as "attacking" germs, "battling" disease, "plotting strategies" against or "defeating" invasive cells, "suffering defeat," or "achieving victory." The prevailing mind-set behind this strategy of confrontation is the antithesis of a needed compassionate approach that values nonviolence. This is especially true for women experiencing domestic violence. Language that

ASK YOURSELF

How Does Language Reflect One's Values?

How do the values reflected in the language of the following statements imply victim blaming?

- Most young, single, poor women get pregnant to increase their welfare benefits.
- If poor, homeless people would take more responsibility for themselves, they could improve their situation. There are jobs out there for people who want to work.
- The highest calling for a woman is to be the family nurturer.
- If an abused woman wanted help, she would just leave the abusive relationship.
- An important part of assessing for domestic violence is to ask what the woman was doing or if she was drinking right before she was hit.
- Resistance to change is a normal part of aging.
- All five senses tend to decline as a person ages.
- Since most low-income women do not comply with therapies, it is not cost-effective to spend too much time with them on health education.
- What did you expect? Look at how her mother behaved.
- People can get ahead if they take advantage of life's opportunities.

supports violence can inadvertently lead to victim blaming, or covertly encourage futile and dangerous retaliation. Indeed, a first step in effective intervention with those experiencing violence is to create a milieu that emphasizes nonviolence. The message has to be clear that violence of any form is wrong and, generally, illegal. This may necessitate a change in how health care providers approach and work therapeutically with people experiencing violence.

SOCIAL ISSUES AND SCHOLARSHIP

Many health care interventions are based, properly, on research; however, nurses need to ask if the underlying research, and therefore the determined therapy, may create problems based on classism, sexism, and racism. For example, many research instruments are not designed for diverse and vulnerable populations, and many intelligence tests are under scrutiny for cultural bias. Studies indicate that racial and ethnic minorities do not participate as readily in research as European Americans (Ashey-Giwa, 2005; Clark, 2009; Villarruel, 2006). Their socioeconomic status and the professional hierarchy often impede minority participation in research studies.

This means that classroom teachings and clinical knowledge may be based on inadequate research for minority populations. It is an ethical responsibility to provide appropriate nursing care to diverse cultural groups. Thus, faculty and students need to be cognizant of the benefits of selected interventions for all population groups and to be cautious in generalizing research findings to diverse population groups without sufficient evidence that they apply to a specific group. Research on vulnerable populations is needed to ensure an adequate database for working with those who are experiencing social issues such as poverty, homelessness, domestic violence, human trafficking, unhealthy aging, and racism.

SUMMARY

This chapter focused on ethical dilemmas that may emerge when providing health care for vulnerable population groups. Ethical decisions related to health care for vulnerable populations confront nurses who work on a daily basis with those experiencing the social conditions of poverty, homelessness, intimate partner violence, human trafficking, unhealthy aging, and racism. Since values affect professional behavior, nurses must analyze personally held values as well as those of the health care agency where they are employed for appropriate consideration of justice, beneficence, nonmaleficence, and autonomy. Nurses who work with vulnerable groups need to utilize these principles in ethical decision making. Nurses must consider the impact and validity of health care interventions and research on vulnerable populations, and must ensure that what nurses teach both in the classroom and to patients is based on research applicable to the populations being served and studied.

CHAPTER HIGHLIGHTS

- Poverty, homelessness, intimate partner violence, human trafficking, aging, and racism affect health in a negative fashion. Limited choices and inappropriate treatment options often interfere with the best health care for these vulnerable populations.

- Applying the concept of justice to vulnerable populations can change the way society and the health care systems provide health care. Addressing the social conditions of the individual with an illness or disease is basic to health care.

- Nonmaleficence and beneficence may clash with autonomy when providing care for vulnerable populations.

- Victim blaming, evident in covert or overt beliefs that all people are accountable for their own situations and responsible for solutions, interferes with health care delivery for vulnerable populations and is evidence of sexism, classism, or racism.

- Advocacy and caring, which are ways to avoid delivering health care that is grounded in sexism, classism, and racism, require letting go of the power relationships that often dominate health care delivery.

- Clearing speech patterns and other behaviors of words and actions that are based on violence is a step toward therapeutic interventions with those who experience violence in their lives.

- Findings from research studies may not be applicable to vulnerable populations if the vulnerable are not part of the study population.

DISCUSSION QUESTIONS AND ACTIVITIES

1. Visit a homeless shelter or shelter for abused women. Interview staff or residents about their health and ability to access health care.

2. Spend a few afternoons volunteering in a soup kitchen. Talk with people who come in for free meals about their health problems and ability to secure health care.

3. Spend some time with a home health nurse or a Meals-on-Wheels volunteer who makes contact with the elderly who live at home alone. Explore the individual's perceptions of quality of life, health dilemmas, and needs.

4. Work with classmates to develop a "health fair" for the homeless, discussing the value of typical activities and materials made available at traditional fairs, while designing a more relevant approach.

5. How many examples of toys, advertisements, acting roles, literature, childrearing practices, and the like can you identify that continue to perpetuate the woman's role as one of caregiver or sexual object? Discuss how the examples contribute to gender inequity for women.

6. Investigate racial and ethnic disparities in health at http://www.cdc .gov/minorityhealth/populations/remp.html; http://www.kff.org/minorityhealth/; and http://womenshealth.gov/minority-health/.

7. Explore information on the issues addressed in this chapter at several of the following websites and report to the class on issues, incidence, prevention, and ethical considerations related to these issues.

> Family Violence Prevention Fund—
> http://www.nnedv.org/resources/nationalorgs/
> 59-national-organizations/9-fvpf.html

> National Network to End Domestic Violence—
> http://www.nnedv.org

Futures Without Violence—
http://www.futureswithoutviolence.org/

Office on Women's Health—
http://www.womenshealth.gov/violence-against-women/

CDC Intimate Partner Violence—
http://www.cdc.gov/ViolencePrevention/index.html

World Health Organization, violence by intimate partners—
http://www.who.int/violence_injury_prevention/violence/
global_campaign/en/chap4.pdf

Violence Against Women Network—
http://www.vawnet.org/

National Coalition Against Domestic Violence—
http://www.ncadv.org/learn/Statistics_115.html

Poverty and health—
http://www.eldis.org/go/topics/resource-guides/health-systems/
health-inequalities#.USUDjWdCx8E

Child Trends Data Bank—
http://www.childtrendsdatabank.org/
http://www.childtrendsdatabank.org/?q=node/229 (Health care
coverage)
http://www.childtrendsdatabank.org/?q=node/221 (Children in
poverty)

National Coalition for the Homeless—
http://www.nationalhomeless.org/
http://www.nationalhomeless.org/factsheets/Health.pdf
http://www.nationalhomeless.org/factsheets/How_Many.pdf
http://www.nationalhomeless.org/factsheets/Whois.pdf
(Ethnicity)
http://www.nationalhomeless.org/factsheets/why.html (Poverty,
domestic violence)
http://www.nationalhomeless.org/factsheets/domestic.pdf
(Domestic violence)

Health of Minority Women—
http://womenshealth.gov/minority-health

World Health Organization (WHO)—
http://www.who.int/ageing/en

Administration on Aging (DHHS)—
http://www.aoa.gov/aoaroot/aging_statistics/index.aspx

Profile of Older Americans—
http://www.aoa.gov/AoARoot/Aging_Statistics/Profile/2011/14.aspx

Minority Elders—
http://www.aoa.gov/AoARoot/Aging_Statistics/Minority_Aging/
index.aspx

Human Trafficking—
http://www.unodc.org/unodc/en/human-trafficking/

National Human Trafficking hotline—
http://www.polarisproject.org/what-we-do/

Recognizing signs of human trafficking—
http://www.polarisproject.org/human-trafficking/
recognizing-the-signs (Signs)
http://www.dhs.gov/xlibrary/training/dhs_awareness_training_
fy12/launchPage.htm (Human trafficking awareness training)

8. Explore international nursing perspectives on current health and social issues at the International Council of Nurses website—http://www.icn.ch/matters.htm.

References

Adler, N. E., & Stewart, J. (2009). Reducing obesity: Motivating action while not blaming the victim. *The Milbank Quarterly, 87*(1), 49–70.

Ashey-Giwa, K. T. (2005). Can a cultural response model for research design bring us closer to addressing participation disparity? Lessons learned from cancer survivorship studies. *Ethnicity & Disease, 15*(1), 130–137.

Barner, J. R., & Carney, M. M. (2011). Interventions for intimate partner violence: A historical review. *Journal of Family Violence, 26*, 235–255.

Blackman, D. J., & Masi, C. M. (2006). Racial and ethnic disparities in breast cancer mortality: Are we doing enough to address the root causes? *Journal of Clinical Oncology, 24*(4), 2170–2178.

Breton, J. H. (2000, November). Treating beyond color: Health issues in minority women. *Advance for Nurse Practitioners*, 65–66, 68, 101.

Chaufan, C., Davis, M., & Constantino, S. (2011). The twin epidemics of poverty and diabetes: Understanding diabetes disparities in low-income Latino and immigrant neighborhoods. *Journal of Community Health, 36*(6), 1030–1043.

Child Trends Data Bank. (2012). Health care coverage. Retrieved February 28, 2012, from http://www.childtrendsdatabank.org/?q=node/297

Clark, P. A. (2009). Prejudice and the medical profession: A five-year update. *Journal of Law, Medicine & Ethics, 37*(1), 118–133.

Dashiff, C., DiMicco, W., Myers, B., & Sheppard, K. (2009). Poverty and adolescent mental health. *Journal of Child and Adolescent Psychiatric Nursing, 22*(1), 23–32.

Davitt, J. K., & Kaye, L. W. (2010). Racial/ethnic disparities in access to Medicare home health care: The disparate impact of policy. *Journal of Gerontological Social Work, 53*(7), 591–612.

Duffy, J., & Hardacre, S. (2005). Why men abuse, why women don't leave: What midwives need to know. *MIDRS Midwifery Digest, 15*(4), 555–559.

Eisler, R. (1987). *The chalice and the blade*. San Francisco: Harper & Row.

Futures Without Violence. (2012). Get the facts. Retrieved February 28, 2012, from http://www.futureswithoutviolence.org/content/action_center/detail/754

Global Initiative to Fight Human Trafficking. (2012). Human trafficking: The facts. Retrieved February 28, 2012, from http://www.unglobal-compact.org/docs/issues_doc/labour/Forced_labour/HUMAN_TRAFFICKING_-_THE_FACTS_-_final.pdf

Idisis, Y., Ben-David, S., & Ben-Nachum, E. (2007). Attribution of blame to rape victims among therapists and non-therapists. *Behavioral Science & the Law, 25*, 103–120.

John, W., & Law, K. (2011). Addressing the health needs of the homeless. *British Journal of Community Nursing, 16*(3), 134–139.

Kushell, M., Gupta, R., Gee, L., & Haas, J. S. (2006). Housing instability and food insecurity as barriers to health care among low income Americans. *Journal of General Internal Medicine, 21*(1), 71–77.

Lillie-Blanton, M., Maleque, S., & Miller, W. (2008). Reducing racial, ethnic, and socioeconomic disparities in health care: Opportunities in national health reform. *Journal of Law, Medicine & Ethics, 36*(4), 693–702.

Little, M. (2000, June 9). Introduction to the ethics of care. Presentation at New Century, New Challenges: Intensive Bioethics Course XXVI, Kennedy Institute of Ethics, Georgetown University, Washington, DC.

Lutz, K. (2005). Abusive experience, perceptions, and associated decisions during the childbearing cycle. *Western Journal of Nursing Research, 27*(7), 802–24.

Macy, R. J., Ferron, J., & Crosby, C. (2009). Partner violence and survivors' chronic health problems: Informing social work practice. *Social Work, 54*(1), 29–43.

McCloskey, L. A., Lichter, E., Williams, C., Gerber, M., Wittenberg, E., & Ganz, M. (2006). Assessing intimate partner violence in health care settings leads to women's receipt of interventions and improved health. *Public Health Reports, 121*(4), 435–444.

Melhado, L. (2005). Women who report abuse during pregnancy have an elevated risk of adverse birth outcomes. *International Family Planning Perspectives, 31*(4), 204.

Mother Teresa Quotes. (2012). Retrieved February 28, 2012, from http://www.great-quotes.com/quotes/author/Mother/Teresa/pg/3

National Coalition Against Domestic Violence. (2012). Pregnancy and domestic violence. Retrieved February 28, 2012, from http://www.ncadv.org/learn/Statistics_115.html

National Coalition for the Homeless. (2012a). Factsheet—Who is homeless? Retrieved February 28, 2012, from http://www.nationalhomeless.org/publications/facts.html

National Coalition for the Homeless. (2012b). Factsheet—Domestic violence. Retrieved February 28, 2012, from http://www.nationalhomeless.org/publications/facts.html

Office on Women's Health. (2012). Violence against women. Retrieved from http://womenshealth.gov/violence-against-women/

Romeo, J. H. (2005). Down and out in New York City: A participant observation study of the poor and marginalized. *Journal of Cultural Diversity, 12*(4), 152–160.

Sapolsky, R. (2005, December). Sick of poverty. *Scientific American,* 93–99.

Tweddale, C. (2006). Trauma during pregnancy. *Critical Care Nursing Quarterly, 29*(1), 53–67.

United Nations Office on Drugs and Crime (UNODC). (2012). Human trafficking. Retrieved February 28, 2012, from http://www.unodc.org/unodc/en/human-trafficking/

U.S. Department of State, Office to Monitor and Combat Trafficking in Persons. (2011). Trafficking in persons report. Retrieved February 28, 2012, http://www.state.gov/j/tip/rls/tiprpt/2011/index.htm

Villarruel, A. M. (2006). Health disparities research: Issues, strategies and innovations. *Journal of Multicultural Nursing and Health, 12*(1), 4–9.

World Health Organization (WHO). (2012a). Aging facts. Retrieved from http://www.who.int/features/factfiles/ageing/ageing_facts/en/index.html

World Health Organization (WHO). (2012b). Violence against women. Retrieved from http://www.who.int/reproductivehealth/publications/violence/en/

World Report on Violence and Health. (2012). Retrieved from http://www.who.int/violence_injury_prevention/violence/world_report/en/

Wright, J. D. (2005). The graying of America: Implications for health professionals. *Case Management Journal, 6*(4), 178–184.

Chapter

17

GENDER ISSUES

"When we are committed to the ideal of concern for all others, it follows that this should inform our social and political policies."

(The Dalai Lama, 1999)

OBJECTIVES

After completing this chapter, the reader should be able to:

1. Describe historical bases of gender issues in nursing.
2. Discuss the relationship between issues of gender and race.
3. Describe factors associated with and the impact of sex discrimination in nursing.
4. Discuss sexual harassment within a nursing context.
5. Discuss communication issues related to gender.
6. Describe nursing issues related to modern sexism.

INTRODUCTION

You will recall from Chapter 1 that gender is one of the most critical factors influencing nursing practice. Throughout history, in nearly every culture, nursing has been a profession of women. Historical texts report that women comprised 95 to 98 percent of early nurses. A recent survey of more than 35 thousand nurses revealed that these numbers are not changing significantly: Currently 92 percent of all nurses in the United States are women (U.S. Department of Labor, 2008). Since the health care system is a small microcosm of the larger society, many gender-related societal issues manifest themselves there. Issues such as pay equity, employment opportunities, sexual harassment, role strain, race relations, and gender stereotyping are but a few examples of gender-influenced conflicts that may be encountered in professional relationships. There are two basic approaches to dealing with these social justice issues. We can simply pretend that these issues do not exist. This approach may result in increased frustration as unresolved feelings and issues play out on the job. Alternatively, we can become aware of the issues and define ways to deal with the realities of our society head-on. This chapter focuses on the latter approach and explores issues concerning gender in the nursing workplace.

HISTORICAL PERSPECTIVES AND OVERVIEW OF GENDER-BASED ISSUES

The American Nurses Association (ANA) defines a nurse as one who applies scientific knowledge; integrates objective data, including the full range of human experiences; and provides a caring relationship that facilitates health and healing (ANA, 1995). Most people perceive a nurse as a person who cares for the disabled or sick, yet there remains controversy concerning the derivation of the title *nurse* and how this title relates to the gender of the person providing care. In her comprehensive work *Woman as Healer,* Achterberg chronicles the journey of women in healing professions. Citing the masculinization of American medicine as one of many issues that challenge nurses, Achterberg (1990) states that although nursing has gained professional status, it suffers because of issues due to nurses functioning under many layers of authority.

As nursing continued to be a predominantly female profession, societal issues that affected women were also reflected in nursing. In a commentary about turn-of-the-century hospitals entitled "The Hospital Hotel," the author noted that nurses were noted for being "well-bred, well-educated specimens of womanhood. . . . highly appreciated, as a rule" (JAMA, 1996, p. 324). Women have been socialized to achieve or be less than they are capable of becoming. This reluctance to achieve is evident in the lack of women in positions of power, especially in the political arena (Hamilton, 1999). Although more recent societal influences have had a positive impact, nursing is still a female-dominated profession with an unfortunate history of oppression that many believe it has yet to overcome.

Throughout the decades, nurses have constantly had to struggle with paternalistic ideology that continues to permeate the profession. **Paternalism** is a gender-biased term that literally means acting in a "fatherly" manner, the traditional view of which implies well-intended actions of benevolent decision making, leadership, protection, and discipline. Coupled with an enduring cultural attitude that diminishes the status of the caring role in society, paternalism has inhibited full actualization of the profession. The negative outcomes of paternalism affect both women and men in the profession.

In what has been termed the *medicalization* of American society, nursing has struggled to overcome the prejudices that have historically embraced the biomedical curative model of health care. As diversified consumers of health care demand more sophisticated and culturally congruent care, nurses are in a prime position to provide cost-effective, high-quality care. If nursing is to be successful in this and other arenas, it must concomitantly address issues of territoriality, power, and authority within its own ranks as well as with other health care professionals.

Many believe that nurses have been forced to work within a framework that focuses on societal expectations of women and what is considered women's work. Williams (1991) found that nearly half of all women work in occupations that are at least 80 percent female, while more than two-thirds of men are employed in occupations that are 80 percent male. Williams chooses as extreme examples the U.S. Marines and nursing to exemplify society's gender stereotypes of certain professions. She writes:

> The military and the nursing profession are intimately linked to stereotypes about gender. Some people may assume that the Marine Corps demands of its soldiers certain "masculine" traits—strength, aggressiveness, emotional detachment; people may also assume that nursing requires "feminine" qualities—nurturing, caring, and passivity. Many believe that men are naturally suited for the Marine Corps and only women for nursing. (1991, p. 1)

Williams (1991) suggests that others may hold different types of offensive stereotypes—for example considering women in the Marine Corps or men in nursing "cross-gender freaks" (p. 1), that is masculine women and feminine men.

GENDER DISCRIMINATION IN NURSING

Women in Nursing

Women have historically worked for lower pay than their male counterparts. Pay equity is generally protected by state laws. However, issues of comparable worth, which have long been associated with traditionally female-dominated professions such as nursing, have not had the same protection. Salaries in nursing remain relatively low compared with other professions that require comparably high levels of skill, education, and responsibility. Some suspect that men in nursing are raising salaries; however, other economic considerations, such as nursing shortages, fair labor legislation, and collective bargaining, may be responsible (Ellis & Hartley, 2003). Although a pay gap exists between men and women in many occupations, the gap is considerably narrower for nurses (Reskin & Padavic, 2002). When compared to other occupations, the fact that nurses have historically earned less may account for this lack of difference. However, the fact that a gap exists at all is striking in that men make up only a small percentage of the nursing profession. Men's dominance in the higher-pay jobs, such as nurse anesthetists, and the patriarchal structure of the health care industry, in which fewer women hold senior management positions, may account for this.

According to sociologist Christine Williams (1995), issues of comparable worth are a real concern for nurses. Williams identifies several hidden advantages to being a man in nursing, particularly in relation to hiring and promotion. Williams's work supports Gilloran's (1995) assertions of gender disequity, as men are typically *tracked* into higher-paying and more prestigious positions. Even in a predominantly female profession, women may be experiencing a form of economic gender discrimination.

Men in Nursing

As has traditionally been the case, relatively few men are registered nurses, but the trend may be changing. Men make up a growing percentage of registered nurses. A 2008 survey revealed that 6.2 percent of nurses licensed before 2000 were men, contrasted with 9.6 percent of nurses who were licensed in the year 2000 or later. These demographics show that the percentage of men who are new graduates is increasing dramatically (U.S. Department of Health and Human Services, 2010). Studies also show a difference in basic education between men and women. Men in nursing are more likely to obtain a higher initial nursing degree while slightly more women than men are likely to obtain a higher final degree. The employment profile of men is also different from that of women. A greater proportion of male nurses work in hospitals, and even though just over 7 percent of employed nurses in 2008 were men, they constituted over 40 percent of nurse anesthetists—a specialty with higher pay (U.S. Department of Health and Human Services, 2010).

ASK YOURSELF

Is There Gender Stereotyping in Nursing?

Nursing schools have failed to narrow the gender gap. Both students and faculty are predominantly female. Even though there are vastly more men in nursing now than in the past, the gender gap remains. William Lecher, president of the American Assembly for Men in Nursing (AAMN), reports that gender stereotyping starts early. When visiting children's classrooms, he hears children say, "You can't be a nurse because you're a man" (Robert Wood Johnson Foundation, 2011).

- In what ways do you think nurses can help dispel this declining but continuing stereotype?

- How would you respond if your son or daughter chose nursing as a profession? Would you encourage him or her? Why or why not?

Sullivan (2000) stresses the value of gender diversity in nursing, noting that men play an important role in the profession. Citing societal stereotyping as one of the major limiting factors for men in nursing, Squires (1995) may be categorizing men even further when he asserts that health care reform that increases responsibility and autonomy will attract more men to the nursing profession. Perhaps what Williams (1995) perceives as hidden advantages for men in nursing adds some credence to Squires's assertions. Despite these and other stereotypes, Squires considers the lure of nursing universal regardless of gender. Noting the challenge, variety, and excitement of nursing, Squires is quick to acknowledge that the road men in nursing have traveled thus far has not been without controversy. The American Assembly for Men in Nursing addresses these issues with its goals to encourage men to become nurses; support men who are nurses to grow professionally; demonstrate the contributions made by men within the nursing profession; and advocate for continued research, education, and dissemination of information about men's health issues and men in nursing (American Assembly for Men in Nursing, 2012).

Gender Issues in Women's Health

Although men may have hidden advantages in nursing, some areas, primarily in women's health, have remained closed to them. Public policies and traditions, taken together, may be illogical. For example, in 1995 California law banned prices based upon gender for services such as haircuts, dry cleaning, or tailoring (Thompson, 1995), while simultaneously upholding a hospital's ban on male nurses in women's health areas (Letizia, 1994). California's Fair Employment and Housing Commission cited "invasion of a woman's privacy" as justification for the exemption, but one nurse called it "the most outlandish ruling" she had ever encountered (Thompson, 1995, p. 9). While some men believe that the perception that men are impeded in nursing today is overblown, others continue to experience discrimination. For example, nursing instructor Sylva Emodi was distraught over the bias that he experienced in a California hospital. Emodi said:

> I remember going to a rotation at a local hospital. The head nurse made it difficult for me to be able to supervise students in labor and delivery, pediatrics and postpartum, I think, because I am a guy. She would say, "You are not a medical doctor, you cannot go into labor and delivery." After a while, I had had enough, so I went to the doctor directly and said, "I need to be here with the students. The students need to see what is going on." The doctor said, "Sure, help yourself. Come on in." (Hilton, 2001)

In previous court proceedings that addressed this issue, the fact that most obstetricians are male was not deemed analogous to the situation of the nurse who is male (Ketter, 1994). Most courts cited that the doctor was chosen by the patient, while the nurse was not. Several state courts addressed this aspect of gender discrimination; however, none sided with the nurse. The Civil Rights Act of 1964 allows for gender-based discrimination if gender "is a bona fide occupational qualification reasonably necessary to the normal operation of that particular business or enterprise" (Ketter, 1994, p. 24). Many men in nursing believe this form of discrimination is reinforced in educational settings when faculty members seek the permission for male student nurses to observe or participate in procedures with female patients, but do not seek the permission of male patients when female students are involved. Some postulate that women are more universally accepted by patients because they are viewed as nurturers (Ellis & Hartley, 2003). Although no data support these assumptions, institutions continue to promote this form of gender discrimination when they proactively provide for the modesty and privacy of their female patients.

Gender and Caring

As the number of men in nursing increases, research directed toward gender-related issues in the profession has emerged. For example, many authors have focused nursing research on caring as it correlates with gender. Research questions related to possible differences in the expression

ASK YOURSELF

Are Male Nurses Perceived as More Competent?

Benokraitis and Feagin (1995) interviewed male nurses. The authors report that physicians view male nurses as more competent than their female counterparts. They also found that female nurses were often ignored, whereas male nurses' opinions were valued.

* Have you observed this behavior in your clinical or classroom settings?
* How could you best deal with this form of modern sexism?

of caring as it relates to the gender of the student, educator, or recipient of care demonstrate the attention these and other issues in nursing have commanded. Recognition of the need to explore gender became evident for Peter and Gallop (1994) in their comparative study designed to examine whether caring uniquely reflected the moral orientation of nursing students. They discovered that differences in caring between medical and nursing students appeared to be related to gender differences. A study exploring the relationship between nurse gender and both nurse and patient perceptions of caring found no significant difference in actual caring between male and female nurses (Ekstrom, 1999). However, from both nurse and patient perspectives, expectations of certain nurse caring behaviors were lower for male nurses.

Ironically, a gender bias in the literature on caring predates much of the actual research. For example, Reverby (1987) offered a historical perspective of caring as it relates to women, but did not address any possible implications in relation to the addition of men to the profession. Chinn (1991) devoted an entire anthology to caring, but did not explore gender in relation to caring, except as it related to economic gains (or lack thereof) for male faculty members in male-dominated academic centers. The exclusion of men by Grigsby and Megel (1995) as they explored the caring experiences of nursing faculty is another example of nursing research that did not include men. Despite an interest in the caring aspect of nursing, Begany (1994) perpetuated a nursing stereotype by equating the positive attribute of caring to images of nurturer or handmaiden.

Some men in nursing may already experience a form of gender discrimination because of the stereotypical belief that all men in nursing are homosexuals. This stereotype is rooted in gender-based role assumptions (such as Begany's) related to the caring attributes that many perceive as feminine. Because nursing has historically been viewed as "woman's work," men in nursing have been categorized as feminine, and have subsequently been labeled as homosexuals. Even though there are hidden opportunities in nursing for men, these advantages may extend only to those who are perceived to have the conventional masculine characteristics, such as a heterosexual orientation (Williams, 1995).

Think About It

Do Men and Women Express Caring in Different Ways?

- *What do you think of Begany's (1994) images of caring? What does caring mean to you?*

- *Williams (1995) believed that organizations are gender biased in how they regard* masculine *behaviors* versus *feminine ones. She suggested the development of gender-sensitive evaluation tools that would acknowledge women's contributions to the profession. If you were appointed to develop such an evaluation tool, what attributes would your tool reward and recognize as unique to women? What justice issues may be involved in using gender-sensitive evaluation processes?*

- *Goals of the American Assembly for Men in Nursing include supporting men already in nursing and educating society about the benefits of male nurses. What do you think are the benefits to patients and society of nurses who are men? How do these differ from the benefits of nurses who are women?*

SEXUAL HARASSMENT IN NURSING

Sexual harassment has been a dominant theme in American nursing. Florence Nightingale countered sexual harassment with the prevailing strategy of the day, which was to gain respect through being a lady (Nightingale, 1859/1992). As noted in Chapter 9, sexual harassment is a form of sex discrimination that violates the Civil Rights Act of 1964. The U.S. Equal Employment Opportunity Commission (EEOC) defines sexual harassment as "unwelcome sexual advances, requests for sexual favors, and other verbal or physical harassment of a sexual nature" (EEOC, 2013). Nurses may not immediately recognize or label behaviors as sexual harassment, and often have difficulty finding appropriate words to describe the experience concisely. Indicators of sexual harassment include the following:

- Invasion of space
- Lack of respect
- Overtly friendly behavior

- Sexually suggestive behavior that is planned or intentional
- Physical or organizational power that supports or protects the harasser while limiting the options of the harassed
- A sexualized workplace where explicit jokes, innuendos, and pictures are common (Madison & Minichiello, 2000)

Nurses need to employ specific strategies to combat sexual harassment in the workplace. Strategies include being assertive, seeking support from other nurses, documenting each incident, filing a complaint or grievance, and initiating legal action. Nurse leaders should develop organization-wide strategies such as education programs focusing on sexual harassment, written procedures to address sexual harassment issues, investigation of all complaints, and counseling for victims.

ASK YOURSELF

Sexual Harassment

Nurses have close contact with many people each day. They discuss intimate matters with patients and families. Occasionally patients make sexual advances toward nurses.

- What types of patient behavior would constitute sexual harassment?
- What is the best way for nurses to react when confronted with sexual advances by patients?
- Is it possible for men in nursing to also face sexual harassment from patients?

We do not need to venture far to find images that reinforce the view that nurses are sexual objects. A quick tour of the *get well* section at your local greeting card shop graphically illustrates this point. Although sexual harassment does not recognize gender boundaries, sexual harassment has predominantly been a problem for women. As more men enter the nursing profession, issues concerning sexual harassment directed toward them or from them may emerge. Research is needed that is directed toward understanding sexual harassment in nursing, how best to address the needs of men in nursing, and implications for the women with whom they work.

MODERN SEXISM

Even though women have made tremendous inroads in the workplace, it is clear that gender inequality is still a major problem. In fact, it may be on the rise in some areas. **Sexism** relates to prejudice, devaluation, stereotyping, or discrimination on the basis of gender. In our predominantly male-oriented health care system, sexism may present itself in many ways. Unfortunately, even within the nursing profession, sexism related to men in nursing also occurs. An example of this is the male colleague who feels he has a hiring edge over women in nursing, because he never needs to be off for maternity leave or to stay home from work to care for sick children.

Heterosexism is a system of beliefs that discriminates against homosexuals on the assumption that heterosexuality is superior and expectable. Nurses must be alert for this form of sexism that marginalizes persons who do not identify as heterosexual. Despite the belief that developing an understanding of these issues may have a tremendous effect upon nursing care, very little attention is given to addressing this and other gender issues within nursing curricula.

SEXUAL ORIENTATION

Lesbians and gay men may be the largest minority group in nursing. Although nobody knows exactly how many of the three million nurses in America are lesbian or gay, there are probably between 100,000 and 200,000 (Zurlinden, 1997). These nurses are likely to be practicing in every state and working in every hospital. Fearing sexual harassment and discrimination from coworkers, superiors, and bureaucratic systems, many remain reluctant to have their sexual orientation known.

Sexual harassment and bigotry is a fact of life for many lesbians and gay men. 40 years after the birth of the modern gay rights movement, a Gallup poll revealed that 43 percent of Americans consider same-gender relationships between consenting adults to be morally wrong (Saad, 2010). This culturally prevalent attitude can range from prejudice to homophobia. Prejudice that is operationalized on the institutional level leads to discrimination. More extreme forms of bigotry include harassment and physical violence. Zurlinden (1997) writes, "Unmasked, homophobia is really hatred, willful ignorance, mean-spiritedness, and narrow-mindedness. People suffering from homophobia do not run screaming in terror when they encounter a lesbian or gay man. Instead, they assume they are justified to be cruel; to discriminate in housing, employment, and education; and to pass laws to prevent gay men and lesbians from enjoying the civil liberties that other Americans take for granted" (p. 11).

Within institutions, bigotry can be insidious, damaging, and difficult to change. Some employers systematically discriminate against lesbians and gay men through hiring, promotion, and disciplinary practices. This may be the result of institutional policy, discriminatory administrative practice, punitive supervisors, or discrimination by coworkers (Zurlinden, 1997).

Discrimination may also take the form of absence of employment benefits available to heterosexuals. Though some employers have agreed to extend spousal benefits such as health insurance, life insurance, and maternity leave to same-gender couples, these are not available in most institutions.

There are also legal implications for nurses who are gay or lesbian. Many states still have laws that forbid particular types of sexual relationships, including same-gender sex. In some states, lesbians and gay men may risk losing their nursing licenses. Being accused of a felony is enough to lead to suspension of a nurse's license in some states; conviction can lead to permanent loss of license (Zurlinden, 1997). Additionally, a number of state boards of nursing have provisions that require good moral character to retain a nursing license. This policy is potentially troublesome, because many people consider same-gender relationships to be morally wrong.

Though discriminatory practices remain, most health care professions have publicly endorsed a nonjudgmental attitude toward sexual orientation. The ANA, American Psychiatric Association, American Psychological Association, National Association of Social Workers, and the American Medical Association all include statements related to nonjudgmental recognition of sexual orientation.

Caring for Lesbian, Gay, Bisexual, and Transgender Patients

Lesbian, gay, bisexual, and transgender (LGBT) patients are more likely to receive substandard health care. Bias exists among some health care providers to the point of open hostility toward LGBT patients. Because LGBT patients are often aware of this bias, they may not reveal their sexual orientation to providers. This leads to deficiencies in access to care, missed opportunities to identify domestic violence, and failure to diagnose diseases that are prevalent in the LGBT community. Nurses should become aware of LGBT health care issues and be sensitive to creating an environment that encourages open dialogue. When talking about sexual relationships, the nurse should use gender-neutral language such as *partner*, assure patients that private information will be kept confidential, and ask specific questions about sexual practices. As with other professional relationships, open communication is the key to providing beneficent and comprehensive health care.

COMMUNICATION ISSUES RELATED TO GENDER

How nurses communicate with each other, their patients, and their colleagues has long been discussed in the nursing literature. Nurses need to address how changing societal roles and expectations relate to the practice of nursing, and determine what research is needed to promote and bring about positive change.

Nurse-Physician Communication

A gender division of labor has been a significant factor in how nurses, who are primarily women, and physicians, who are primarily men, relate to each other in health care settings. Communication with physicians remains an area of primary concern for many nurses. Since poor nurse-physician communication has been shown to lead to unfavorable patient outcomes, strategies to improve communication are imperative (Page, 2004).

Many nurses use less-than-straightforward methods to manage conflict among themselves or between nurses and physician colleagues. Staff nurses are most comfortable using avoidance, while nurse managers tend to use compromise as their primary method of conflict management (Valentine, 1995). These methods may be reinforced by nursing educators, who also employ avoidance as their primary conflict management tool.

Problem communications between nurses and physicians may result in harm to patients when nurses are not able to convince physicians of deteriorating patient conditions. Andrews and Waterman (2005) describe situations in which nurses know that patients' conditions are deteriorating, yet cannot convince physicians. Andrews and Waterman attribute the problem, in part, to differences in nurses' and physicians' styles. While nurses may sense subtle changes in patients' conditions, physicians are unconvinced until there are hard and objective changes. According to Tannen (2001), the primary reason for these and other communication conflicts relates to identifying and understanding gender differences in communication.

With females comprising nearly 50 percent of students entering medicine, and males comprising 12 percent of students entering nursing school,

Think About It

Do Men and Women Communicate Differently?

Tannen (2001) asserts that men and women communicate from such differing frames of reference that their communication could be considered a cultural clash of sorts.

- *What has your experience been in this area?*
- *What communication concerns with fellow students, faculty, patients, or physicians have you experienced in your program of study?*
- *How would you rate the nurse-physician communication in your clinical agencies? Describe why.*
- *Describe potential gender-based differences in communication.*

perhaps the patriarchal system of health care will shift. The implications this may have for nursing remain unknown. Several studies focus on the traditional nurse-doctor relationship. None to date has examined the interactions of nurses, male or female, with physicians who are female.

Communicating with Patients

Through informal dress and communications, nurses may in fact be sending powerful negative messages to their patients and medical colleagues. The tone of familiarity expressed by nurses who use their first names with patients may translate sociologically into persistent stereotypic themes and become a mechanism of social control. While superior nursing care may reduce these stereotypes, deliberative communications strategies are needed to accelerate professional recognition (Campbell-Heider & Hart, 1993).

Successful interpersonal communications with patients is central to the practice of nursing. In relation to sensitive issues and sexuality, Propst (1996) found that registered nurses' communication practices are lacking. Only half of the respondents in her sample of women's health nurses discussed issues concerning sexuality with their patients. This indicates that, even in a specialty practice area such as women's health, nurses are not immune to communication issues when sensitive topics are involved.

GENDER AND RACE

Issues concerning race are closely linked to gender as they relate to access to educational preparation, employment opportunities, and wage inequities (Amott & Matthaei, 1996). Amott and Matthaei additionally discuss class as it relates to gender and race in their extensive review *Race, Gender, and Work: A Multicultural Economic History of Women in the United States*. Based on their premise that race, gender, and class are intrinsically interconnected, Amott and Matthaei believe that the explanatory power of each concept, in itself, is limited, but together they may broaden our understanding of the lives of women who enter nursing. Both Achterberg (1990) and Amott and Matthaei concur that the takeover of medicine by white men, who forced midwives and other women healers out of health care, coincided with the development of nursing.

Most minority groups are represented in nursing, though the racial and ethnic profile of registered nurses is substantially different from that of the U.S. population as a whole (U.S. Department of Health and Human Services, 2010). Satcher and Pamies (2006) reported that the number of minority students increased in most health professions schools, with nursing showing a very promising increase. In the decade between 1994 and 2004, the percent of minority nursing students rose from 13 percent to 18.5 percent, while the number of minority registered nurses rose from 13 percent to 17 percent during the same time. The 2008 National Sample Survey of Registered Nurses showed a slight decline of registered nurses from 2001 to 2008 (U.S. Department of Health and Human Services, 2010). The largest group of nurses represented in the 2008 survey was White (83 percent), compared to 66 percent of the population as a whole. In 2008, registered nurses came from diverse racial and ethnic backgrounds as follows: 4.6 percent were African American; 5.8 percent were Asian or Pacific Islander; 3.6 percent were Hispanic; 0.3 percent were American Indian/Alaskan Native; and 1.7 percent were from two or more racial backgrounds. Although the numbers of Asian and Hispanic nurses are increasing in certain geographic areas, African Americans continue to comprise the largest minority group of nurses. Interestingly, African Americans (14.6 percent) were more likely to have their highest preparation at the master's or doctorate level compared to 13.4 percent among White, non-Hispanics; 10.5 percent among Hispanics; and 8.3 percent among Asian/Native Hawaiian/Pacific Islander, non-Hispanic nurses (U.S. Department of Health and Human Services, 2010).

A rich history of the African American nurse experience in the United States is depicted by Lewenson (1996) as she describes the establishment of educational programs for African American nurses in the late 1800s and the 43-year history of the National Association of Colored Graduate Nurses (NACGN) (1908–1951). The NACGN eventually integrated with the ANA, because the ANA did not discriminate as many state organizations did when African American nurses tried to join.

Racism, the assumption that members of one race are superior to those of another, was an everyday experience for African American nurses at the turn of the century. Despite Title VII of the Civil Rights Act of 1964, many African Americans continue to experience racism. After experiencing racism on the job, Nicole Cole, an African American nurse, poignantly describes her thoughts:

> I told my children to work hard and be the best at whatever they decided to do, and they would achieve success. But in the back of my mind, I don't know if I truly believed that sentiment. I know the world is cruel and being black is like having a target you can't hide. Whether the title is "valedictorian," "Miss America," or "Secretary of State," there are still people out there who differentiate you by the color of your skin. "You know, the black one"—I've uttered those words myself. (Cole, 2011)

There are good reasons for Cole's perceptions. Historically, African American nurses have very different employment experiences than Whites. They have been disproportionately employed in institutions that serve African

Americans and in public as opposed to private organizations (Satcher & Pamies, 2006). These employment demographics may partially explain the wide salary gap experienced by racial minorities. In one New York study, minority nurses earned an average of $6,000 less than White counterparts with the same level of education and experience (McGinnis & Moore, 2009). Discussion related to transcultural nursing is raising awareness of cultural diversity and disparities in the nursing workforce.

Strategies for improving racial equality in the nursing profession include incorporating race equality issues in school of nursing curricula; educating staff in equal opportunity and antiracist strategies; and the recruitment, selection, and career progression of minority faculty. Swinney and Dobal (2008) describe a program designed to increase the number of ethnic minority and disadvantaged nurses by targeting predominantly Hispanic and African American communities. The goals of the project are to recruit students to nursing, support and retain students in nursing, and provide stipends and scholarship. The program increased the number of ethnic minority and disadvantaged students by 30 percent in 3 years. This program and others like it are important. If nursing is a reflection of society at large, issues of racial inequalities within the broader context of society must also be confronted.

SUMMARY

Nursing has been faced with gender issues since the early days of the profession. Nursing role and status have been colored by societal expectations of women and paternalistic ideology permeating the health care arena. Considerations of gender can be related to lower salaries for nurses compared with primarily male professions, communication patterns with physicians and patients, perceptions of abilities to carry out nursing's caring imperative, and stereotypical expectations of how nurses should look and act. While men in the profession face the challenge of dealing with societal stereotypes, they are also often tracked into higher-paying and more prestigious positions. Issues concerning discrimination based on sexual orientation occur on many fronts and may be underrecognized. Awareness of these issues enables nurses of both genders to be alert for inequities and to develop strategies for change.

CHAPTER HIGHLIGHTS

- Controversy exists regarding how the title of the person caring for the sick relates to the gender of the person providing care. Both women and men in nursing must deal with social stereotyping regarding expected roles and behaviors.

- Societal expectations of women and paternalistic ideology throughout history have led to discrimination in nursing, though gender discrimination may exist for both women and men in different nursing
  settings.

- Issues concerning race and gender are closely related and must be
  addressed in nursing.

- Issues of comparable worth relative to gender are of concern in
  nursing, particularly in areas of salary and positions of prestige and
  responsibility.

- Nurses need to be alert to, and employ strategies to combat, sexual
  harassment.

- Gender-based differences in styles and patterns of communication
  can affect all areas of nursing practice, requiring attentiveness to
  effective communication with patients and colleagues in order to
  foster better patient outcomes.

- Sexism, occurring in both subtle and overt ways, continues to be an
  issue in nursing, and harassment and discrimination based on sexual
  orientation may be underrecognized.

DISCUSSION QUESTIONS AND ACTIVITIES

1. One frequently cited political action strategy is to build coalitions with
   powerful persons of like mind. If nurses in your community are to become empowered, with whom would they build coalitions?

2. In what ways does your school or curriculum address issues of improving racial equality in the nursing profession?

3. Read an article on how nursing students learn to care. Do men learn
   about or express caring differently than women? How does this relate
   to your experiences as a student nurse? How does this relate to Begany's (1994) images of nurturer or handmaiden?

4. What stereotypes of nurses are present in your community or the national media? What types of *get well* cards are in your local card shop?
   What do you think it will take to change these and other stereotypes
   about nurses?

5. What is the gender makeup of your local nursing administration?
   How many women are in positions of authority or power within your
   health care setting? What are their salary ranges? How do their salaries compare with those of men in positions of similar responsibility?

6. Observe gender-based communication patterns between nurses
   and physicians. Consider your own style of communication with

same-gender and other-gender friends and colleagues. What patterns do you identify? How might these patterns affect your professional interactions? Are there areas that need to be modified in order to promote more effective communication?

7.   Explore various websites to determine guidelines regarding sexual harassment that are offered by the ANA, the Canadian Nurses Association, and other professional organizations at http://www.cna-nurses.ca and http://www.ana.org.

REFERENCES

Achterberg, J. (1990). *Woman as healer*. Boston, MA: Shambhala.

American Assembly for Men in Nursing. (2012). About us. Retrieved from http://aamn.org/aamn.shtml

American Nurses Association. (1995). *Nursing's social policy statement* [Brochure]. Washington, DC: Author.

Amott, T., & Matthaei, J. (1996). *Race, gender, and work: A multicultural economic history of women in the United States* (2nd ed.). Boston, MA: South End Press.

Andrews, T., & Waterman, H. (2005). Visualizing deteriorating conditions. *Grounded Theory Review, 4*(2), 63–94.

Begany, T. (1994). Your image is brighter than ever. *RN, 57,* 28–35.

Benokraitis, N. V., & Feagin, J. R. (1995). *Modern sexism: Blatant, subtle, and covert discrimination* (2nd ed.). Englewood Cliffs, NJ: Prentice-Hall.

Campbell-Heider, N., & Hart, C. (1993). Updating the nurse's bedside manner. *Image, 25,* 133–139.

Chinn, P. L. (1991). *Anthology on caring*. New York: National League of Nursing Press.

Cole, N. M. (2011). From hate to hope: A nursing journey. *Minority Nurse.* Retrieved from http://www.minoritynurse.com/african-american-black-nurses/hate-hope-nursing-journey.

Dalai Lama. (1999). *Ethics for the new millennium*. New York: Penguin Putnam.

Ekstrom, D. N. (1999). Gender and perceived caring in nurse-patient dyads. *Journal of Advanced Nursing, 29*(6), 1393–1401.

Ellis, J., & Hartley, C. (2003). *Nursing in today's world* (8th ed.). Philadelphia: Lippincott.

Equal Employment Opportunity Commission. (2013). Sexual harassment. Retrieved from http://www.eeoc.gov/laws/types/sexual_harassment.cfm

Gilloran, A. (1995). Gender differences in care delivery and supervisory relationship: The case of psychogeriatric nursing. *Journal of Advanced Nursing, 21*, 652–658.

Grigsby, K., & Megel, M. (1995). Caring experiences of nurse educators. *Journal of Nursing Education, 34*, 411–418.

Hamilton, P. (1999). *Realities of contemporary nursing* (2nd ed.) Menlo Park, CA: Addison-Wesley.

Hilton, L. (2001, May 14). A few good men: Male nurses defy stereotypes and discrimination to find satisfaction in a female-dominated profession. *Nurse Week.* Retrieved July 18, 2006, from http://www.nurseweek.com/news/features/01-05/men.html

JAMA. (1996). The hospital hotel. *Journal of the American Medical Association, 275*, 324.

Ketter, J. (1994, April). Sex discrimination targets men in some hospitals. *The American Nurse, 26*, 1, 24.

Letizia, B. (1994, December). Ban on male nurses in labor and delivery is upheld. *RN, 57*, 16.

Lewenson, S. (1996). *Taking charge: Nursing, suffrage, and feminism in America, 1873–1920.* New York: National League of Nursing Press.

Madison, J., & Minichiello, V. (2000). Recognizing and labeling sex-based and sexual harassment in the health care workplace. *Journal of Nursing Scholarship, 32*(4), 405–410.

McGinnis, S. L., & Moore, J. (2009). An analysis of racial/ethnic pay disparities among hospital nurses in New York City. *Policy, Politics, & Nursing Practice, 10*(4), 252–258.

Nightingale, F. (1859/1992). *Notes on nursing: What it is, and what it is not.* London: Harrison & Sons.

Page, A. (Ed.). (2004). *Keeping patients safe: Transforming the work environment of nurses.* Committee on the Work Environment for Nurses and Patient Safety, Institute of Medicine. Washington, DC: National Academy Press.

Peter, E., & Gallop, R. (1994). The ethic of care: A comparison of nursing and medical students. *Image, 26*, 47–51.

Propst, M. (1996). Registered nurses' practice and perspective toward sexuality in women's health. *Southern Nursing Research Society Abstracts*, 83.

Reskin, B., & Padavic, I. (2002). *Women and men at work* (2nd ed.). Thousand Oaks, CA: Pine Forge Press.

Reverby, S. (1987). A caring dilemma: Womanhood and nursing in historical perspective. *Nursing Research, 36*, 5–10.

Robert Wood Johnson Foundation. (2011). Nurse leaders, IOM report call for push to increase diversity in nursing. Retrieved from http://www.rwjf.org/newsroom/product.jsp?id=71931

Saad, L. (2010). Americans' acceptance of gay relations crosses 50% threshold. Gallup Politics. Retrieved from http://www.gallup.com/poll/135764/americans-acceptance-gay-relations-crosses-threshold.aspx

Satcher, D., & Pamies, R. J. (2006). *Multicultural medicine and health disparities.* New York: McGraw-Hill.

Squires, T. (1995). Men in nursing. *RN, 58,* 26–28.

Sullivan, E. J. (2000). Men in nursing: The importance of gender diversity. *Journal of Professional Nursing, 16*(5), 253–254.

Swinney, J. E., & Dobal, M. T. (2008). Embracing the challenge: Increasing workforce diversity in nursing. *Hispanic Health Care International, 6*(4), 200–204. DOI: 10.1891/1540-4153.6.4.200

Tannen, D. (2001). *You just don't understand: Women and men in conversation.* New York: Harper Collins.

Thompson, J. (1995, February). Banning male RNs from L & D is blatantly unfair [Letter to the editor]. *RN, 58,* 9.

U.S. Department of Health and Human Services. (2010). Registered Nurse Population: Findings from the 2008 national sample survey of registered nurses. Retrieved from http://bhpr.hrsa.gov/healthworkforce/rnsurveys/rnsurveyfinal.pdf

U.S. Department of Labor. (2008). Quick facts on registered nurses. Retrieved from http://www.dol.gov/wb/factsheets/Qf-nursing-08.htm

Valentine, P. (1995). Management of conflict: Do nurses/women handle it differently? *Journal of Advanced Nursing, 22,* 142–149.

Williams, C. (1995). Hidden advantages for men in nursing. *Nursing Administration Quarterly, 19,* 63–70.

Williams, C. L. (1991). *Gender differences at work: Women and men in non-traditional occupations* (reprint edition). Berkeley, CA: University of California Press.

Zurlinden, J. (1997). *Lesbian and gay nurses.* Clifton Park, NY: Delmar.

Chapter

18

TRANSCULTURAL AND SPIRITUAL ISSUES

God is a spirit, a mystery beyond human understanding, and therefore we can only approach that mystery through metaphor. Our metaphors come, of course, from human and cultural understandings of the good, the loving, the just. . . . More surely than anything else, we are defined by our stories—the cultural myths we hear from our earliest days.

(Sewell, 1991, pp. 237, 261)

OBJECTIVES

At the end of this chapter, the reader should be able to:

1. Describe factors associated with cultural sensitivity within nursing.

2. Discuss the influence of culture on health and health care decisions.

3. Identify approaches for dealing with transcultural issues in nursing.

4. Discuss issues related to the use of complementary therapies by patients.

5. Identify legal considerations related to transcultural issues.

6. Discuss the relationship between spirituality and health.

7. Describe issues associated with spirituality and religion.

8. Identify the nursing role in addressing patients' spiritual concerns.

9. Discuss considerations regarding nurturing one's spirit.

INTRODUCTION

The influence of culture, religion, and spirituality are major factors in the development of values. Because nurses deal with people from varied cultural and spiritual backgrounds, they must be alert for issues relating to these areas. This chapter presents general considerations regarding culture and spirituality and discusses related issues that may arise when caring for patients.

TRANSCULTURAL ISSUES

We live in a multicultural society, alive with diversity. Such diversity of people and backgrounds provides a richness to our lives, yet it challenges our abilities to appreciate, rather than judge or fear, differences. **Diversity** is encountered wherever there are differences among people such as gender, age, socioeconomic position, sexual orientation, health status, ethnicity, race, or culture. Because dealing with diversity is an essential component of nursing care, nurses are expected to demonstrate competence in providing culturally appropriate care. **Cultural competence** (Engebretson, 2013; Jeffreys, 2010) includes **cultural awareness** and **cultural sensitivity**. Cultural awareness includes knowledge about the values, beliefs, behaviors, and the like of cultures other than one's own. Cultural sensitivity is the ability to incorporate the patient's cultural perspective into nursing assessments and to modify nursing care in order to be as congruent as possible with the patient's cultural perspective.

Culture teaches us to understand a particular perception of reality. Because of this, the same phenomenon may be viewed differently by people from different cultures. For example, the *man in the moon* that most people in this country have been taught to "see" is identified in other cultures as a *frog in the moon,* a *woman in the moon,* or a *rabbit in the moon* (Tafoya, 1996). Another way of appreciating different perspectives is to consider what we see when we are in the valley, compared with what we see from halfway up the mountain or the view from the top of the mountain. Different perceptions of the same reality derive from the perspectives from which it is viewed. One view of reality is not more correct than the other; the different views merely come from different perspectives.

Understanding Culture

Self-awareness is a key factor in dealing with transcultural issues. The best starting point for becoming sensitive to the culture of another is to understand our own culture and its influence on our perceptions and behaviors.

Culture refers to the totality of lifeways of a group of interacting individuals, consisting of learned patterns of values, beliefs, behaviors, and customs shared by that group (Engebretson, 2013; Leininger & McFarley, 2005; Ray, 2010). These *learned patterns* are transmitted from one generation to the next in formal ways, such as through educational settings, and in informal ways, such as through role modeling. Unique cultural expressions can be observed within many groups of interacting individuals—for example, the culture of the deaf community, prison culture, or the culture of health care. When we recognize that each of us is part of a culture and identify the values, beliefs, and behaviors that we hold dear, we become clearer about our own cultural perspective. It is important to in this process be alert to our own **ethnocentrism**, reflected in our tendency to judge behaviors of someone from another culture by the standards of our own culture.

ASK YOURSELF

How Do You Deal with Diversity?

Consider a situation in which you were afraid of or judged someone you did not know because she or he was different from you.

- What was it about the person or situation that triggered your judgment or fear?
- Why do you think you reacted to the person or situation the way you did?
- How and from whom did you learn to react in this way?
- What has helped you to understand diversity and overcome fear?
- How can nurses learn to appreciate rather than fear diversity among colleagues and patients?

In its *Position Statement on Cultural Diversity in Nursing Practice,* the American Nurses Association (ANA) (1991) stated that ethnocentric approaches to nursing practice were ineffective in meeting the health and nursing needs of diverse cultural groups, and encouraged nurses in all settings to be knowledgeable about cultures and their impact on interactions with health care. Developing cultural sensitivity implies understanding the behaviors and values of another culture within the context of that culture, without imposing our own cultural values on others. Cultural sensitivity includes avoiding **stereotyping**, which is expecting all persons from a particular group to behave, think, or respond in a certain way based on preconceived ideas. Every culture contains variation, and some people within the group may not ascribe to all beliefs and values attributed to that culture.

Ask Yourself

How Might Ethnocentrism Affect Nursing Care?

Consider the varied meanings the following behaviors may have depending upon the cultural context in which they occur: direct eye contact may connote honesty or intrusion, a firm handshake may be viewed as confidence or as hostility, and frequent bathing may be considered to be necessary or unhealthy.

- How might behaviors such as these be judged by people within the dominant culture in this country?
- How do practices and expectations within health care settings reflect ethnocentrism regarding behaviors such as these?
- How might ethnocentrism or stereotyping affect interaction with others, especially within a nursing setting?

Cultural Values and Beliefs

Because culture is one of the key organizing concepts of nursing, nurses need to be knowledgeable about

> how cultural groups understand life processes; how cultural groups define health and illness; what cultural groups do to maintain wellness; what cultural groups believe to be the causes of illness; how healers cure and care for members of cultural groups; and how the cultural background of the nurse influences the way in which care is delivered. (ANA, 1991)

Cultural values and beliefs guide our thinking, being, and doing in patterned ways. Beliefs about health and practices related to health and healing are some of the patterns influenced by culture that are significant in providing health care. Such beliefs and practices manifest in both direct and subtle ways, and sensitivity to them can affect patient outcomes and satisfaction with care. It is helpful to recognize a distinction between **disease**, which is the biomedical explanation of sickness, and **illness**, which is a personal response to the disease that flows from how our culture teaches us to be sick. Transcultural issues are often present in nursing situations, but may not be identified as such. Instead, patients may be labeled as stoic, uncooperative, noncompliant, strange, or "crazy" because of choices they make, and their health and care may be compromised. Madeline Leininger (1991), a pioneer in the area of transcultural nursing, delineated principles of transcultural care, human rights, and ethical considerations that offer guidance for nurses in dealing with transcultural issues. These principles, listed in Figure 18–1, continue to offer a framework for providing culturally sensitive care. In light of these principles, many nursing practices derived from the Western biomedical model may benefit from reevaluation.

1. Human beings of any culture in the world have a right to have their cultural care values known, respected and appropriately used in nursing and other health care services.

2. Human cultures have diverse and universal modes of caring and healing practices that need to be recognized and used by professional nurses to function effectively and therapeutically with people of different cultures.

3. Care is the essence of nursing and a basic human need for growth, healing, well-being, recovery, and survival.

4. Cultural care is a critical component influencing human health, well-being, and recovery from illnesses or disabilities.

5. Every culture has at least two major types of health care systems namely, the *folk (generic, lay or indigenous) care system* and the *professional care system* which influence their health outcomes, and the transcultural nurse is challenged to use this knowledge to guide nursing care decisions and actions.

6. All professional nurses are challenged to respect common human needs and humanistic aspects of people care worldwide, and also the divergent care expressions, meanings, and practices.

7. Transcultural nurses are expected to respect Western and non-Western cultures who often have different values, beliefs, and norms to assess and understand human beings.

8. Transcultural nursing principles and practices are the arching framework for all nursing care practices which differ from nursing practices that rely on traditional medical symptoms, diseases and treatment regimes.

9. Since transcultural nursing focuses upon *comparative cultural care* values, beliefs and practices of cultures, the nurse is expected to work with individuals, families, groups, cultures, subcultures and institutions that reflect cultural care variabilities.

10. Nurses with transcultural knowledge are expected to respond appropriately to *culture care differences* and *similarities* in order to ease or ameliorate a human condition or lifeway, and to help clients face death.

11. Ethical and moral differences and similarities exist among human cultures which necessitates that nurses recognize, respect and respond appropriately to such variabilities.

12. It is essential that transcultural nurses be open-minded and willing to learn from cultural informants about their human values, beliefs, needs and practices in order to make appropriate nursing care plans, judgments and actions.

13. The ability of the nurse to listen, use silence and envision the client's or family's human condition or cultural circumstance with its positive or less positive features is important in transcultural nursing.

FIGURE 18–1   Transcultural Care Principles, Human Rights, and Ethical Considerations

14. Transcultural nursing often requires that nurses communicate with clients in their native language to know, learn and understand individuals, families and groups of different cultures.

15. Transcultural nurses are challenged to identify what constitutes ethical or moral principles and norms of cultures and not assume that all cultures are alike.

16. Transcultural nurses are expected to guide other nurses who have not been prepared in transcultural nursing in order to prevent marked ethnocentrism, cultural imposition practices, and inappropriate ethical and moral judgments about clients.

17. Transcultural nursing reflects that individuals or groups of a designated culture are active participants and decision makers in culture care practices in order to develop and maintain creative and effective professional care practices.

18. Clients of diverse or similar cultures have a right to have their caring lifestyles and expressions known and used in transcultural nursing in order to promote client health or well-being.

19. Transcultural nursing takes into account the world view, environmental context, ethnohistory, social structure features (including the religious, kinship, philosophic, economic, political, technological and cultural values), language, expressions, gender and age differences of people.

20. Transcultural nursing is concerned with the assessment of caregiver and care-receiver expressions, beliefs and lifeways that often go beyond nurse-client dyadic relationship to that of care relationships with families, groups, institutions and communities in order to facilitate congruent care practices and to avoid unfavorable culture care conflicts, stress and negligent care practices.

21. Since ethical, moral and legal systems of human values and rights exist in all cultures, it is the task and responsibility of transcultural nurses to discover these dimensions with key and general informants and in diverse cultural contexts.

22. Human care rights tend to be covert and embedded in the social structure, cultural values and world view of clients, and so the transcultural nurse is challenged to discover these dimensions mainly through qualitative research methods.

23. Transcultural nurses recognize that cultures are complex, dynamic and change over time and in varying ways.

24. Transcultural nurses recognize that many cultures and subcultures in the world have not been studied and yet nurses are expected to care for all peoples including minorities.

25. Transcultural nursing is a major breakthrough for new nursing knowledge and practices that do not follow the traditional nursing or medical disease, symptom and illness models.

Leininger, M. (1991). *Journal of Transcultural Nursing, 3,* 21–23. Reprinted with permission of the *Journal of Transcultural Nursing.*

FIGURE 18–1   *(continued)*

Incorporating cultural assessment into care with patients is an important part of a comprehensive nursing assessment. This assessment facilitates better understanding of sometimes overlooked factors that influence health behaviors and decisions. Cultural assessment helps nurses to appropriately identify and understand the meaning of behaviors that might otherwise be judged negatively or be confusing to the nurse (Campinha-Bacote, 2007; Engebretson, 2013; Giger & Davidhizar, 2007). We recognize that each person is culturally unique, and that not all persons in a particular cultural group believe or respond similarly. Cultural assessment includes exploration of cultural phenomena that are evident in all cultural groups: communication, personal space, social organization, time, environmental control, and biological variation (Engebretson, 2013; Giger & Davidhizar, 2007). Such exploration enables nurses to identify areas where modifications in care can be incorporated so that care is more culturally congruent. Although the process may also reveal divergent beliefs that are difficult to accommodate within the current health care system, acknowledging differences may help the patient and family to feel more comfortable within the system. For example, when assessing eating patterns and food preferences, the nurse might discover that the patient commonly eats only two meals a day, consisting of burritos in the morning and rice and beans in the evening. Typical hospital food and a three-meals-a-day pattern might not be appetizing for this patient. The patient's nutrition may suffer, and she may perceive that she is not being fed. By arranging for the patient to have culturally similar foods at similar times, the nurse provides more culturally congruent care.

Case Presentation

Cultural Differences

Brenda White is a home health nurse caring for 72-year-old Mrs. Cortez, who is living with her daughter and family while recovering from a stroke. Part of the care involves working with the patient on coordination and strengthening exercises. Brenda has found Mrs. Cortez to be very cooperative and uncomplaining in doing the exercises under her direction, indicating that she would do what was needed to get well. One day Brenda's supervisor, Maria Lopez, tells her that the agency has received a complaint from Mrs. Cortez's family that Brenda is being too rough on the patient. Brenda responds that she does not understand this, because Mrs. Cortez has never complained. Brenda further explains that she was trying to have the patient work to her maximum capability and to give her instructions in a clear and direct manner. Ms. Lopez says that in her culture elders are considered very precious and are treated with gentleness and respect. Perhaps the family perceived that Brenda's direct ways indicated disrespect for their mother, even though the patient did not indicate this.

Think About It

How Can Nurses Develop Cultural Competence?

- *How is cultural diversity evident in this situation?*
- *Where is there evidence of a lack of cultural competence?*
- *What might Brenda do to make her care more culturally sensitive?*
- *How do you think you would respond in a similar situation?*
- *How can nurses develop cultural competence?*

Culture and the Health Care System

Concepts of health and healing, of right and wrong, of what is proper and what is not, are rooted in culture. Cultures have different explanatory models regarding health and illness that reflect their beliefs about the causes, symptoms, and treatments of illness and their response to dying and death. Our explanatory model helps us to recognize, respond to, interpret, cope with, and make sense of illness and other life experiences (Engebretson & Headley, 2013).

Transcultural issues arise when nurses, patients, and families hold differing views of what is important or necessary regarding health, recovery, illness, or the dying process. Providing culturally competent nursing care may help to address concerns before they become serious ethical issues. Addressing cultural issues within some areas of the contemporary health care system can be a challenge. In spite of growing emphasis on cultural competence, this system often includes the attitude that the health care provider knows what is "best for the patient," as viewed from the health care provider's perspective.

The health care provider's perspective generally derives from a combination of two cultural orientations. The primary cultural orientation is the biomedical model, and the secondary cultural orientation is the provider's personal cultural background. If the patient's perspective is different from this model and is not considered, dilemmas may emerge. Consider, for example, a situation in which the physician, who is schooled in the Western biomedical model, views death as "the enemy" to be overcome at all costs. The patient, who comes from a Native American culture, views death as a part of life that one prepares for by being in harmony with one's surroundings. Medical or surgical interventions that may prolong the patient's life a few weeks, which would be very important in the physician's world view, may be low on the list of considerations for this patient. Another patient who believes the suffering from his illness is a way of atoning for his sins may resist taking pain medication that health professionals deem important for his recovery.

The health care system is a different culture from that of most of the patients served by the system. The medical language and the values, norms, behaviors, rituals, and overall environment are generally unfamiliar to those who seek its services. Even people who belong to the same dominant culture in society as their health care providers are often strangers when they enter the institutions of the system. For those who do not belong to the dominant culture, negotiating the system can be a formidable task. Lack of understanding of the language, procedures, expectations, and other elements of the dominant culture can lead to miscommunication, unclear decisions, and a sense of powerlessness or lack of control. Ethical or legal dilemmas may arise due to misunderstandings. Consider again the case of Mrs. Cortez. Misunderstanding of the nurse's intent might lead the family to decide to terminate nursing care or to bring legal action against the nurse because of their perception that their mother is being mistreated. Another example is a mentally alert 90-year-old Appalachian woman who, after her doctor of 35 years retired, sought care from a new young physician. After a few visits she stopped going to see him, even though she was having serious health problems, because, in her perception, he did not do anything for her. Essentially, he did not talk with her nor spend the kind of time with her that her former physician had, and instead he gave her medicines that she felt made her sick and that she did not need.

When considering values such as autonomy, beneficence, justice, or the right to self-determination, we ask from whose perspective these values are understood—that of the nurse or that of the patient. This same question is appropriate regarding definitions of health. For example, some cultures place a higher emphasis on working together and loyalty to the group than on the self-reliance and individualism valued within the broader culture in the United States (Andrews, 2011; Bednarz, Schim, & Doorenbos, 2010; Chater & Tsai, 2008). Health care decisions in these cultures may be made by a group such as the family, community, or society, rather than by the individual. Cultural assessment provides insight into the congruence, or lack thereof, between patients' and nurses' values and understandings of health. Consider, for example, a situation in which the nurse believes that health includes being able to be a productive member of society and that health problems provide opportunities for one to grow and become more self-actualized. The patient, on the other hand, believes that his work-related injury is an act of *fate* and focuses on being free of pain and able to "get around." If the differing perceptions of health are not recognized and addressed, efforts to have the patient participate in rehabilitation and job retraining or to utilize nonpharmacological measures for pain control may meet with much resistance and patient dissatisfaction.

Complementary Therapies

Culture guides one's choice of when to go for health care, what kind of care to seek, to whom to go for care, and how long to participate in care. It is common knowledge that many people who utilize conventional health care settings also utilize alternative or complementary therapies. Such therapies may derive from traditions in the patient's own culture, or may be borrowed from traditions of another culture. Complementary therapies (also known as integrative therapies) include a wide variety of modalities, such as relaxation techniques, healing touch and other energy-based healing techniques, spiritual healing, biofeedback, nutritional practices, herbal treatments, massage and other body work, meditation, prayer, homeopathy, acupuncture, and biofeedback.

These therapies are often used concurrently with conventional therapies, but they may be chosen in lieu of conventional therapies. In order to have a broad picture of the many factors affecting a patient's health and healing, we need to be aware of various therapies being utilized by the patient. We should incorporate discussion of complementary therapies into nursing assessment in an open way, since patients may be hesitant to bring up the subject. We do not need to use or support such therapies in order to become knowledgeable about them. Complementary therapies often derive from paradigms that differ from, and may not make sense in, the conventional medical model, yet may be very useful in the healing process. When patients are interested in complementary therapies, we can assist them in determining whether there are risks associated with their use. If there are significant risks involved, and the patient is committed to using the therapy, we can work with other health team members to minimize risks and maximize benefits. When there is not a strong commitment to the nonconventional modality, we can encourage ongoing discussion of known risks and benefits related to various options (Adams, Cohen, Eisenberg, & Jonsen, 2002; Barnett, 2007). When conventional health care providers can work with traditional systems and their healers, the overall care becomes more culturally congruent.

The principle of patient self-determination directs us to honor the right of persons to use both conventional and complementary therapies to address their health care needs. Respect for persons calls us to be open to views other than our own, and to appreciate that there are many paths to healing. Complementary modalities should never be discounted merely because they are not understood within the Western biomedical frame of reference. We need to respect convictions that derive from belief systems that are different from our own, and to be open to the contributions to health offered by other explanatory models. A nonjudgmental approach that respects differing values and beliefs and is sensitive to ethnocentric bias enhances the opportunity to explore jointly the efficacy of all options with the patient.

The area of informed consent presents some important questions relative to complementary therapies. Since listing alternative treatments is an important element of an informed consent, consider whether it is an ethical duty for practitioners of bioscientific medicine to include discussion of complementary therapies in discussion of therapeutic alternatives. Similarly, do you think that practitioners of other healing modalities should make certain that their clients are aware of biomedical alternatives? Those who offer complementary therapies should explain the intervention and discuss risks, expected effects and benefits, and treatment options prior to initiating therapy. It is prudent to apprise other health team members of the use of complementary therapies, because these therapies can affect conventional interventions in varying ways.

Practitioners of both conventional and complementary therapies need to be alert to potential threats to patient autonomy that flow from practitioner attitudes. When we assume that patient values and thought processes are the same as ours, we may believe that what we suggest is the only reasonable course of action. When patients choose another course of action, we may question their decision-making capacity or label them as unreasonable. In conventional practice, this is evident in references to nonconventional therapies as quackery or non-scientific, in trying to dissuade patients from using them, and even in deriding the patient for making such choices. Remember that a patient's choice of an option that may seem unreasonable from our perspective does not necessarily mean that the patient has not thought it through. Such differences often merely reflect a difference in values.

Factors important for the healing process are often culturally prescribed. For example, the involvement of family in the care of a sick member may be very important in some cultures. It can be quite distressing for nursing staff on a hospital unit when multiple family members "camp out" in a patient's room or the nearby hallway, or bring food from home that is not on a patient's diet. Providing culturally congruent care in such situations may include relaxing visiting regulations and collaborating with the family regarding appropriate foods from home. If the needs of one patient are different from those of the roommate, dilemmas may arise that require diplomatic interventions by the nurse.

Think About It

How Should Nurses Deal with Complementary Therapies?

Conventional medicine and medical practitioners tend to be skeptical of healing modalities that have not been subjected to empirical scientific study; thus, discussion of nonconventional modalities is not included in lists of alternatives for patients, nor are these modalities generally available in most conventional health care settings.

- *What do you think about this attitude toward complementary therapies?*

- *What experiences have you had with complementary therapies?*

- *How might attitudes toward complementary therapies affect the ability of nurses to provide culturally congruent care for their patients?*

- *What are the ethical implications related to limiting a patient's access to complementary therapies and practitioners within conventional health care institutions?*

- *How have you experienced complementary therapies within nursing practice?*

Legal Considerations Related to Transcultural Issues

Cultural misunderstandings can provide fertile ground for litigation. Communication—verbal, nonverbal, and written—is always of utmost importance. When a patient's first language is different from our own, we must determine the extent of the patient's understanding of our language as well as the extent of our understanding of the patient's language. When the patient uses another language (including sign language), having an interpreter fluent in the patient's language is essential. If the interpreter is a member of the patient's family, the translation may be filtered through the perspective of the family member. Consider, for example, an elderly Cambodian man who is in the hospital and not doing well. His grandson serves as interpreter. The grandson was born in this country and is embarrassed by his grandfather's "old" ways. When the man says that he needs a particular traditional herbal tea each afternoon in order to get well (which is available in a local international foods store), the grandson translates this generically as "tea." Even though the nurse responds by making sure that the patient has tea each afternoon, the patient's needs are not met.

The language in which we explain procedures and the language of consent forms present other issues. Be sure that the patient or family member is able to read the language in which the form is written, and that all terms used are understood. Indeed, we need to assess the patient's literacy level, even if the form is in English. If the form needs to be interpreted for the patient, it is essential that the interpreter understands the procedure and that an appropriate person is available to clarify any areas of uncertainty. People may indicate that they understand when they do not, in order to avoid offending the nurse or being considered ignorant. One way of dealing with this is having patients describe in their own words what they have been told.

ISSUES RELATED TO SPIRITUALITY AND RELIGION

Spirituality is a universal human experience that transcends culture, although it may be conditioned and shaped by cultural experiences. A basic part of nursing practice is being attentive to spirituality and recognizing the individual as a body-mind-spirit being who experiences health concerns in all these dimensions. In the midst of advances in technology and scientific discoveries that have increased our understanding of the nature of illness and disease, awareness of the role of spirituality in health and healing has diminished. Perhaps the limited scientific knowledge of former times made the role of the spirit and the intangible forces deriving from that spirit more apparent. Many persons were cared for in their homes, even in the case of serious illness. Touching, praying, and presence were a natural part of such environments. Historically, institutions such as hospitals were often staffed by religious orders concerned for both spiritual and physical needs.

Healing and health care have long been connected with the spirituality of a people. With indigenous peoples, healing rituals frequently are spiritual in nature. People seeking medical care continue to incorporate spiritual and religious rituals and practices into their care for self and others. It is noteworthy that the words *health, holy,* and *whole* all derive from the same old-Saxon word *Hal* and Greek word *Holos,* both meaning "whole." By their nature, then, health and healing are associated with that which is holy and whole. A question to ponder is whether contemporary health care culture, now vested in technology, managed care, medical home, mergers, and the like, can once again incorporate spirituality within its vision of healing.

Approaching Spirituality

By nature, humans are body-mind-spirit beings. The uniqueness of each person a nurse encounters encompasses the spiritual as well as physical, mental, and emotional manifestations of that person. **Spirituality** is the animating force, life principle, or essence of being that permeates life and is expressed and experienced in multifaceted connections with self, others, nature, and God or Life Force (Burkhardt, 1994; Burkhardt & Nagai-Jacobson, 2002, 2013; Rykkje, Eriksson, & Råholm, 2011). Meaning and purpose in life and life events flow from the spirit and are manifested in open or private ways. All persons are spiritual, whether they ascribe to a religious orientation or deny the existence of the Divine. Beliefs and values are molded and shaped by our spirituality as well as by societal and cultural conditioning.

Nursing espouses a holistic, body-mind-spirit view of persons. Understanding that persons are indeed body-mind-spirit beings, we recognize that spirituality is part of every encounter whether we are conscious of it or not. Holistic nursing care impels us to address the spiritual as well as physical and mental concerns of patients. We strive to become more aware of our own and others' spirituality in order to bring this essential aspect of care consciously into every nursing interaction.

Because spirituality is at once universal and yet often very personal and private, we may find this area difficult to approach. Developing competence in addressing spiritual needs is an important area of nursing practice. The recommendations for integrating spirituality into care that were derived from the Consensus Conference on Improving the Quality of Spiritual Care in Palliative Care (Puchalski et al., 2009) apply to nursing care in all settings. These recommendations include:

- Making spiritual care integral to all patient-centered health care system models of care;

- Basing spiritual care models on honoring the dignity of all people and providing compassionate care;

- Treating spiritual distress or religious struggle with the same urgency or importance as treating other medical or social problems;

- Considering spirituality as a patient vital sign that is routinely screened; and

- Implementing interdisciplinary spiritual care models that include board-certified chaplains in clinical settings. (Puchalski et al., 2009, p. 891)

Recognizing that spirituality is both basic to health and an essential component of nursing care enables us to listen for language, observe behavior, and gather information related to spiritual concerns in every encounter with patients and families.

Spirituality assessment can provide us with information about how patients view life, death, health, and health concerns. Such assessment provides insight into important connections, beliefs, practices, or rituals that may influence a person's choices or affect healing. Processes that incorporate open-ended questions and allow patients to tell their stories facilitate spirituality assessment (Burkhardt & Nagai-Jacobson, 2002, 2013; Liehr & Smith, 2008; Nagai-Jacobson & Burkhardt, 1996; Puchalski, 2007–2008). Although expression of spiritual concerns may include talk of God or faith, patients communicate their spiritual needs and concerns in many other ways as well. They may express questions related to the meaning of present or past experiences, fears or worries about what is happening, or how they will find the strength they need. They may talk about important relationships, the need for reconciliation, experiences of peace or anxiety, or the desire to put their lives in order. Religious articles may be evident, or the nurse may observe the patient engaging in practices such as prayer or meditation.

Opportunities to explore spirituality with patients are present in many situations. Effective spirituality assessment requires us to attend with our whole beings to indicators of spirituality occurring within routine interactions with patients. One process for spiritual assessment is the *FICA Spiritual History Tool* (Puchalski, 2007–2008). This process incorporates open-ended questions regarding four key elements of spirituality:

- **F**aith, belief, meaning—whether the person considers self to be spiritual or religious and what is meaningful to the person;

- **I**mportance and influence of these in one's life and what might be supportive in times of stress;

- **C**ommunity—spiritual and other groups to which the person belongs and that provide meaning and support to the person;

- **A**ddress/action in care—how would the person like the health practitioner to address the above in care?

This spirituality assessment guide is available at http://www.gwumc.edu/gwish/clinical/fica-spiritual/index.cfm.

Spirituality and Religion

Although spirituality may be expressed through religious beliefs and practices, it is not synonymous with these terms. **Religion** is the codification of beliefs and practices concerning the Divine and one's relationship with the Divine that are shared by a group of people. Religion may be quite intertwined within a dominant culture, as with Judaism in Israel or Hinduism in India, or it may be a counterculture, as with the Amish in the United States. Some religions, such as many Christian sects, include people from different cultures. Religious teachings generally include rules regarding right and wrong and guidelines for dealing with issues related to these areas.

Think About It

Recognizing Spiritual Concerns

Spiritual issues reflect core experiences that often defy explanation. Such experiences may relate to suffering, forgiveness, hope, love, or mystery. In the midst of care with patients, nurses often hear comments or questions or observe behaviors reflective of spiritual concerns. Consider the following examples:

A patient or family member says,

> *"I don't know why God is doing this to me (or her)."*
>
> *"I should have locked the gate."*
>
> *"Will you pray for me?"*
>
> *"I don't know why, but having surgery worries me."*
>
> *"I wish I had been willing to go to the beach when he wanted to."*
>
> *"I think I need to trust God and not take chemotherapy. God wants me to trust Him completely."*
>
> *"Without my income I don't know how my family will make it."*
>
> *"We told him not to buy that motorcycle."*
>
> *"Do you believe in miracles?"*

Patients or family members may be observed:

> *Reading a sacred text.*
>
> *Wearing religious jewelry or articles of clothing.*
>
> *Praying or meditating.*
>
> *Staring out a window with a worried or pensive expression.*

In each of the above examples

- *How are spiritual concerns reflected in these comments or behaviors?*

- *What personal beliefs or experiences might affect your feelings and responses to comments or behaviors such as these?*

- *Describe aspects of each comment or behavior that might raise questions or concerns for you.*

- *How would you respond to each of these comments or behaviors? In which circumstances would you feel more comfortable or less comfortable?*

Because religious beliefs and teachings flow from a particular world view, rules and values can be quite variable among different religions. A minor consideration within one religion or sect may constitute a serious dilemma in another. Norms for proper dress for women is one example.

For instance, although most Christian denominations have few, if any, restrictions regarding how women dress, some Christian sects teach that women should wear only skirts or dresses and neither use makeup nor cut their hair. Amish women dress in a particular fashion, and orthodox Muslims and Jews have strict rules regarding how women are to dress in public.

What is considered right or wrong within a particular religion is not always congruent with the ethical perspectives of the greater society. Consider, for example, an infant girl brought to a hospital in the United States with severely infected wounds from trauma to her labial area following a clitorectomy procedure performed by her father. From the perspective of the nurse and the institution, this might be viewed as severe mutilation, constituting abuse—whereas the family would consider this an important religious practice. Another example is the Jehovah's Witness belief that blood transfusions are prohibited, and the ensuing dilemma when a transfusion is medically indicated as a life-saving measure.

ASK YOURSELF

How Does Spirituality Affect Your Nursing Practice?

- What religious or spiritual beliefs or practices are important to you?
- How has your spirituality or religious perspective been influential in your choice of nursing as a profession?
- How do you think your spirituality or religious perspective might affect or be incorporated into your nursing practice?

Religiosity refers to beliefs and practices that are the expressive aspects of religion. These include, among others, prayer, ritual, dietary practices, modes of dress, and study of sacred texts. Awareness of religious practices and beliefs that are important to patients and families enables nurses to incorporate religious needs into care planning. Familiarity with the beliefs and practices of different religions that may affect health care is important in order to be better able to incorporate particular needs into patient care (Andrews & Hanson, 2011). This information provides a basis from which nurses can explore with patients what is necessary to support or meet their spiritual needs, taking care not to presume a need until it is verified with the patient. For example, a Catholic patient may not wish to have a priest called, a Jewish patient may have no problem with eating ham, or a patient who lists no religious affiliation may practice daily meditation.

Although many people express their spirituality through religion, spiritual expression is not limited to this context. Many people will note that they believe in God but do not go to church. Instead, they pray on their own, or experience the Divine through nature, or relate to a Higher Power or Universal Being that is found in all of life. We must plan nursing care according to how each patient expresses and experiences spirituality.

Creating Sacred Space

Addressing religious concerns within a health care setting does not require us to share the same religious perspective as our patients. What is necessary is that we create an environment that is open to a variety of religious and spiritual expression. Creating sacred space in the midst of science and technology can challenge our creativity. Nursing care may include providing the quiet a patient needs for meditation, arranging a private space for a particular ritual, contacting an appropriate spiritual support person, or ensuring that specific dietary requirements are met.

Praying with or reading sacred scripture to patients may be included in nursing care, providing it is based on an assessment of the patient's spiritual needs and done with the patient's permission and within the context of the patient's tradition. The literature provides evidence for the therapeutic value of prayer and that prayer can be an important intervention (Breslin & Lewis, 2008; Dossey, 2001; Helming, 2011; Narayanasamy & Narayanasamy, 2008). As with any therapeutic intervention, obtaining permission from patients before praying for them is an important part of nursing care. Unsolicited prayer by health practitioners may make patients or family members uncomfortable or reflect a goal different from that of the patient, and may be considered unethical (French & Narayanasamy, 2011; Narayanasamy & Narayanasamy, 2008). For nurses who are so inclined, it is good to include prayer for patients in their personal prayer, with an openness to what is for the patient's highest good. Overall we need to be aware of acting out of our own spiritual or religious perspectives while taking care not to impose our views on another.

Dilemmas Related to Religious Beliefs

When patients refuse conventional medical treatments based on religious beliefs or spiritual perspective, dilemmas can arise. Patients who decide to rely on prayer for healing, rather than chemotherapy for treatment of cancer, for example, may be considered irrational, and their competence to make decisions may be questioned. If an adult refuses a blood transfusion due to religious beliefs, after all risks have been explained, it is considered an informed decision. If a parent refuses a transfusion for a child based on the same belief, it may be taken to court as neglect or abuse. A woman who refuses to leave a dangerously abusive marriage because of religious convictions may find that frustrated health care providers are less responsive to her cries for help.

Case Presentation

When Religious Beliefs and Medical Care Conflict—Part 1

Suella is a 33-year-old, unmarried woman who belongs to a Holiness church that includes the practice of snake handling. Three days ago she was bitten twice during a church service. Following the service she stayed with the preacher, who prayed with her for healing as is the custom in this church. The religion does not believe in taking antivenom. Suella's parents and siblings, who do not belong to the same church, brought her to the hospital in renal failure. Upon admission she was alert but lethargic, and repeatedly informed nurses that she did not want any blood, dialysis, feeding tube, or life support. She kept saying "My King will take care of me," insisting that her reliance was on God, and that she did not want antivenom. Upon her move to the intensive care unit, the attending physician documented the conversation with the patient, indicating that she did not want blood, dialysis, feeding tubes, cardiopulmonary resuscitation (CPR) or life support. The attending physician also consulted a renal physician, who ordered dialysis. A nurse who was getting ready to do the second dialysis treatment read the attending physician's note and recognized the ethical dilemma.

Think About It

Dealing with Conflicts Between Religious Beliefs and Medical Care

- *What should the nurse do in this situation?*
- *How do you think you would react to this patient's decisions?*
- *What principles would guide you in dealing with dilemmas arising from religious convictions?*
- *What personal religious or spiritual practices are important to your health?*
- *What personal convictions might affect your health care decisions?*

Nurturing Spirit

Caregiving is influenced by a nurse's spiritual, as well as physical and emotional, well-being. The ability to attend to spirituality with another requires that nurses first attend to their own spirits (Burkhardt & Nagai-Jacobson, 2002, 2013). Self-awareness, which includes appreciation of ourselves as

Case Presentation

When Religious Beliefs and Medical Care Conflict—Part 2

The nurse in this situation requested an ethics consult, and members of the hospital's ethics committee talked with the patient. Although the patient was lethargic, she could nod and reply "yes" and "no" when questioned. The patient reaffirmed her same wishes as noted on admission. When asked if she knew what would happen without treatment she stated, "I'll die." The primary physician spoke to the patient again in the presence of an ethics member, at which time she once again reiterated her previous wishes. The physician discontinued all dialysis and set up a meeting with the family, after which the family spoke to the patient. Later that day the patient said she changed her mind and now wanted everything done. Ethics committee members were again called. When they asked the patient why she changed her mind, she responded, "My family." Further exploration of what "everything" meant to the patient revealed that she was willing to have dialysis, blood, and tube feedings, but no CPR or intubation.

Think About It

When Family Members Have Different Religious Beliefs

- *How would you, as the nurse, feel about following this patient's new directives?*
- *Do you see any new dilemmas resulting from the current situation?*
- *Is there any evidence of coercion in this situation? If so, how would you respond to that?*
- *How would your own spiritual perspective influence your care for this patient and family?*

unique body-mind-spirit beings, underlies our recognition of this same wholeness in others.

Just as sustenance and care are necessary for the health of body and mind, so too does the spirit require nurture. Caring for our spirit includes mindfulness and taking time to attend to our inner being. The spirit can be nurtured in many ways, and we must each discover what our own spirit needs in order to thrive. Prayer, meditation, music, religious worship, or shared ritual may be important. The spirit may be nurtured through special time with friends or family, or by giving ourselves alone time at home, in nature, or in some other sacred space. Attending to our need for rest, play, or creative activity are other ways to care for spirit. The spirit can be nurtured in a very profound way through sharing our stories. As we become more adept at nurturing our spirits, we are better able to recognize and support this process with patients and families.

SUMMARY

Attentiveness to spiritual and cultural aspects of care with patients is an important part of holistic nursing care. The diversity of cultures and spiritual expressions within our society requires that nurses be able to identify concerns and issues in these areas and address them competently and confidently. Familiarity with the values, beliefs, and practices of various cultures and religions is a useful adjunct to careful cultural and spiritual assessments with patients. Self-awareness regarding our own cultural and spiritual values, beliefs, and expressions is necessary in order to address these areas with patients. Such awareness allows us to act from our own spiritual or cultural perspectives, while taking care not to impose these views on others. In this way care planning can more readily flow from assessments that identify issues and needs regarding the patient's cultural and spiritual expressions and experiences.

CHAPTER HIGHLIGHTS

- Since culture influences beliefs and behaviors regarding health and healing, cultural assessment is integral to a comprehensive nursing assessment.

- Providing effective nursing care within the diversity of our multicultural society requires cultural competence on the part of nurses. Cultural competence can help prevent dilemmas from arising when there are differences in cultural perspective between patient and nurse.

- The culture of health care institutions may vary greatly from that of the people served by these systems. Values such as autonomy, beneficence, or the right to self-determination need to be considered from the cultural perspectives of patient, family, and health care providers.

- Complementary/integrative therapies are used by many people seen in conventional health care settings. Nursing care is enhanced when nurses are aware of various therapies being utilized by patients. Knowledge of and working with traditional healing systems and healers can help nurses promote more culturally congruent care.

- Communication is a key factor in providing culturally congruent and spiritually sensitive care and in averting associated legal and other dilemmas.

- Health and healing are associated with that which is holy and whole. Spirituality has long been a component of healing and health care, since, by nature, humans are body-mind-spirit beings.

- Grounded in a holistic view of persons, nursing care includes spirituality assessment and interventions addressing spiritual needs, recognizing that religious or spiritual perspective may influence health care choices.

- Expressions of spirituality are many and varied and may include, but are not limited to, the context of religion. Religious values are not always congruent with the ethical perspectives of the greater society.

- Providing spiritual care requires that nurses be attentive to both their own spirits and the spiritual concerns of patients and create an environment that is open to a variety of religious and spiritual expressions. Nurses need to be aware of acting from their own cultural, spiritual, or religious perspectives, while not imposing these views on others.

DISCUSSION QUESTIONS AND ACTIVITIES

1. Consider how your cultural, spiritual, or religious values affect personal choices regarding health and healing. Discuss this with other students, noting similarities and differences.

2. What aspects of the culture of the health care system are difficult for you as a nurse? Identify personal conflicts and the beliefs and values underlying them.

3. Recall a time when you or someone you know experienced a conflict with persons within the health care system. What values, beliefs, or understandings contributed to this conflict?

4. Discuss with other students nonconventional therapies, or folk remedies, that you or someone you know have used. Why was the therapy used? How did you know about the therapy? Was it used in place of, or along with, conventional therapies? What was the outcome? Research a complementary therapy through the National Center for Complementary and Alternative Medicine (http://www.nccam.nih.gov).

5. List 10 things that nurture you spiritually. Consider how often you have done these in the past day, week, or month. Make a plan to include at least one each day for the next week.

6. Choose a religious tradition or complementary therapy with which you are unfamiliar. Explore this tradition or therapy through readings and discussions with members, practitioners, or persons who have practiced the religion or utilized the therapy. Share your findings with classmates.

7. Discuss how nurses can create sacred space within health care settings.

8. Discuss patient health care choices or behaviors that are based on religious beliefs that might present a dilemma for you. Consider how you would approach the situation in a professional manner and describe the ethical stance that would guide your decisions.

9. Expand your knowledge of cultural competency, diversity, and spiritual care by exploring some of the following websites:

http://www.nursingworld.org/MainMenuCategories/EthicsStandards/Ethics-Position-Statements

http://www.innovations.ahrq.gov/CulturalCompetence.aspx

http://nccc.georgetown.edu/ (National Center for Cultural Competence)

http://www.hrsa.gov/culturalcompetence/index.html

http://www.tcns.org/index.html (Transcultural Nursing Society)

http://www.tcns.org/TCNStandardsofPractice.html (Standards of Practice for Culturally Competent Nursing Care)

https://cccm.thinkculturalhealth.hhs.gov/ (USDHHS Office of Minority Health)

http://www.gwumc.edu/gwish/clinical/fica-spiritual/index.cfm (Institute for Spirituality and Health, George Washington University)

http://www.spiritualityandhealth.duke.edu/

http://www.ish-tmc.org/ (Institute for Spirituality and Health, Texas Medical Center)

http://www.csh.umn.edu/modules/index.html (Free online learning— integrative therapies)

http://www.spiritualityhealth.com

http://www.ahna.org/

REFERENCES

Adams, K. E., Cohen, M. H., Eisenberg, D., & Jonsen, A. R. (2002). Ethical considerations of complementary and alternative medical therapies in conventional medical settings. *Annals of Internal Medicine, 137*(8), 660–664.

American Nurses Association. (1991, October 22). Ethics and human rights position statements: Cultural diversity in nursing practice. Author. Retrieved February 13, 2012, from http://www.nursingworld.org/MainMenuCategories/EthicsStandards/Ethics-Position-Statements/prtetcldv14444.html

Andrews, M. M. (2011). Cultural diversity in the health care workforce. In M. M. Andrews & J. S. Broyle (Eds.), *Transcultural concepts in nursing care* (6th ed., pp. 297–326). Philadelphia: Lippincott, Williams & Wilkins.

Andrews, M. M., & Hanson, P. A. (2011). Religion, culture, and nursing. In M. M. Andrews & J. S. Broyle (Eds.), *Transcultural concepts in nursing care* (6th ed., pp. 355–407). Philadelphia: Lippincott, Williams & Wilkins.

Barnett, H. (2007). Complementary and alternative medicine and patient choice in primary care. *Quality in Primary Care, 15*, 207–212.

Bednarz, H., Schim, S., & Doorenbos, A. (2010). Cultural diversity in nursing education: Perils, pitfalls, and pearls. *Journal of Nursing Education, 49*(5), 253–260.

Breslin, M. J., & Lewis, C. A. (2008). Theoretical models of the nature of prayer and health: A review. *Mental Health, Religion & Culture, 11*(1), 9–21.

Burkhardt, M. A. (1994). Becoming and connecting: Elements of spirituality for women. *Holistic Nursing Practice, 8*, 12–21.

Burkhardt, M. A., & Nagai-Jacobson, M. G. (2002). *Spirituality: Living our connectedness.* Clifton Park, NY: Delmar.

Burkhardt, M. A., & Nagai-Jacobson, M. G. (2013). Spirituality and health. In B. M. Dossey & L. Keegan, *Holistic nursing: A handbook for practice* (6th ed., pp. 721–749). Burlington, MA: Jones & Bartlett Learning.

Campinha-Bacote, J. (2007). *The process of cultural competence in the delivery of healthcare services: The journey continues.* Cincinnati, OH: Transcultural C.A.R.E. Associates.

Chater, K., & Tsai, C. T. (2008). Palliative care in a multicultural society: A challenge for Western ethics. *Australian Journal of Advanced Nursing, 26*(2), 95–100.

Dossey, L. (2001). *Healing beyond the body.* London: Times Warner.

Engebretson, J. C. (2013). Cultural diversity and care. In B. M. Dossey & L. Keegan (Eds.), *Holistic nursing: A handbook for practice* (6th ed., pp. 677–702). Burlington, MA: Jones & Bartlett Learning.

French, C., & Narayanasamy, A. (2011). To pray or not to pray: A question of ethics. *British Journal of Nursing, 20*(18), 1198–1204.

Giger, J. N., & Davidhizar, R. E. (2007). *Transcultural nursing: Assessment and intervention* (5th ed.). St. Louis, MO: Mosby.

Helming, M. B. (2011). Healing through prayer: A qualitative study. *Holistic Nursing Practice, 25*(1), 33–44.

Jeffreys, M. (2010). *Teaching cultural competence in nursing and health care* (2nd ed.). New York: Springer Publishing.

Leininger, M. (1991). Transcultural care principles, human rights, and ethical considerations. *Journal of Transcultural Nursing, 3,* 21–22.

Leininger, M., & McFarley, M. R. (2005). *Culture care diversity and universality: A worldwide nursing theory* (2nd ed.). Burlington MA: Jones & Bartlett Learning.

Liehr, M. P. R., & Smith, M. J. (2008). Story theory. In M. J. Smith & P. R. Liehr (Eds.), *Middle range theory for nursing* (2nd ed.). New York: Springer.

Nagai-Jacobson, M. G., & Burkhardt, M. A. (1996). Viewing persons as stories: A perspective for holistic care. *Alternative Therapies in Health and Medicine, 2,* 54–58.

Narayanasamy, A., & Narayanasamy, M. (2008). The healing power of prayer and its implications for nursing. *British Journal of Nursing, 17*(6), 394–398.

Puchalski, C. M. (2007–2008). Spirituality and the care of patients at the end-of-life: An essential component of care. *Omega, 56*(1), 33–46.

Puchalski, C. M., Ferrell, B., Virani, R., Otis-Green, S. Baird, P., Bull, J., . . . Sulmasy, D. (2009). Improving the quality of spiritual care as a dimension of palliative care: The report of the Consensus Conference. *Journal of Palliative Medicine, 12*(10), 885–904.

Ray, M. A. (2010). *Transcultural caring dynamics in nursing and health care.* Philadelphia, PA: F. A. Davis.

Rykkje, L., Eriksson, K., & Råholm, M. (2011). A qualitative metasynthesis of spirituality from a caring science perspective. *International Journal for Human Caring, 15*(4), 40–53.

Sewell, M. (Ed.). (1991). *Cries of the spirit: A celebration of women's spirituality.* Boston: Beacon Press.

Tafoya, T. (1996, May). Embracing the shadow: Mending the sacred hoop. Paper presented at the South Texas AIDS Training (STAT) for Mental Health Providers: The Human, Transcultural, and Spiritual Dimensions of HIV/AIDS, San Antonio, TX.

Part

V

The Power to Make
A Difference

Part V discusses the importance of empowerment of nurses and patients. To deal with the complex issues facing nursing today, nurses are required to exercise integrity, accountability, and courage. Nurses have the responsibility, authority, and power to make principled choices. Additionally, empowerment of patients is an important element of nursing care that derives from an appreciation that patients have the ability to discern their needs and make decisions about their lives and health. Being a facilitator of empowerment requires nurses to relinquish power and embrace the patient as an equal partner. Nurses can facilitate empowerment by working directly with patients and through addressing social, political, and environmental factors affecting empowerment of individuals and communities. In the midst of an ever-changing and challenging health care environment, in which issues of power and control continue to affect patient care, it is imperative that nurses be both empowered and competent enablers of patient empowerment.

Chapter

19

EMPOWERMENT FOR NURSES

Copper Woman warned Hai Nai Yu that the world would change and times might come when Knowing would not be the same as Doing. And she told her that Trying would always be very important.

(Cameron, 1981, p. 53)

OBJECTIVES

After completing this chapter, the reader should be able to:

1. Discuss the effect of mind-set on expectations regarding nursing practice and ethical stances.

2. Describe metaphors for nursing and discuss their impact on nursing ethics.

3. Explain the impact on nursing practice of perceptions about nursing from within and from outside the profession.

4. Describe the concepts of power and empowerment.

5. Discuss personal empowerment and its importance within nursing.

6. Discuss the relationship among professional empowerment, principled behavior, and nursing practice.

7. Describe the role of diversity in empowerment.

8. Discuss the influence on professional practice of nursing's vision of nursing.

INTRODUCTION

Dealing in a principled way with issues facing nursing requires integrity, accountability, and courage. Discussion of issues in this book are grounded in the belief that (1) nurses have the power to make choices and to act in responsible and principled ways, and (2) nurses have the authority to make decisions and recommendations regarding activities that are within the scope of their practice. The parameters of nursing's power and authority, however, are not always clear. Many nurses feel constrained by the systems within which they work and by persisting paternalistic attitudes that promote disempowerment. This chapter discusses the concept of empowerment as a process through which nurses are enabled to clarify and claim their ability to make decisions regarding issues related to nursing practice. Elements of personal empowerment are addressed, and factors associated with professional empowerment are considered. The principles regarding empowerment for nurses that are discussed in this chapter apply as well to empowering patients, which is the focus of Chapter 20.

INFLUENCES ON NURSING'S PERCEPTIONS OF PRINCIPLED PRACTICE

Nurses, patients, and other health care providers may vary greatly in their perceptions of ideals for nursing and nursing practice. These perceptions influence expectations and decisions regarding care, authority, and accountability. Expectations regarding good nursing care or taking an ethical stance flow from such perceptions. We recognize that factors in our internal and external environments affect both personal and professional decision making. External environment factors include the norms, ideals, and expectations of patients, families, other health care providers, and the professional and social systems within which we interact. The internal environment includes our *mind-set* or inner world of personal beliefs and perceptions.

Influence of Mind-Set

Our attitudes, views, and beliefs about the health care system influence how we identify and respond to ethical issues and dilemmas in practice. For example, when nurses view health care in terms of medical cases focused on the cure of disease, the physician is seen as the dominant authority. In this view of health care, following the physician's orders (whether or not the nurse agrees with them) and loyalty to the physician and institution are considered the legitimate and ethical focus of nursing activities. This mind-set is contrary to the independent, ethical practice of nursing that requires nurses to be accountable for their own actions and decisions. If nurses view health care as a commodity in which nursing and medical care are sold to patients by institutions, the nurse's primary responsibility is to the employing institution. Within this view, needs of individual patients may be subordinated to the utilitarian goal focused on the good of the greatest number of people, or the institutional goal of making a profit. Nurses who hold this view may not challenge the rightness or wrongness of nursing actions provided they are congruent with the goals and policies of the institution. This mind-set finds fertile ground in large institutional settings and managed care arenas. When nurses view health care as a basic human need and a right for each person, the nurse's primary responsibility is to the patient. The legitimate and ethical focus of nursing activities within this mind-set must include attention to patient rights, safety, and overall well-being.

Metaphors of Nursing

Metaphors help us to understand a concept by comparing two things that are different, yet share common characteristics. People often use *metaphors* to focus attention on particular aspects of reality in order to enhance understanding of roles, events, and experiences. Metaphors may also influence our perceptions of these events and experiences. For example, likening nurses to *angels in white* calls attention to the nursing roles of caring, protecting, and serving; yet viewing nurses as angels may set up the expectation that they should be somewhat distant and above human frailties. Metaphors that have been associated with nursing reflect different ideas about nursing roles and responsibilities in health care. These metaphors also suggest different approaches to determining an appropriate ethical stance for nursing care delivery.

The military metaphor for nursing that was common from the late nineteenth into the mid-twentieth century is associated with obedience to higher authority; a view of disease as the enemy; discipline; respect for those of higher rank; uniform dress; and, above all, loyalty. Loyalty to patients was considered part of being loyal to the institutions and to the physicians under whom nurses worked. Ethical imperatives that flow from this metaphor include following physician orders, even if the nurse questions the appropriateness of these orders; upholding the patient's faith in the physician, even if the nurse questions the doctor's competence; and being loyal to health care colleagues, even at the expense of the patient.

In the early history of nursing, following the physician's order without question would have absolved the nurse from guilt, even in the event of a harmful outcome for the patient. Today, however, this is not the case.

Nursing's move from vocation to profession requires that nurses be more personally accountable for their actions. Court rulings have held nurses legally responsible for their decisions and actions. Legal decisions, changes in the health care delivery system, and feminist awareness within the nursing profession have encouraged the transition from the metaphor of loyal soldier to that of patient advocate. Beginning in the 1960s and 1970s, a significant revision in nursing's self-image included the legal metaphor of patient advocacy and the academic metaphor of rational thought regarding ethical dilemmas (Milton, 2009; Sharoff, 2009). Greater emphasis on consumerism and patient rights, coupled with growing dissatisfaction with increased costs and depersonalization of health care, helped to open the door for nurses to expand their roles as patient advocates. As advocates for patient rights, nurses are responsible to those who require nursing care. This obliges nurses to be alert to situations in which patients may be endangered by incompetent, unethical, or illegal practices by any member of the health care team or the health care system, and to take appropriate actions to safeguard the patient (American Nurses Association [ANA], 2001). Current nursing codes and standards that stress responsibility to patients through collegial membership in the health care team reflect ethical imperatives flowing from the metaphor of advocacy.

Loyalty remains a valued virtue for nurses within the advocacy metaphor. Although ideally the nurse's first loyalty is to the patient, circumstances of conflicting loyalty may occur. Loyalty to colleagues and to employers is also important, and nurses may at times be faced with making difficult decisions between advocacy for patients or loyalty to colleagues. Such situations require personal integrity, knowledge, and courage on the part of the nurse.

Nursing's self-image is evident in the metaphors nurses use to describe their roles and their practice. These images illuminate the complexities and ambiguities of nursing practice as well as the influence of social, organizational, and cultural constraints on nurses. How nurses picture nursing and the vision they hold of their role in health care influences their ability to practice in a holistic, patient-focused way. Personal self-image affects how we live in the world, relate to ourselves and others, think, act, behave, and make decisions. Influences on nursing self-image evident in nursing literature include personal thoughts and experiences, social and environmental feedback, reference groups, roles and value of women in society, and media and other public images of nurses (Fletcher, 2007). Constraints engendered by negative self-images prompt nurses to feel unable to practice nursing in a way that is consistent with their values. Awareness of various factors that influence self-image empowers nurses to work to counter negative influences and to enhance their professional self-image (Fletcher, 2007; Gordon, 2010).

Think About It

How Does Mind-Set Affect Perceptions?

You are the vice president for nursing at a large medical center. Recently one of the physicians, who holds a lot of power in the system and is generally very open and easy to work with, expressed considerable displeasure about the refusal of a particular nurse to carry out a medical order and then deciding to refer her concerns about certain physician practice decisions to the ethics committee. The physician says that you should fire the nurse for insubordination. You are aware that the nurse's decisions were reasonable, in the patient's interest, and based on sound principles and standards of nursing practice. You are also aware that the physician in question is well known nationally and brings a lot of money to the hospital.

- *How would you respond to the physician?*
- *Where do you see potential for conflicting loyalties in this situation?*
- *Discuss how differing perceptions of nursing might affect this situation.*
- *Describe what you see as the most realistic outcome in this situation. What about the ideal outcome?*

How Nursing Is Perceived by Others

Factors such as mind-set and metaphors influence our perceptions of and choices regarding principled behavior. The perceptions of others also affect our considerations regarding appropriate or ethical nursing actions. Although nursing as a profession has now claimed the metaphor of advocate in lieu of that of loyal soldier, there are nurses within the profession who have not fully embraced the change. Operationalizing the advocacy role may put nurses at risk in some institutions and situations, as demonstrated in cases such as that of Jolene Tuma discussed in Chapter 11, and in cases of whistle-blowing discussed later in this chapter. Although nursing has made a paradigm shift regarding its role and responsibilities, awareness of nursing's current professional imperatives is often lacking among patients, families, physicians, and health care administrators. The role of nursing as perceived by many outside of the profession remains embedded in the loyal soldier metaphor, and mind-sets that view health care as a collection of medical cases or as a commodity. As a result, many physicians still expect nurses to follow their bidding and take offense when nurses challenge their decisions or actions. The hierarchical, patriarchal system remains the norm in many health care institutions. Since physicians are perceived to be of higher rank, their influence often holds more sway than that of nurses who may challenge them. Although patients and families often have more continual and direct contact with nurses, they may not fully understand that the nurse is their advocate. Instead, they often function from the mind-set that the physician is the captain of a ship on which the nurse is a member of the crew. Images in the media that depict nurses in ancillary, subordinate roles also affect perceptions of patients and others regarding expectations of nurses.

Understanding Power and Empowerment

Nurses have the power to make a difference by acting in principled ways in all areas of their lives and practice. However, as has been evident throughout the discussions in this book, many factors mitigate against nurses claiming this power. Nurses need to develop skills in dealing with these factors in order to function fully in their legitimate roles within health care. Nurses must be aware of values, beliefs, and other factors affecting personal decision making, and must expand their knowledge of ethical principles, contextual factors, legal considerations, and other issues facing nursing. Understanding **power** and **empowerment** can help in developing strategies for action in this regard.

Although the word *power* is often understood in terms of strength, force, or control, dictionary definitions of the term, derived from its Latin root *potere*, refer as well to the ability to do or act, which includes the capability of doing or accomplishing something. To have power, then, implies having the ability to do or act; and to *empower* would be to facilitate the ability of another person to do or to act.

Seeking a better understanding of both the concept of empowerment and how empowerment (or its lack) affects nurses and patients has been a topic in the nursing literature for many years. Intrapersonal, interpersonal, and environmental factors all play a role in empowerment. Self-esteem; personal values and perceptions; sense of self in relation to others; and an environment that allows access to information, resources, and support are some factors that influence empowerment. Empowerment is understood to be a participative process, or a partnership between a nurse and patient, that supports patient well-being and facilitates changing unhealthy behaviors (Ellis-Stoll & Popkess-Vawter, 1998; Hewitt-Taylor, 2004; Shearer & Reed, 2004; Williamson, 2007). This partnership is viewed by some as a social process of recognizing, promoting, and enhancing patients' abilities to meet their own needs, solve their own problems, and mobilize the necessary resources in order to feel in control of their own lives (Connelly, Keele, Kleinbeck, Schneider, & Cobb, 1993; Fulton, 1997; McCarthy & Freeman, 2008). Another understanding of empowerment is the capacity of disenfranchised people to understand and become active participants in the matters that affect their lives, suggesting that a personal attitude that affirms change as possible is important for empowerment to occur (Bolton & Brookings, 1998). Empowerment may be viewed as a philosophy or worldview flowing from a belief in each person's inherent worth and a belief in the process of self-discovery that involves creating a vision, taking risks, making choices, and behaving in authentic ways (Gurka, 1995). Empowerment requires respect for an individual's personal beliefs and goals and trust in the person's ability to make decisions, take action, and be accountable for the actions. Although sharing knowledge through education is important for empowerment, the literature clearly indicates that emotional and social support is essential as well.

In-depth analyses of the concept of empowerment suggest that it is both process and outcome, taking different forms within different people and contexts (Ellis-Stoll & Popkess-Vawter, 1998; Gibson, 1991; McCarthy & Freeman, 2008; Rodwell, 1996; Ryles, 1999). Because of this, empowerment needs to be defined by the people concerned. Empowerment is a transactional process involving relationship with others. This relationship includes mutually beneficial interactions aimed at strengthening rather than weakening; power sharing through mutual sharing of knowledge, resources, and opportunities; and respect for self and others. Empowerment is nurtured by collaborative efforts that focus on solutions rather than problems, and on strengths, rights, and abilities rather than deficits. Empowerment derives from a feminine perspective of *power with* or *power to,* which implies sharing responsibility, knowledge, and resources; collaboration for goal achievement; incorporating diversity; valuing the contributions of each person; and valuing the process. In contrast, the masculine view of *power over* incorporates a sense of paternalistic control, struggle for and protection of limited resources, separation of leaders and followers, expediency, and results even at the expense of persons (Chinn, 2013).

Empowerment can seem like a rather abstract term, and you may be wondering what being empowered looks and feels like. Certainly, two people in the same circumstances can have different experiences of empowerment. Nurse scholars use a variety of descriptive terms when discussing people who are empowered. These terms include: positive self-concept, personal satisfaction, self-efficacy, sense of mastery regarding self and the environment, sense of control, sense of connectedness, self-development, feeling of hope, the ability to make changes, self-determination, action orientation, authority, autonomy, capability of social intercourse, caring, choosing, self-confidence, courage, decision-making ability, emancipatory power, endurance, expertise, freedom, influence, instrumental exercise of power, participation, resilience, rights, self-control, solidarity, strength, sturdiness, taking a position, assertiveness, coercion, enabling, and freedom to make choices (Bolton & Brookings, 1998; Connelly et al., 1993; Ellis-Stoll & Popkess-Vawter, 1998; Fulton, 1997; Hartrick & Schreiber,

1998; Jones, O'Toole, Hoa, Chau, & Muc, 2000; Kuokkanen & Leino-Kilpi, 2000; Laschinger, Wong, & Greco, 2006; Manojlovich, 2007; McCarthy & Freeman, 2008; Rodwell, 1996; Ryles, 1999). Although not all of these attributes are necessarily part of every experience of empowerment, they provide markers that help us identify the process and presence of empowerment.

Empowerment implies choice on the part of those being empowered. We cannot empower another, because to presume to do so removes the element of choice. Empowerment requires both inner motivation and environmental factors that support the process. This process requires self-awareness, positive self-esteem, a commitment to self and others, and the desire and ability to make decisions. Responsibility and accountability for our actions and having the authority to act are implicit in the ability to choose.

Through the empowerment process, we can enable others to develop awareness of areas that need change; foster a desire to take action; and share resources, skills, and opportunities that support the change. Self-empowerment derives from self-awareness and resources more than services provided to persons (Rodwell, 1996). Enhanced self-esteem, personal satisfaction, a sense of connectedness, the ability to set and reach goals, a sense of control over life and change processes, and a sense of hope and direction are all outcomes of empowerment.

ASK YOURSELF

What Makes You Feel Empowered?

- Consider a situation in which you felt empowered. Describe factors contributing to your sense of empowerment.

- Recall a time when you felt disempowered. What contributed to this sense? How might you have felt more empowered in the situation?

PERSONAL EMPOWERMENT

Nursing's power to make a difference in care with patients derives from many factors. In order to serve as credible models of empowerment for others, we must demonstrate congruence between values and behaviors in our own lives. Personal integrity implies an ability to be honest with and care for ourselves, as well as respond to the needs of others. Often nurses, and especially women, have learned to value care for others before or instead of care for self. A true value for human life must include value for our own lives as well. The biblical adage is "Love thy neighbor *as* thyself," not *instead* of thyself or *before* thyself (Leviticus 19:18). We must attend to ourselves and treat ourselves with the same respect and dignity with which we treat others. Personal empowerment begins with actions that support the meeting of our own needs and self-actualization. It is from our personal stores of creativity, empowerment, and health that we are able to inspire, teach, and assist others in achieving their potential.

In principle, many nurses would agree with the concept of care for self; however, actions often conflict with this acknowledged belief. Nurses often agree to work additional hours even when they are exhausted; consume large amounts of caffeine and sugar to boost waning energy; go home to care for children, spouse, and friends; and collapse into bed only to get up and do it all again the next day because they feel limited power to do otherwise. What causes a person to behave in a way that conflicts with his or her stated values? Often the person has learned conflicting messages. A belief in caring for ourselves may conflict with a learned belief that caring for others is more admirable or more important than caring for ourselves.

Some people feel very little control over any area of their lives. Others may feel empowered to make decisions in some situations but not in others—for example, a person may actively make decisions in the home environment while feeling like a pawn of the system at work. The sense of power that nurses have in their personal lives may affect their perception of empowerment in the professional arena. Burnout, job dissatisfaction, and limited professional commitment affect the quality of patient care, and are often associated with feelings of powerlessness (Leiter & Laschinger, 2006; Manojlovich, 2007; Ning, Zhong, Libo, & Qiujie, 2009; O'Brien, 2011). Attributes of empowerment noted in the previous section reflect important considerations for self-empowerment on both personal and professional levels.

The ability to facilitate empowerment in others requires us to attend to personal empowerment. This means valuing ourselves as we listen inwardly to our own senses as well as carefully listening to others, consciously taking in and forming strength (Chinn, 2013). Self-awareness is necessary, since self-perception has a direct link to quality of patient care (Fletcher, 2007). Such awareness requires attentiveness to factors that influence our thoughts, feelings, actions, and reactions in the present circumstance and reflective consideration of such influences on past experiences. Empowerment involves taking ownership of our inner lives and recognizing that we have full control over our thoughts, feelings, and actions.

Owning our thoughts involves recognizing old or repetitive thought patterns and changing those that are no longer supporting a creative, actualizing life. Self-critical, judgmental, and negative thinking are particularly confining. Old thinking can be updated with new knowledge. Questioning the origin of particular thoughts can reveal ideas that were true at one time but now are no longer true. For example, a child who was always told that she did not know enough to make a decision, and that mother knew best, may become an adult who still consults her mother before making decisions. Seeking alternative views of situations and learning logical or critical thinking skills are other ways to restructure thought patterns.

Feelings are transient signals that alert us to what is supportive or offensive in a situation. Owning feelings means acknowledging and investigating the internal source of the message, rather than blaming other persons or situations for our feelings. People may experience different feelings in similar situations. For example, a death can elicit feelings of sadness, despair, hope, relief, joy, and others, depending upon the unique inner response of each person. Feelings and the reactions they elicit are in the person, not in the event.

We need to name and take ownership of personal values and to claim our ability to make choices. When experiencing a lack of control in life, we should identify both internal and external barriers to having control, consider whether we want control, and explore what we need to do and are willing to risk in order to take control. Consciously acting based upon a clear evaluation of the current situation, rather than acting automatically, is one way to own our behavior. Taking ownership of behavior requires being able to see options. Believing that there are no options can result in feeling powerless, trapped, or victimized. Even when we do not believe we can change a current unacceptable situation immediately, we can make a plan for change and set that plan into motion one step at a time. A *victim* waits and hopes something or someone else will change; makes excuses for not taking action (time, cost, fatigue, and the like); blames people, places, or things for the situation; and is trapped and unaware of options. An *empowered person* decides to be accountable for personal responses, makes plans, considers options, develops strategies for change, and acts on plans by doing what is necessary to succeed.

Personal empowerment requires growth of personal strength and power, and includes the ability to enact our own will and love for ourselves in the context of love and respect for others. This can only happen when individuals express respect and reverence for all forms of life and appreciate that the energy of the self is interconnected with the energy of the Earth (Chinn, 2013). A commitment to personal growth and self-care, developing a positive sense of self, awareness of strengths and abilities as well as limitations, and drawing on our supports and sources of connectedness foster this process. Empathy with others, appreciation of diversity, tolerance, flexibility, and willingness to compromise empower a person.

Enacting personal moral agency requires that we trust ourselves and our knowledge and abilities and be courageous in taking risks. **Moral courage** reflects a high degree of personal empowerment. Moral courage means the willingness to stand up for personal core values and ethical beliefs, even when we stand alone (Lachman, 2007; Murray, 2010). Implicit in moral courage is being willing to do what is right even when faced with the risk of ridicule, social rejection, shame, unemployment, and emotional anxiety. Lachman (2007) suggests that moral courage requires the ability to determine the right thing to do, how to handle one's fears, and the course of action needed to maintain one's integrity. This implies thoughtful consideration of the issues inherent in the situation and the risks involved. Empowerment requires being true to ourselves and our values when faced with morally distressing situations. Congruence among our being, knowing, and doing reflects personal integrity. This means that our actions flow from our essence, and our choices derive from what we know to be good and true.

PROFESSIONAL EMPOWERMENT

Professional empowerment is built upon the foundational elements of personal accountability and support of nursing colleagues. In order to deal in a principled way with issues and dilemmas arising within health care settings, nurses must feel personally and professionally empowered to act on sometimes difficult choices. Many factors affect nursing actions in the professional arena, including personal attitudes and self-concept; the structural and functional interrelatedness of health care systems; political, economic, and social forces; and interactions with patients and colleagues. Barriers to empowerment exist within the community of nursing and are also imposed from external sources.

Empowerment requires nurses to become knowledgeable about and address system issues as well as interpersonal issues. Such issues include recognizing the need for changing the power base within the current health care system; moving from a paternalistic, hierarchical model of control toward one that values collaboration; and the power of the collective. Developing and supporting processes for nurses to become involved in shared decision making and in forming institutional policies is part of this process (Edmonson, 2010; Mathes, 2005).

The effect of nurses' empowerment in the health care environment can have personal, institutional, and patient care implications. In terms of nursing management and health systems, some authors view empowerment as a method for delegating authority and sharing power, and a strategy for improving the productivity of nurses. The literature suggests a link between nurses' perceptions of job satisfaction, their work effectiveness, and workplace empowerment, and that empowered nurses are more likely to initiate and sustain independent behaviors that increase work effectiveness (Laschinger, Leiter, Day, & Gilin, 2009; Ning et al., 2009). Factors that have a positive impact on empowerment include access to the structures of information, support, and resources (Laschinger et al., 2009; Purdy, Laschinger, Finegan, Kerr, & Olivera, 2010). Studies indicate that workplace empowerment relates to job satisfaction, nurse retention, and better patient care (Laschinger et al., 2009; Ning et al., 2009; Purdy et al., 2010). In contrast, feelings of powerlessness are associated with job dissatisfaction, low levels of professional commitment, and burnout, which are barriers to quality patient care (Laschinger et al., 2009; Ning et al., 2009; O'Brien, 2011). Nurses who are burned out and dissatisfied are more inclined to give only the most routine care. Only an empowered workforce can be effective in today's health care system with its innovations of patient-focused care, case management, and shared governance (Edmonson, 2010; Hader, 2005; Mathes, 2005). Inherent in this perspective is a sense that each person is free to make choices and that those who are empowered, both internally and by the system, feel more in control of their lives; are able to act in appropriate, meaningful ways; and are able to do what they truly want to do.

When nurses feel disempowered in their work settings, they can choose the *victim* stance, which relinquishes power to the system, or they can challenge the system. Dealing with the system requires skills in conflict management, negotiation, and effective communication, as well as moral courage. Challenging the system can take many forms. Being a change agent begins with the nurse's personal presence and attitude. For example, one nurse described how her commitment to caring for the whole person was challenged when she began working in a Level III trauma center. Feeling constantly criticized by coworkers as she incorporated emotional and spiritual support into her care, she made the choice to act out of her values as a holistic nurse and return a loving spirit to the injustice of their criticism. She noted that this choice came as a great challenge, and that it was often difficult to go to work under the scrutiny focused in her direction. However, she used each opportunity of conversation with coworkers to suggest that they work together to unite the staff with an attitude of mutual caring, support, and nurturance. Her presence was reflected in her choice to stand in her power and speak her truth. Although this was not easy, living her values contributed to a change in attitude within the whole staff, particularly regarding how they supported and cared for each other.

Nurses can address social and economic constraints on nursing and health care through their involvement in professional organizations and through becoming politically active. Participation on institutional boards or committees that focus on patient care and professional practice concerns is another way to challenge the system, as is speaking out about unsafe or questionable practices. Informing authorities within or outside of one's work setting about practices or situations that are unethical, unsafe, questionable, or unlawful, particularly when these practices are being overlooked by others, may be considered to be **whistle-blowing**.

Unity in Diversity

Empowerment incorporates divergent and conflicting solutions to problems based on value in support of others rather than in divisiveness (Chinn, 2013; Falk-Rafael, 2005; Mathes, 2005). It implies embracing diversity and moving away from fear of that which is different to appreciation of the strength derived from and unity contained in diversity. Nurses need to recognize that systems exert control, in part, by fostering divisiveness among workers in order to deter unity of opposition to system policies. When nurses unite with and support colleagues who challenge harmful or potentially harmful practices, they are personally and professionally empowered.

Advocating for and making every effort to protect the rights, health, and safety of patients is a nursing responsibility that is clearly delineated in the *ANA Code of Ethics for Nurses* (ANA, 2001). Challenging unjust, unprofessional, or unethical practices is not an easy decision, and may entail risk for nurses. Nurses who identify dangerous situations within their work settings that pose a serious threat to patient or staff health, safety, or rights need to follow appropriate channels within the organization to rectify the situation. When every effort has been made to have the situation corrected, and the danger still persists, a nurse may decide to "blow the whistle" on the person or institution. Whistle-blowers are those who attempt to expose wrongdoing within an organization through warning the public about negligence, professional misconduct or incompetence, or other factors that may endanger patients or staff (Lachman, 2008; Ray, 2006). Situations that prompt whistle-blowing can involve ethical dilemmas related to a conflict between loyalty to coworkers or the institution and loyalty to patients, or benefit of the action (to the patient) versus risk to the nurse. Whistle-blowing is considered a last resort in advocating for patients and their safety. A nurse who feels that being a whistle-blower is the necessary course of action needs to be clear that it is being done for the correct moral reason and needs to be aware of potential consequences of the action (Jackson et al., 2010; Lachman, 2008; Ray, 2006). Feeling empowered to take a stand requires personal integrity and support from others. Support that enables nurses to be true advocates for patients may come from colleagues, from professional organizations, and from the legal protection of *whistle-blower laws.* Most states have enacted or introduced **whistle-blower** legislation or regulations in recent years, and federal regulations also provide legislative protection for whistle-blowers. For nurses who are considering taking action or speaking out, Tressman (2000) offers these suggestions:

- Determine through personal reflection and consultation with others if you are ready, both personally and professionally, to take action.

- Consult a lawyer.

- Contact your state nurses' association for information about the status of whistle-blower legislation in your state, and for guidance in the whistle-blower process.

- Use a journal to document instances that give you concern and that compromise care, creating a paper trail that includes dates, times, and outcomes of unsafe or inappropriate care. Make a copy of all documentation.

- Fill out "assignment despite objection" forms when you are working in situations that are unsafe.

- Speak only the truth, state only the facts, and follow the institution's chain of command to the letter before contacting an outside agency.

- If you decide to contact an outside agency, send all documents via certified mail with a return receipt.

- Be professional when dealing with the administration and refrain from making it personal. Presuming that administrators with integrity will act on your concerns quickly, do not wait too long for results.

- Build leadership skills and unity among your colleagues.

- Work with your state nurses' and national nurses' associations to help pass or strengthen whistle-blower laws in your state and nationally. (p. 22)

Nurses need to be willing to struggle with difficult questions and arrive at decisions that flow from their internal values and perspective, rather than looking for the *right* answer from an external source. Empowerment implies accountability for our own choices and actions. Jameton (1984) reflects that people pretend they are forced to do things when they are not. He gives the example of a nurse who instructs a patient to take a medication because the physician ordered it, noting that both patient and nurse pretend that they must act because of the physician's order, although each could make another choice. Reflecting that nurses who choose to work in systems such as hospitals are accountable for their actions despite the existence of systemic problems affecting health care, Jameton (1984) writes,

> If one fails to resist exploitation, incompetence, and corrupt practices, one becomes responsible for them. If one resists them, one enters into conflict with conventional conceptions of behavior for employees and thereby risks reprisals. One has to choose between complicity and self-sacrifice, or enter the uncomfortable middle ground of irony. Ethics does not give a clear answer as to which one must choose. Instead, one is free to move in the direction of the kind of world one personally desires to create. (p. 289)

We must decide whether we prefer a world in which we are empowered in the professional arena, or one in which we are controlled by others. The choices we make influence the outcome.

Re-Visioning Nursing

Empowerment within the profession requires a renewed vision of nursing. As nurses, we need to redefine nursing according to our own vision, rather than accepting the definition imposed by the dominant groups in health care such as physicians and institutions. When nurses draw pictures of their vision of nursing, what emerges are images of caring, light, comfort, and love. These images reflect the heart of the vision of nursing within nurses. Making choices based on the vision and values of the profession fosters congruence between nursing's knowing and doing, which strengthens personal and professional effectiveness. In contrast, nurses who work in situations in which they feel a lack of synchronicity with their values often experience burnout, become nasty, take on attributes and values of the dominant group, and look for someone to blame (behaviors reflective of oppressed groups). Remaining in a victim role involves a choice to give away our power and allow someone else to define our reality. Redefining nursing according to nursing's own vision is an act of empowerment.

Empowerment involves risk and commitment and requires both courage and compassion. Curtin (1996) illustrates this through a parable about a baby eagle that fell from its nest and broke its wing. The eagle was found by a mountain climber who took it home, nursed the wing, and put the eagle in with the chickens. Not knowing what to eat, the eagle followed the chickens pecking the feed on the ground. As he grew larger and stronger he continued to peck like the chickens, forgetting that he was an eagle. A friend of the climber noted that the eagle should be flying in the mountains with other eagles. The climber responded that the eagle had a good situation with free food and a warm coop, and would not fly away even if he could. The friend offered to teach the eagle to fly and took him to the barn roof, told him he was an eagle, and explained that he could fly freely. The eagle heard this but remembered what happened the last time he tried to fly. Seeing the chickens below, he remembered the food and shelter, and would not fly. The friend decided to take the eagle to the mountains, taught him how to flap his wings, encouraged his efforts, and told him repeatedly that he was an eagle and could fly. Finally the eagle took the risk and flew, delighting in the experience; but as he flew over the chicken yard, he remembered that he was hungry and returned to peck for food with the chickens. The friend disparaged the eagle for continuing to act like a chicken when he could be free. A new plan was devised. The friend crept up to the eagle, put a hood over his head, and carried him to an area where there were other eagles. The eagle saw their nests and watched them hunt, eat, and fly. The friend showed the eagle the beauty of his homeland, encouraged him to hunt and fly, and reminded him that he was an EAGLE. After several days the eagle got the idea, and when the friend took him to the top of the highest mountain, he took off and soared high, never looking back, and never eating chicken feed again, because he was an EAGLE, and he knew it. (Summarized from Curtin, 1996.)

Curtin relates the insights of this parable to empowerment for nurses. The story demonstrates that empowerment is not easy for either the one trying to empower or the one being empowered, but that it is important not to give up. We must also realize that empowerment costs money, time, and effort.

> It (empowerment) isn't easy. Telling the eagle to fly wasn't enough. It isn't easy. Changing the eagle's environment and even teaching him to fly wasn't enough. It isn't easy. You have to start at the beginning and recreate an attitude in a new environment. It's tough on the eagle too. The eagle was frightened: he had been hurt. The eagle knew the old, safe ways of pecking and free grain and warm nest. And he could have that with no effort! It was hard for the eagle to believe that the easy way sooner or later would destroy him. And it was really tough on the eagle when [the friend] blamed him for being what he'd been taught to be all his life. (Curtin, 1996, p. 210)

Curtin notes that neither freedom nor risk are easy, and that they are not for everyone. It is important, however, not to "blame the chickens for what they are. It's unfair—and it's a waste of time. But never give up on the eagles. They can fly—and they will" (p. 210). Empowerment for nurses means recognizing *who* we are, knowing that—like the eagle—we have both the ability and the freedom to fly!

SUMMARY

Empowerment is a multifaceted concept. Awareness of attitudes about nursing's role in health care and factors that shape these attitudes enables nurses to identify more effectively that which supports or diminishes both personal and professional empowerment. Attentiveness to personal empowerment, which includes integrity, accountability, and courage, is foundational for addressing empowerment issues within the profession. No one can empower another. However, we can facilitate the inner process of empowerment when knowledge and resources are offered within an environment of mutual respect and support. Empowerment for nurses requires remembering *who* we are, recognizing that *knowing* must be the same as *doing*, and following our own vision of nursing.

CHAPTER HIGHLIGHTS

- Mind-set regarding health care influences how nurses identify and respond to ethical issues and dilemmas in practice settings.

- Nursing's contemporary self-perception reflects the legal metaphor of patient advocate rather than the military metaphor of loyal soldier. Each of these metaphors implies different ethical imperatives for nursing.

- Current nursing codes and standards of practice reflect ethical imperatives that flow from the advocacy metaphor.

- Empowerment, which is both process and outcome, derives from a feminine perspective of *power to* or *power with*, reflecting a supportive partnership based on mutual love and respect that enables people to change situations given the necessary resources, knowledge, skills, and opportunities. Empowerment comes from within a person and involves choice; we cannot empower another.

- The ability to deal with health care issues and dilemmas in a principled way derives from personal and professional empowerment and requires attentiveness to intrapersonal, interpersonal, and systems issues.

- Personal empowerment requires self-awareness and is characterized by maintaining personal integrity in the midst of a loving response to the choices of others. Self-concept and sense of power in a nurse's personal life affects nursing care and a nurse's ability to enable empowerment in others.

- Recognizing unity in diversity and incorporating divergent views and solutions empowers nurses and others.
- Defining nursing according to nursing's own vision is an act of empowerment that implies accountability for our own choices and actions, with awareness that each choice helps create the kind of world and environment within which nurses must practice.

DISCUSSION QUESTIONS AND ACTIVITIES

1. Talk with both retired and practicing nurses about ethical imperatives that guide (or guided) their nursing practice. Identify mind-set and metaphors reflective of these imperatives.

2. Where in your life do you feel most personally empowered? Discuss the circumstances surrounding your feelings of empowerment with other students.

3. Review Chapters 4 and 5 and reflect on how your values and current phase of development affect your sense of personal empowerment.

4. Describe a situation in which you took ownership for your own thoughts, feelings, or actions. Describe a time when you found yourself blaming others or assuming a victim stance. Describe a situation in which you felt you acted with moral courage. Discuss with classmates factors prompting each stance and how you felt in each situation.

5. Discuss differences in others that might engender fear or caution in you and limit your ability to embrace the diversity.

6. What aspects of empowerment do you think are most important in nursing practice settings? Which are the most challenging? Support your perspective.

7. Interview practicing nurses regarding personal and professional power, including situations where they feel empowered to make decisions, where they derive authority to make decisions, and in which they have experienced dilemmas around the issue of power. Ask them to describe their ideal image of nursing and compare that to their current reality.

8. Illustrate your vision of nursing and develop strategies for making nursing's self-vision better known to others. Implement one strategy.

9. Explore issues related to whistle-blowing in your state or province, including the status of whistle-blower legislation. Discuss the ethical basis for whistle-blowing.

REFERENCES

American Nurses Association (ANA). (2001). *Code of ethics for nurses with interpretative statements*. Silver Spring, MD: American Nurses Publishing.

Bolton, B., & Brookings, J. (1998). Development of a measure of intrapersonal empowerment. *Rehabilitation Psychology, 43*(2), 131–142.

Cameron, A. (1981). *Daughters of copper woman*. Vancouver, BC: Press Gang.

Chinn, P. (2013). *Peace and power: Building communities for the future* (8th ed.). New York: Jones & Bartlett.

Connelly, L. M., Keele, B. S., Kleinbeck, V. M., Schneider, J. K., & Cobb, A. K. (1993). A place to be yourself: Empowerment from the client's perspective. *IMAGE: Journal of Nursing Scholarship, 25*(4), 297–303.

Curtin, L. (1996). *Nursing into the 21st century*. Springhouse, PA: Springhouse.

Edmonson, C. (2010). Moral courage and the nurse leader. *Online Journal of Issues in Nursing, 15*(3). Item Number: 2010889995.

Ellis-Stoll, C. C., & Popkess-Vawter, S. (1998). A concept analysis on the process of empowerment. *Advances in Nursing Science, 21*(2), 62–68.

Falk-Rafael, A. (2005). Speaking truth to power: Nursing's legacy and moral imperative. *Advances in Nursing Science, 28*(3), 212–223.

Fletcher, K. (2007). Image: Changing how women nurses think about themselves. Literature review. *Journal of Advanced Nursing, 58*(30), 207–215.

Fulton, Y. (1997). Nurses' views on empowerment: A critical social theory perspective. *Journal of Advanced Nursing, 26*, 529–536.

Gibson, C. H. (1991). A concept analysis of empowerment. *Journal of Advanced Nursing, 16*, 354–361.

Gordon, S. (2010). Nursing and health policy perspectives. *International Nursing Review, 57*(4), 403–404.

Gurka, A. M. (1995). Transformational leadership: Qualities and strategies for the CNS. *Clinical Nurse Specialist, 9*, 169–174.

Hader, R. (2005). How do you measure work force integrity? *Nursing Management, 36*(9), 32–37.

Hartrick, G., & Schreiber, R. (1998). Imaging ourselves: Nurses' metaphors of practice. *Journal of Holistic Nursing, 16*(4), 420–434.

Hewitt-Taylor, J. (2004). Challenging the balance of power: Patient empowerment. *Nursing Standard, 11*(18), 33–37.

Jackson, D., Peters, K., Andrew, S., Edenborough, M., Halcomb, E., Luck, L., . . . Wilkes, L. (2010). Understanding whistleblowing: Qualitative insights from nurse whistleblowers. *Journal of Advanced Nursing, 66*(10), 2194–2201.

Jameton, A. (1984). *Nursing practice: The ethical issues.* Englewood Cliffs, NJ: Prentice-Hall.

Jones, P. S., O'Toole, M. T., Hoa, N., Chau, T. T., & Muc, P. D. (2000). Empowerment of nursing as a socially significant profession in Vietnam. *Journal of Nursing Scholarship, 32*(3), 317–321.

Kuokkanen, L., & Leino-Kilpi, H. (2000). Power and empowerment in nursing: Three theoretical approaches. *Journal of Advanced Nursing, 31*(1), 235–241.

Lachman, V. D. (2007). Whistleblowers: Trouble makers or virtuous nurses? *MEDSURG Nursing, 17*(2), 126–134.

Lachman, V. D. (2008). Whistleblowing: Role of organizational culture in prevention and management. *Dermatology Nursing, 20*(5), 394–396.

Laschinger, H. K. S., Leiter, M., Day, A., & Gilin, D. (2009). Workplace environment, incivility, and burnout: Impact on staff nurse recruitment and retention outcomes. *Journal of Nurse Management, 17,* 302–311.

Laschinger, H. K. S., Wong, C., & Greco, P. (2006). The impact of staff nurse empowerment on person-job fit and work engagement burnout. *Nursing Administration Quarterly, 30*(4), 358–367.

Leiter, M. P., & Laschinger, H. K. S. (2006). Relationships of work and practice environment to professional burnout: Testing a causal model. *Nursing Research, 55*(2), 137–146.

Manojlovich, M. (2007, January 1). Power and empowerment in nursing: Looking back to inform the future. *Online Journal of Issues in Nursing, 12*(1). Item number: 2009526637.

Mathes, M. (2005). On nursing, moral autonomy, and moral responsibility. *MEDSURG Nursing, 14*(6), 395–398.

McCarthy, V., & Freeman, L. H. (2008). A multidisciplinary concept analysis of empowerment: Implications for nursing. *Journal of Theory Construction and Testing, 12*(2), 68–74.

Milton, C. L. (2009). Common metaphors in nursing ethics. *Nursing Science Quarterly, 22*(4), 318–322.

Murray, J. S. (2010, September 1). Moral courage in healthcare: Acting ethically even in the presence of risk. *Online Journal of Issues in Nursing, 15*(3). Item Number: 2010889996.

Ning, S., Zhong, H., Libo, W., & Qiujie, L. (2009). The impact of nurse empowerment on job satisfaction. *Journal of Advanced Nursing*, *65*(12), 2642–2648.

O'Brien, J. L. (2011). Relationship among structural empowerment, psychological empowerment, and burnout in registered staff nurses working in outpatient dialysis centers. *Nephrology Nursing Journal*, *38*(6), 475–481.

Purdy, N., Laschinger, J. H. S., Finegan, J., Kerr, M., & Olivera, F. (2010). Effects of work environments on nurse and patient outcomes. *Journal of Nursing Management*, *18*, 901–913.

Ray, S. L. (2006). Whistleblowing and organizational ethics. *Nursing Ethics*, *13*(4), 438–445.

Rodwell, C. M. (1996). An analysis of the concept of empowerment. *Journal of Advanced Nursing*, *23*, 305–313.

Ryles, S. M. (1999). A concept analysis of empowerment: Its relationship to mental health nursing. *Journal of Advanced Nursing*, *29*(3), 600–607.

Sharoff, L. (2009). Expressiveness and creativeness: Metaphorical images of nursing. *Nursing Science Quarterly*, *22*(4), 312–317.

Shearer, N. B. C., & Reed, P. G. (2004). Empowerment: Reformulation of a non-Rogerian concept. *Nursing Science Quarterly*, *17*(3), 253–259.

Tressman, S. (2000). Speaking out: Two nurses tell their stories. *The American Nurse*, *32*(4), 1–2, 22.

Williamson, K. M. (2007). Home health care nurse's perceptions of empowerment. *Journal of Community Health Nursing*, *24*(3), 133–153.

Chapter

20

FACILITATING PATIENT EMPOWERMENT

The most common way for people to give up power is by thinking that they don't have any.

(Walker, 2012)

OBJECTIVES

After completing this chapter, the reader should be able to:

1. Discuss the meaning of patient empowerment.

2. Discuss the nursing role in empowerment of patients.

3. Describe nurse attitudes that facilitate empowerment.

4. Identify nursing knowledge and skills basic to empowerment.

5. Describe factors that enhance or block patient empowerment.

6. Discuss approaches to fostering empowerment with patients.

INTRODUCTION

The concept of empowerment relates to the principle of autonomy and to the nursing role of patient advocate. Fostering empowerment in others requires nurses to be attentive to both personal and professional empowerment. This chapter focuses on nursing's role in facilitating empowerment of patients. Understanding of power and empowerment, discussed in Chapter 19, applies to patients as well as nurses. The discussion of empowerment in this chapter flows from these same understandings.

PATIENTS AND EMPOWERMENT

The concept of empowering patients has emerged as nursing has directed its ethical focus to advocacy for patients. Adherence to principles discussed throughout this book, particularly respect for persons, autonomy, justice, and beneficence, makes it incumbent upon nurses to involve patients in making decisions about their health and care. Some patients have both the desire and skills to take charge of their lives, some have desire but need to improve their skills, while others have limitations in ability and desire. Negotiating within a system that has traditionally placed decision-making authority and power primarily within the hands of physicians requires skill, support, and a strong sense of personal empowerment. Factors discussed in Chapter 19 regarding personal empowerment for nurses apply as well to patients. Patient empowerment is both a process and outcome in which nurses have an active role.

NURSES AND PATIENT EMPOWERMENT

Speaking of empowering another suggests that power is a commodity given by one person to another. Such a view of empowerment strips patients of their ability to choose. Empowerment as described in nursing literature is a dynamic, interactive, and reciprocal process that is an inherent facet of the nurse-patient relationship (McCarthy & Freeman, 2008). Facilitating the empowerment process requires a paradigm shift away from the paternalistic attitude of knowing what is best for the patient. Taking into account cultural diversity regarding the locus of responsibility for health, we recognize and accept that patients are essentially responsible for their own health and have the ability to discern what they need, make decisions, and direct their own destinies. In order to make appropriate decisions, however, people may need information and support.

Empowerment is a social process arising from reciprocal interactions among people through which the ability to meet needs, solve problems, and mobilize resources is recognized and enhanced (Gibson, 1991; Manojlovich, 2007; McCarthy & Freeman, 2008). As a process of assisting people in asserting control over the factors that affect their health, empowerment links autonomy with accountability in a way that promotes greater access to needed resources (Gibson, 1991; McCarthy & Freeman, 2008). In light of this understanding of empowerment and nursing's focus on patient advocacy, nurses are called on to facilitate the empowerment process with patients, families, and communities. Certain attitudes, knowledge, and skills are basic to fulfilling this role.

Attitudes of Nurses That Facilitate Empowerment

A view of the nurse as a partner, facilitator, and resource rather than merely one who provides services for patients is basic to facilitating empowerment with patients (Laschinger, Gilbert, Smith, & Leslie, 2010; Shearer, 2007). Nurses must learn to surrender their need for control, developing instead attitudes of collaboration and mutual participation in decision making. This requires self-reflection on the part of the nurse, through which the nurse confronts personal values and the subtle—and not so subtle—benefits gained from being in a position of power. It is essential that nurses make a commitment to being with patients as they struggle with their questions and issues and seek meaning in the process. Relinquishing control also means that nurses need to accept decisions made by patients and families, even when they are different from what the nurse might do or suggest. Respect for persons, which includes valuing others and mutual trust, is key (Henderson, 2003; Hewitt-Taylor, 2004; Ho, Berggren, & Dahlborg-Lyckhage, 2010; Laschinger et al., 2010; Shearer, 2007).

Nursing Knowledge and Skills Necessary for Facilitating Empowerment

Information presented throughout this book provides a foundation for facilitating the empowerment process. Attention to ethical principles and processes of decision making fosters empowerment. Awareness of the development of values and their impact on choices allows nurses to clarify their own perspectives, so as to foster integrity and avoid imposing personal values on others. Knowledge of social, cultural, political, economic, and other forces affecting a person's options and health choices is essential.

Empowerment is an interactive process. As in many other areas of nursing, effective communication is necessary for facilitating empowerment.

The ability to listen with our whole being and to trust intuitive as well as intellectual understandings is important. Reflective listening allows us to help people recognize their own strengths, abilities, and personal power. Active listening also helps people to develop awareness of root causes of problems and to determine their readiness to take action for change. When it seems that the patient does not want to be empowered, nurses can provide interventions in a style of empowerment rather than control (Ho et al., 2010). This means approaching patients with an attitude of trust in their ability—at some place within themselves—to know what they need, as well as incorporating behaviors such as offering choices about aspects of care over which they can have control.

Having the opportunities and resources necessary for understanding and changing our world is part of the empowerment process. Nurses must have knowledge of factors affecting a patient's health and health care decisions in order to help provide or share the necessary resources. Such knowledge includes awareness of patient and family values and decision-making style; cultural context; social, political, and economic influences on our options; and health care system constraints. We also recognize that individual responsibility for health is necessarily tempered by social and environmental factors. Nurses need to focus health promotion efforts on the macro social level, attending to conditions that control, influence, and produce health or illness in people (Hewitt-Taylor, 2004; Manojlovich, 2007; Oudshoorn, 2005; Shearer, 2007). Efforts as individuals, within professional organizations, and within communities, aimed at providing access to health care for all, provide a broad base of support for empowerment.

Approaching patients as equal partners is key to patient empowerment. Skillful collaboration and negotiation that incorporate power sharing and mutually beneficial interactions facilitate empowerment. Relinquishing professional power returns power to the patient.

ENHANCING PATIENT CAPACITY FOR DECISION MAKING

The ability to make decisions regarding our lives and destinies requires a basic level of cognitive functioning and sense of control over life and change processes. Empowerment originates in self-esteem; is developed through love, a sense of connectedness, responsibility, and opportunities for choice; and is supported through perceived meaning and hope in life (Manojlovich, 2007; McCarthy & Freeman, 2008).

Helping patients to know who they are facilitates empowerment. Since empowerment flows from a deep understanding of self, the process of self-discovery enables patients to decide what they want to do, based on an appreciation of who they are. Supporting patient empowerment may require facilitating a patient's self-awareness on many levels, such as identifying personal values, the sources of these values, where and with whom they feel connected, and where and how they experience control in life. Utilizing the decision-making process discussed in Chapter 7 can facilitate empowerment with patients.

Determining whether a person functions primarily from a sense of internal or external locus of control can be useful. **Locus of control** refers to beliefs about the ability to control events in our lives. People who believe that they are able to influence or control things that happen to them are considered to have an **internal locus of control**. On the other hand, people who feel that forces outside of themselves direct or rule their lives—whether these be generalized forces such as fate, or other persons who are perceived as more powerful—are considered to have an **external locus of control**. Persons who are internally motivated are more likely to perceive themselves as having power to make choices and control their lives, and to be motivated to make necessary changes. Those who are externally motivated tend to be more fatalistic, expecting their lives to be controlled by powerful others, and less likely to enact personal power (Brincks, Feaster, Burns, & Mitrani, 2010).

ASK YOURSELF

How Does Locus of Control Affect Empowerment?

- Reflect on how you have thought through significant decisions in your life. Do you consider that you are more internally or more externally motivated? Give specific examples to support your self-assessment.

- In working with patients, what would you consider indications of internal and external locus of control?

- How would your approach to facilitating empowerment be different with persons who exhibit internal locus of control compared to those with external locus of control?

Barriers to Empowerment

Empowerment involves a willingness to take risks and move beyond that which is known, and perhaps comfortable, to the unknown. It often requires a change in self-perception, developing a different vision of who we are. This can stimulate anxiety and fear. Nurses need to recognize such barriers and appreciate that not everyone wants to take the risks and assume the responsibility that empowerment demands. Paternalistic attitudes and sociocultural role expectations within the health care system have fostered reliance on health care providers to determine what patients need for health.

Other barriers include patient lack of knowledge of resources or strategies that promote empowerment, dependency, apathy, mistrust, being labeled by staff, and the nurse's unwillingness to share decision-making power with patients (Connelly, Keele, Kleinbeck, Schneider, & Cobb, 1993; Henderson, 2003; Hewitt-Taylor, 2004). Social, cultural, economic, or political factors can present barriers such as limited resources, control of knowledge about options, locking people into traditional roles and expectations, social labeling that stereotypes and devalues certain people or behaviors, and restriction of access to resources. Professionals' lack of empowerment and their inability to relinquish power to patients affect patient empowerment as well. Honoring patient decisions may be very threatening to nurses who do not appreciate that patients know what they need.

Fostering Patient Empowerment

We can facilitate empowerment in others by being role models of self-empowerment. As noted previously, a belief that patients have the right and ability to make choices regarding their health, and other areas of their lives, is basic to empowerment. Patients need to be given opportunities for choice regarding small as well as major decisions. This means that there needs to be participatory decision making, involving collaboration and negotiation, in all areas of health care. For example, involving patients in making decisions about when they will bathe, what foods to include in their diet, or when to take their medications is as important to empowerment as their participation in decision making regarding life-support measures. Because of social, environmental, and other factors, some people have had limited opportunities for making choices and may need education, practice, and nurturing in this area. Offering options and developing strategies to enhance the patient's ability to set and reach goals are important parts of the nursing role. Connelly et al. (1993) suggest that choosing implies having both the freedom and the courage to choose from different options. Support is an important part of the encouraging process.

Support can take many forms. We provide support by determining what patients identify as empowering to them and by encouraging these choices, behaviors, or attitudes. Caring relationships, in which experiences are shared and patients are accepted for who they are, offer support. Having at least one other person who supports a choice made or a stance that a person takes enhances the likelihood that the person will follow through on the decision.

Considering options and making choices implies having both knowledge and availability of needed resources. Facilitating empowerment may require us to provide or help patients discover how to access resources. In some instances this may mean becoming politically and socially active regarding health care issues affecting vulnerable populations. We need to develop strategies that enhance a patient's ability to acquire necessary knowledge. This may mean working with patients or communities to identify both health concerns and socioculturally relevant approaches to dealing with these concerns. We foster empowerment by promoting processes that encourage mutually respectful exchange of ideas and analysis of concerns and potential solutions. Success in achieving goals must be defined from the perspective of the patient or community.

Think About It

Outcomes of Patient Empowerment

Upholding the view that patients know what they need opens nurses to the probability that some patients will make decisions that are not consistent with what the nurse or other health team members think is best. Such decisions may have a relatively minor impact on a patient's or family's health and well-being or may be judged to have potentially serious outcomes for the patient or family.

- *What factors need to be considered when dealing with decisions involving differing values between patients and nurses?*

- *Give examples of situations in which patient empowerment might pose an ethical dilemma for you.*

- *If you feel a patient is making an unwise decision, how would you respond?*

- *Discuss your views regarding any limits or constraints on patient empowerment.*

SUMMARY

Patient empowerment is an important element of nursing care that derives from an appreciation that patients have the ability to discern their needs and make decisions about their lives and health. Facilitating empowerment requires that nurses learn to relinquish power and embrace the patient as an equal partner. Self-awareness, respect for others, and effective communication skills serve as foundations for the process. Empowerment requires both knowledge about and availability of resources, support, and opportunities for choice. Nurses can facilitate empowerment by working directly with patients and through addressing social, political, and environmental factors affecting empowerment of individuals and communities. In the midst of an ever-changing and challenging health care environment in which issues of power and control continue to affect patient care, facilitating patient empowerment is an essential part of nursing care.

CHAPTER HIGHLIGHTS

- Patient empowerment, which is both a process and an outcome, relates to ethical principles and flows from nursing's focus on patient advocacy.

- Facilitating patient empowerment requires recognition and acceptance that patients have the ability to discern what they need, to make decisions, and to direct their own destinies.

- Empowerment is interactive and requires of nurses self-knowledge of personal values and needs for control, mutual trust and respect, effective communication and reflective listening skills, and a willingness to accept patient decisions regardless of whether the nurse thinks they are best.

- Fostering patient empowerment requires knowledge of social, political, cultural, economic, and environmental factors affecting a person's options and health choices and may involve addressing health promotion efforts on the macro social level.

- Empowerment is fostered through self-discovery; enhanced self-esteem; a sense of connectedness; support; opportunities for choice; and having needed resources, knowledge, and skills.

- Empowerment strategies that mesh with a person's or a community's sociocultural context are more effective.

DISCUSSION QUESTIONS AND ACTIVITIES

1. Describe a personal experience as a patient within the health care system in which you felt that you were empowered. What contributed to the empowerment process for you?

2. Describe a patient or family with whom you have worked who exhibited empowerment. Give specific examples of evidences of empowerment from your perspective.

3. Observe practicing nurses in a clinical setting and describe attitudes and behaviors that foster or block empowerment with patients.

4. Discuss factors within the health care system that inhibit patient empowerment.

5. Describe the relationship between patient empowerment and principled behavior in nursing.

6. Describe a situation in which you believe you fostered empowerment with a patient or family. How did you facilitate the process? Describe the outcome.

7. What would indicate to you that a patient might not want to be empowered? How would you approach and work with this patient?

REFERENCES

Brincks, A. M., Feaster, D. J., Burns, M. J., & Mitrani, V. B. (2010). The influence of health locus of control on the patient-provider relationship. *Psychology, Health & Medicine, 15*(6), 720–728.

Connelly, L. M., Keele, B. S., Kleinbeck, S. V. M., Schneider, J. K., & Cobb, A. K. (1993). A place to be yourself: Empowerment from the client's perspective. *Image, 25,* 297–303.

Gibson, C. H. (1991). A concept analysis of empowerment. *Journal of Advanced Nursing, 16,* 354–361.

Henderson, S. (2003). Power imbalance between nurses and patients: A potential inhibitor of partnership in care. *Journal of Clinical Nursing, 12,* 501–508.

Hewitt-Taylor, J. (2004). Challenging the balance of patient empowerment. *Nursing Standard, 18*(22), 33–37.

Ho, A. Y. K, Berggren, A., & Dahlborg-Lyckhage, E. (2010). Diabetes empowerment related to Pender's health promotion model: A meta-synthesis. *Nursing & Health Sciences, 12,* 259–267.

Laschinger, H. K. S., Gilbert, S., Smith, L. M., & Leslie, K. (2010). Towards a comprehensive theory of nurse/patient empowerment: Applying Kanter's empowerment theory to patient care. *Journal of Nursing Management, 18,* 4–13.

Manojlovich, M. (2007, January 1). Power and empowerment in nursing: Looking back to inform the future. *Online Journal of Issues in Nursing, 12*(1): Manuscript 1. DOI: 10.3912/OJIN.Vol12No01Man01

McCarthy, V., & Freeman, L. H. (2008). A multidisciplinary concept analysis of empowerment: Implications for nursing. *Journal of Theory Construction and Testing, 12*(2), 68–74.

Oudshoorn, A. (2005). Power and empowerment: Critical concepts in the nurse-client relationship. *Contemporary Nurse, 20*(1), 57–66.

Shearer, N. B. C. (2007). Toward a nursing theory of health empowerment in homebound older women. *Journal of Gerontological Nursing, 12,* 38–45.

Walker, Alice. (2012). Retrieved from http://www.great-quotes.com/quote/94632

Appendix

A

ONLINE RESOURCES

CODE OF ETHICS FOR NURSES

American Nurses Association

www.ana.orgd

www.nursingworld.org/codeofethics

THE PATIENT CARE PARTNERSHIP

Understanding Expectations, Rights and Responsibilities

American Hospital Association

www.aha.org

CODE OF ETHICS FOR REGISTERED NURSES

Canadian Nurses Association

www.cna-aiic.ca

THE ICN CODE OF ETHICS FOR NURSES

International Council of Nurses

www.icn.ch

Glossary

Accountability The state of being answerable to someone for something one has done.

Active voluntary euthanasia An act in which the physician both provides the means of death for a patient, such as a lethal dose of medication, and administers it.

Activism A passionate approach to everyday activities that is committed to seeking a more just social order through critical analysis, provocation, transformation, and rebalancing of power.

Act-utilitarianism A basic type of utilitarianism that suggests people choose actions that will, in any given circumstance, increase the overall good.

Administrative law The branch of law that consists mainly of the legal powers granted to administrative agencies by the legislature, and the rules that the agencies make to carry out their powers.

Advance directives Instructions that indicate which health care interventions to initiate or withhold, or that designate someone who will act as a surrogate in making such decisions, in the event that a person loses decision-making capacity.

Advocacy The act of supporting, speaking for, defending, or interceding on behalf of another.

Allocative policies Policies designed to provide net benefits to some distinct group or class of individuals or organizations, at the expense of others, in order to ensure that public objectives are met.

Anonymity A situation in which even the researcher cannot link information with a particular participant in a study.

Appeals to conscience Personal and subjective beliefs, founded on a prior judgment of rightness or wrongness, that are motivated by personal sanction, rather than external authority.

Assault The unjustifiable attempt or threat to touch a person without consent that results in fear of immediately harmful or threatening contact.

Assent Agreeing to or concurring with a decision or proposal (such as a child agreeing with a parent's decision related to participating in a research protocol).

Assisted suicide A situation in which patients receive the means of death from someone, such as a physician, but activate the process themselves.

Authority The state of having legitimate power and sovereignty.

Autonomy An ethical principle that literally means self-governing. It denotes having the freedom to make independent choices.

Axiology The branch of philosophy that studies the nature and types of values.

Battery The unlawful touching of another or the carrying out of threatened physical harm, including every willful, angry, and violent or negligent touching of another's person, clothes, or anything attached to his or her person or held by him or her.

Belmont Report Policies developed by the U.S. National Commission for the Protection of Human Subjects of Biomedical and Behavioral Research (1978) regarding ethical principles for research with human subjects.

Beneficence The ethical principle that requires one to act in ways that benefit another. In research, this implies the protection from harm and discomfort, including a balance between the benefits and risks of a study.

Breach of duty A failure to perform a promised act or obligation.

Bullying Acting in an intimidating, badgering, or demeaning way toward another or others—often with the intent to exert power over the other.

Cartesian philosophy A widespread belief during the Renaissance related to Descartes's proposals that the universe is a physical thing, that all therein is analogous to machines that can be analyzed and understood, and that the mind and body are separate entities.

Case law The basis of the judicial system, also known as common law.

Categorical imperative The Kantian maxim stating that no action can be judged as right that cannot reasonably become a law by which every person should always abide.

Causation A legal term denoting a causal relationship between an action and the resulting harm or injury.

Character ethics Theories of ethics, sometimes called virtue ethics, that are related to the concept of innate moral virtue.

Cheating Dishonesty and deception regarding examinations, projects, or papers.

Civil law (Also called private law) The law that determines a person's legal rights and obligations in many kinds of activities involving other people.

Cloning The process of using biotechnology to create a genetically identical copy of a cell or organism.

Code of nursing ethics Explicit declaration of the primary goals and values of the profession that indicate the profession's acceptance of the responsibility and trust with which it has been invested by society.

Coercion Actual or implied threat of harm or penalty for not participating in a research project, or offering excessive rewards for participation in the project.

Common law A system of law, also known as case law, based largely on previous court decisions. In this system, decisions are based upon earlier court rulings in similar cases, or precedents. Over time, these precedents take on the force of law.

Communitarian theories Theories of justice that place the community, rather than the individual, the state, the nation, or any other entity, at the center of the value system; that emphasize the value of public goods; and that conceive of values as rooted in communal practices.

Compassion A focal virtue combining an attitude of active regard for another's welfare with an imaginative awareness and emotional response of deep sympathy, tenderness, and discomfort at the other person's misfortune or suffering.

Competence A person's ability to make meaningful life decisions. A declaration of incompetence involves legal action with a ruling by a judge that the person is unable to make such life decisions.

Complementary therapies Therapeutic interventions that derive from traditions other than conventional Western medicine that are used by patients with or without the knowledge of conventional medical practitioners.

Confidentiality The ethical principle that requires nondisclosure of private or secret information with which one is entrusted. In research, confidentiality refers to the researcher's assurance to participants that information provided will not be made public or available to anyone other than those involved in the research process without the participant's consent.

Consent Agreeing to or approving of a request, proposal, or decision.

Consequentialism A theory of ethics, sometimes called utilitarianism.

Constitutional law A formal set of rules and principles that describe the powers of a government and the rights of the people.

Contract An agreement between two or more people that can be enforced by law.

Contract law A type of law that deals with the rights and obligations of people who make contracts.

Cosmology A branch of philosophy that describes the structure, origin, and processes of the universe.

Covert values Expectations that are not in writing that are often identified only through participation in, or controversies within, an organization or institution.

Criminal law A type of law that deals with crimes or actions considered harmful to society.

Cultural awareness Knowledge about values, beliefs, behaviors, and the like of cultures other than one's own.

Cultural competence Skill in dealing with transcultural issues, which is demonstrated through cultural awareness and cultural sensitivity.

Cultural sensitivity The ability to incorporate a patient's cultural perspective into nursing assessments, and to modify nursing care in order to be as congruent as possible with the patient's cultural perspective.

Culture The total lifeways of a group of interacting individuals, consisting of learned patterns of values, beliefs, behaviors, and customs shared by that group.

Damages Monetary compensation awarded by a court to an individual who has been injured through the wrongful actions of another person.

Decision-making capacity The ability of a person to understand all information about a health condition, to communicate understanding and choices, and to reason and deliberate, as well as the possession of personal values and goals that guide the decision.

Declaration of Helsinki Principles issued by the World Medical Assembly in 1964 to guide clinical research; revised in 1975.

Defamation Harm that occurs to a person's reputation and good name, diminishes others' value or esteem of that person, or arouses negative feelings toward the person by the communication of false, malicious, unprivileged, or harmful words.

Defendant The person sued or accused in a court of law.

Deontology Related to the term *duty*, deontology is a group of ethical theories based upon the rationalist view that the rightness or wrongness of an act depends upon the nature of the act, rather than the consequences that occur as a result of it.

Dilemma A problem that requires a choice between two options that are equally unfavorable and mutually exclusive.

Discernment A focal virtue of sensitive insight, acute judgment, and understanding that results in decisive action.

Disease The biomedical explanation of sickness.

Distributive justice Application of the ethical principle of justice that relates to fair, equitable, and appropriate distribution in society, determined by justified norms that structure the terms of social cooperation. Its scope includes policies that allot diverse benefits and burdens such as property, resources, taxation, privileges, and opportunities.

Diversity The experience within nursing of differences among colleagues and patients in areas such as gender, age, socioeconomic position, sexual orientation, health status, ethnicity, race, or culture.

Do not resuscitate (DNR) orders Written directives placed in a patient's medical chart indicating that cardiopulmonary resuscitation is to be avoided.

Durable power of attorney Allows a competent person to designate another as a surrogate or proxy to act on her or his behalf in making health care decisions in the event of the loss of decision-making capacity.

Duty of care An overarching legal principle that calls for the nurse to act as an ordinary, prudent, reasonable nurse would act in similar circumstances.

Egalitarian theories Theories of justice that promote ideals of equal distribution of social benefits and burdens and that recognize the social obligation to eliminate or reduce barriers that prevent fair equality of opportunity.

Empirical Knowledge gained through the processes of observation and experience.

Empowerment A helping process and partnership, enacted in the context of love and respect for self and others, through which individuals and groups are enabled to change situations and are given the skills, resources, opportunities, and authority to do so. It involves creating a vision, taking risks, making choices, and behaving in authentic ways.

Ethic A personal consciousness of the moral importance that guides personal action in particular situations.

Ethic of caring An approach to ethical decision making grounded in relationship and mutual responsibility, in which choices are contextually bound and strategies are focused on maintaining connections and not hurting anyone.

Ethic of justice An approach to ethical decision making, based on objective rules and principles, in which choices are made from a stance of separateness.

Ethic of responsiveness An approach that demonstrates respect for persons and a desire to do good for this particular patient on this particular day. The nurse with this quality responds with sensitivity to the concerns, needs, and preferences of each patient.

Ethical dilemma Occurs when there are conflicting moral claims.

Ethical principles Basic and obvious moral truths that guide deliberation and action. Major ethical principles include autonomy, beneficence, nonmaleficence, veracity, confidentiality, justice, fidelity, and others.

Ethical treatment of data Implies integrity of research protocols and honesty in reporting findings.

Ethics A formal process for making logical and consistent decisions based upon moral beliefs.

Ethnocentrism Judging behaviors of someone from another culture by the standards of one's own culture.

Eugenics Meaning "good birth," eugenics is based in the belief that some human traits are more desirable for society than others, and that society should weed out what proponents consider to be undesirable traits. Proponents of eugenics advocate policies that encourage so-called "genetically superior" people to have children, while discouraging so-called "genetically inferior" people from having children, through practices such as forced sterilization.

Euthanasia Causing the painless death of a person in order to end or prevent suffering.

Expertise The characteristic of having a high level of specialized skill and knowledge.

External locus of control The belief that forces outside of oneself direct or rule one's life, whether these be generalized forces such as fate or other persons who are perceived as more powerful.

External standards of nursing practice Guides for nursing care that are developed by non-nurses, legislation, or institutions.

Faith A generic feature of the human struggle to find and maintain meaning flowing from an integration of ways of knowing and valuing.

False imprisonment The unlawful, unjustifiable detention of a person within fixed boundaries, or an act intended to result in such confinement.

Felonies Serious crimes that carry significant fines and jail sentences. Examples of felonies include first- and second-degree murder, arson, burglary, extortion, kidnapping, rape, and robbery.

Fidelity An ethical principle related to the concept of faithfulness and the practice of promise keeping.

Forgery Includes fraud or intentional misrepresentation.

Formalism A term often used to refer to deontology.

Foreseeability The legal concept that a person has the ability to reasonably anticipate that damage or injury may result from certain acts or omissions.

Fraud A deliberate deception for the purpose of securing an unfair or unlawful gain.

Full disclosure Indicates that a research participant must be fully informed of the nature of a study, anticipated risks and benefits, time commitment, expectations of the participant and the researcher, and the right to refuse to participate.

Genetic diagnosis A process of biopsy of embryos to determine the presence of genetic flaws and gender prior to implantation.

Genetic engineering The ability to genetically alter organisms for a variety of purposes, particularly to promote their health and strength.

Genetic screening A process for determining whether persons are predisposed to certain diseases, and whether couples have the possibility of giving birth to a genetically impaired infant.

Grassroots lobbying Lobbying efforts that involve mobilizing a committed constituency to influence the opinions of policy makers.

Guardian *ad litem* A court-appointed guardian for a particular action or proceeding; such a guardian may not oversee all of the person's affairs.

Health policies Authoritative decisions focusing on health that are made in the legislative, executive, or judicial branches of government and are intended to direct or influence the actions, behaviors, or decisions of others; their lifestyles and personal behaviors; and improvements in the availability, accessibility, and quality of their health care services.

Human trafficking Modern-day slavery that involves the acquisition, harboring, and trade of persons through force, threats, deception, or other forms of coercion with the aim of exploiting them for forced labor, for their organs, and for sexual services.

Illness A personal response to disease flowing from how one's culture teaches one to be sick.

Incivility A term for social behavior that lacks respect, is rude, impolite, discourteous, and offensive.

Informed consent A process by which patients are informed of the possible outcomes, alternatives, and risks of treatments and are required to give their consent freely. This implies legal protection of a patient's right to personal autonomy by providing the opportunity to choose a course of action regarding plans for health care, including the right to refuse medical recommendations and to choose from available therapeutic alternatives. *In research*, this refers to consent to participate in a research study after the research purpose, expected commitment, risks and benefits, any invasion of privacy, and ways that anonymity and confidentiality will be addressed have been explained.

Injury A wrong or damage done to another person, which may be physical or emotional harm as well as damage to reputation or dignity, loss of a legal right, or breach of contract.

Integrity Refers to adherence to moral norms that is sustained over time. Implicit in integrity is trustworthiness and a consistency of convictions, actions, and emotions.

Intentional torts Willful or intentional acts that violate another person's rights or property.

Internal locus of control The belief that one is able to influence or control things that happen in one's life.

Internal standards of nursing practice Standards of nursing practice that are developed within the profession of nursing.

Intervening factors Elements that appear in the situation in such a way as to interfere with, alter, or obstruct action.

Invasion of privacy Includes intrusion on the patient's physical and mental solitude or seclusion, public disclosure of private facts, publicity that places the patient in a false light in the public eye, or appropriation of the patient's name or likeness for the defendant's benefit or advantage.

Journals Personal written records kept on a periodic or regular basis containing factual material and subjective interpretations of events, thoughts, feelings, and plans.

Judicial decisions Authoritative court decisions that direct or influence the actions, behaviors, or decisions of others.

Justice An ethical principle that relates to fair, equitable, and appropriate treatment in light of what is due or owed to persons, recognizing that giving to some will deny receipt to others who might otherwise have received these things.

In research, justice implies the rights of fair treatment and privacy, including anonymity and confidentiality.

Kantianism A deontological theory of ethics based upon the writings of the philosopher Immanuel Kant.

Lateral (horizontal) violence Incivility, shaming, humiliating, damaging, and belittling behavior directed toward peers or colleagues.

Law The system of enforceable principles and processes that governs the behavior of people in respect to relationships with others and with the government.

Libel Printed defamation by written words and images that injure a person's reputation or cause others to avoid, ridicule, or view the person with contempt.

Libertarian theories Theories of distributive justice that propose that the just society protects the rights of property and liberty of each person, allowing citizens to improve their circumstances by their own effort.

Living wills Legal documents developed voluntarily by persons, giving directions to health care providers related to withholding or withdrawing life support if certain conditions exist.

Lobbying The art of persuasion—attempting to convince a legislator, a government official, the head of an agency, or a state official to comply with a request—whether it is convincing them to support a position on an issue or to follow a particular course of action.

Locus of control Beliefs about the ability to control events in one's life.

Loyalty Showing sympathy, care, and reciprocity to those with whom we appropriately identify; working closely with others toward shared goals; keeping promises; making mutual concerns a priority; sacrificing personal interests to the relationship; and giving attention to these over a substantial period of time.

Malpractice The form of negligence in which any professional misconduct, unreasonable lack of professional skill, or nonadherence to the accepted standard of care causes injury to a patient or client.

Managed care An integrated form of health care delivery and financing that represents attempts to control costs by modifying the behavior of providers and patients.

Material rules Rules by which distributive justice decisions regarding entitlement are made.

Medical futility Situations in which medical interventions are judged to have no medical benefit, or in which the chance for success is low.

Misdemeanor A criminal offense of a less serious nature than a felony, usually punishable by a fine or short jail sentence, or both.

Modern era A somewhat arbitrary term often used in common language to refer to present or recent time. The term is used in this text and many others to refer to the historical period immediately following the Renaissance, generally thought to include the late sixteenth through the late eighteenth centuries.

Moral courage The willingness to stand up for personal core values and ethical beliefs, even when we stand alone.

Moral development A product of the sociocultural environment in which one lives and develops that reflects the intellectual and emotional process through which one learns and incorporates values regarding right and wrong.

Moral distress The reaction to a situation in which there are moral problems that seem to have clear solutions, yet one is unable to follow one's moral beliefs because of external restraints. This may be evidenced in anger, frustration, dissatisfaction, and poor performance in the work setting.

Moral integrity A focal virtue that relates to soundness, reliability, wholeness, an integration of character, and fidelity in adherence to moral norms sustained over time.

Moral outrage A state that occurs when someone else in the health care setting performs an act the nurse believes to be immoral. In cases of moral outrage, the nurse does not participate in the act and therefore does not feel responsible for the wrong, but feels powerlessness to prevent it.

Moral particularism Moral particularism utilizes the principles and rules of other moral theories, embracing the uniqueness of cases, the culturally significant ethical features, and ethical judgment in each particular case.

Moral philosophy The philosophical discussion of what is considered to be good or bad, right or wrong.

Moral reckoning Moral reckoning is a three-stage process that includes a stage of ease, a situational bind, resolution, and reflection. It may include other processes such as moral distress, moral agony, and moral outrage.

Moral thought Individuals' cognitive examination of right and wrong, good and bad.

Moral uncertainty A state that occurs when one senses that there is a moral problem, but is not sure of the morally correct action; when one is unsure what moral principles or values apply; or when one is unable to define the moral problem.

Moral values Preferences or dispositions reflective of right or wrong, should or should not, in human behavior.

Naturalism A view of moral judgment that regards ethics as dependent upon human nature and psychology.

Necessity In general, necessity refers to the fact of being required or indispensable. As a defense to battery, necessity refers to touching a person with the purpose of helping them in an emergency, even though consent was not obtained.

Negligence The omission to do something that a reasonable person, guided by those ordinary considerations that ordinarily regulate human affairs, would do, or doing something that a reasonable and prudent person would not do.

Noncompliance Denoting an unwillingness on the part of the patient to participate in health care activities that have been recommended by health care providers.

Nonmaleficence An ethical principle related to beneficence that requires one to act in such a manner as to avoid causing harm to another, including deliberate harm, risk of harm, and harm that occurs during the performance of beneficial acts.

Nuremberg Code A set of principles for the ethical conduct of research against which the experiments in the Nazi concentration camps could be judged.

Nurse practice acts Legislative statutes within each state that define nursing, describe boundaries of practice, establish standards for nurses, and protect the domain of nursing.

Nursing process A model commonly used for decision making in nursing.

Obligation Being required to do something by virtue of a moral rule, a duty, or some other binding demand, such as a particular role or relationship.

Overt values Values of individuals, groups, institutions, and organized systems that are explicitly communicated through philosophy and policy statements.

Palliative care A comprehensive, interdisciplinary, and total care approach, focusing primarily on comfort and support of patients and families facing illness that is chronic or not responsive to curative treatment.

Parentalism A nongender term that parallels the meaning of paternalism, while avoiding gender bias.

Partisan Adherence to the ideology of a particular political party.

Paternalism A gender-biased term that literally means acting in a "fatherly" manner, the traditional view of which implies well-intended actions of benevolent decision making, leadership, protection, and discipline that, in the health care arena, manifest in the making of decisions on behalf of patients without their full consent or knowledge.

Patient Self-Determination Act A federal law requiring institutions such as hospitals, nursing homes, health maintenance organizations, and home care agencies receiving Medicare or Medicaid funds to provide written information to adult patients regarding their rights to make health care decisions.

Philosophy The intense and critical examination of beliefs and assumptions.

Plagiarism Taking another's ideas or work and presenting them as one's own.

Plaintiff The term used for the complaining or injured party in a lawsuit.

Policy formulation A phase of the policy-making process that includes such actions as agenda setting and the subsequent development of legislation.

Policy implementation A phase of the policy-making process that follows enactment of legislation and includes taking actions and making additional decisions necessary to implement legislation, such as rule making and policy operation.

Policy modification A phase of the policy-making process that exists to improve or perfect legislation previously enacted.

Political Relates to the complex process of policy making within the government.

Political issues Those issues that are regulated or influenced by decisions within either the executive, judicial, or legislative branch of government.

Political parties Organized groups with distinct ideologies that seek to control government.

Power The ability to do or act; the capability of doing or accomplishing something.

Practical dilemma A situation in which moral claims compete with non-moral claims.

Practical imperative The Kantian maxim requiring that one treat others always as ends and never as a means.

Precautionary principle When an activity raises threats of harm to human health or the environment, precautionary measures should be taken even if some cause-and-effect relationships are not fully established scientifically.

Precedents Court rulings upon which subsequent rulings in similar cases are based. Over time these precedents take on the force of law.

Principles Basic and obvious truths that guide deliberation and action.

Privacy Privacy refers to the right of an individual to control the personal information or secrets that are disclosed to others.

Private law (Also called civil law) The law that determines a person's legal rights and obligations in many kinds of activities involving other people.

Problem A problem is a discrepancy between the current situation and a desired state.

Profession A complex, organized occupation preceded by a long training program geared toward the acquisition of exclusive knowledge necessary to provide a service that is essential or desired by society, leading to a monopoly that provides autonomy, public recognition, prestige, power, and authority for the practitioner.

Professional codes of ethics Explicit, discipline-specific rules of behavior for members of a profession that are developed to protect the people the profession serves, ensure the competence of members, and safeguard the integrity and trustworthiness of the discipline.

Public law Law that defines a person's rights and obligations in relation to government, and describes the various divisions of government and their powers.

Quality of life A subjective appraisal of factors that make life worth living and contribute to a positive experience of living.

Racism The assumption that members of one race are superior to those of another.

Rationalism A view of moral judgment that regards truth as necessary, universal, and superior to the information received from the senses, having an origin in the nature of the universe or in the nature of a higher being.

Regulatory policies Policies that are designed to influence the actions, behaviors, and decisions of others through directive techniques.

Religion The codification of beliefs and practices concerning the Divine and one's relationship with the Divine that are shared by a group of people.

Religiosity Beliefs and practices that are the expressive aspects of religion.

Respect for autonomy An ethical principle that denotes the ethical obligation to honor the autonomy of the other persons.

Respect for human dignity Implies the rights of patients to full disclosure and self-determination regarding participation in research and in making health care choices.

Respect for persons An attitude by which one considers others to be worthy of high regard.

Right to fair treatment Assures equitable treatment of participants in the research selection process, during the study, and after the completion of the study.

Right to privacy The right to be left alone or to be free from unwanted publicity. In *research*, this is the right of research participants to determine when, where, and what kind of information is shared, with an assurance that information and observations are treated with respect and kept in strict confidence.

Rules or regulations Policies that are established to guide the implementation of laws and programs.

Rule-utilitarianism A type of utilitarianism that suggests people choose rules that, when followed consistently, will maximize the overall good.

Self-awareness Conscious awareness of one's thoughts, feelings, physical and emotional responses, and insights in various situations.

Sexism The assumption that members of one sex are superior to those of the other.

Sexual harassment All unwelcome sexual advances, requests for sexual favors, and other conduct of a sexual nature.

Situational bind A moral problem in a particular situation in which core beliefs come into irreconcilable conflict with social or institutional norms or other claims.

Slander Defamation that occurs when one speaks unprivileged or false words about another.

Spirituality The animating force, life principle, or essence of being that permeates life and is expressed and experienced in multifaceted connections with self, others, nature, and God or Life Force.

Stage of ease A time after the novice period, in which the professional has confidence in technical skill and a sense of comfort with rules and expectations in the workplace. Internal and external values and expectations are congruent.

Stakeholders Persons with interest in a given situation.

Standards of nursing practice Written documents outlining minimum expectations for nursing care.

Statutes or laws Legislation that has been enacted by legislative bodies and approved by the executive branch of government.

Statutory (legislative) law Formal laws written and enacted by federal, state, or local legislatures.

Stem cell Considered a "master cell" that can grow into a variety of other cells—a cell that is unspecialized (does not yet have a specific function), and has the capacity to divide and replace itself and to differentiate into various types of specialized cells.

Stereotyping Expecting all persons from a particular group to behave, think, or respond in a certain way based on preconceived ideas.

Sympathy Sharing, in imagination, of others' feelings.

Theory A proposed explanation for a class of phenomena.

Tort A wrong or injury that a person suffers because of someone else's action, either intentional or unintentional. The action may cause bodily harm; damage a person's property, business, or reputation; or make unauthorized use of a person's property.

Trustworthiness A focal virtue that results in recognition by others of one's consistency and predictability in following moral norms.

Unintentional torts Torts that occur when an act or omission causes unintended injury or harm to another person.

Utilitarian theories Theories of distributive justice that distribute resources based on the premise of the greatest good for the greatest number of people. These theories place social good before individual rights.

Utilitarianism A moral theory holding that an action is judged as good or bad in relation to the consequence, outcome, or end result derived from it.

Utility The property of usefulness in any object, whereby it tends to produce benefit, advantage, pleasure, good, or happiness or prevent mischief, pain, evil, or unhappiness.

Values Ideals, beliefs, customs, modes of conduct, qualities, or goals that are highly prized or preferred by individuals, groups, or society.

Values clarification Refers to the process of becoming more conscious of and naming what one values or considers worthy.

Values conflict Internal or interpersonal conflict that occurs in circumstances in which personal values are at odds with those of patients, colleagues, or the institution.

Veracity Truth telling.

Victim blaming Holding the people burdened by social conditions accountable for their own situations and responsible for needed solutions.

Virtue ethics Theories of ethics, usually attributed to Aristotle, that represent the idea that an individual's actions are based upon innate moral virtue.

Whistle-blowers Persons who alert the public about serious wrongdoing created or concealed within an organization, such as unsafe conditions, incompetence, or professional misconduct.

Whistle-blowing Speaking out about unsafe or questionable practices affecting patient care or working conditions. This should be resorted to only after a person has unsuccessfully used all appropriate organizational channels to right a wrong, and has a sound moral justification for taking this action.

Index

A

abortion, 317–318, 390
academic honesty, 330–331
accountability
  authority and, 143
  explanation of, 139
  mechanisms of, 139–143
  unity and, 144
Achterberg, Jeanne, 9, 13, 22, 450, 461
active voluntary euthanasia, 319–320
activism, 402
act-utilitarianism, 41, 42
administrative law, 194
advance directives
  decision-making capacity and, 306–308
  durable power of attorney as, 305–306
  explanation of, 304–305
  living wills as, 305
  nursing role and responsibilities
    regarding, 310, 312
  Patient Self-Determination Act
    and, 308
Advanced Practice Registered Nurses
  (APRN), 209
advocacy, 67–68
Africa, 379–380
Agency for Healthcare Research and Quality
  (AHRQ), 399
AIDS. *See* HIV/AIDS
Alexander the Great, 365–366
allocative policies, 394
altruism, 239–240
American College of Physicians, 377
American Hospital Association (AHA), 74
American Medical Association (AMA)
  American Nurses Association and, 24
  background of, 372
  code of ethics, 75
American Nurses Association (ANA).
    See also Code of Ethics for Nurses
    (American Nurses Association)
  American Medical Association and, 24
  on cultural diversity, 470, 471
  definition of nursing, 450
  development of code of ethics by, 132
  on health care reform, 396
  on human rights and prevention of
    discrimination, 248
  on lateral violence and bullying, 243
  lobbying function of, 401
  model nurse practice acts of, 142
  Nursing's Social Policy Statement, 7
  on nutrition and hydration, 273

  on patient decision making, 308
  on privacy and confidentiality, 219
  on research, 333
  on responsibilities of nurses, 233, 320
  on standard of care, 140, 201
  on third-party reimbursement, 394
Americans with Disabilities Act of 1990
  (ADA), 248, 250–251
Amott, T., 461
ancient cultures
  health care delivery in, 365–366
  philosophy and, 12–13
  religious influences and, 9–11
  role of women in, 10, 11
Andrews, T., 460
anonymity, 336
a priori method of fixing belief, 112–113
Aquinas, Thomas, 14, 17
Aristotle, 12–14, 48–49, 52, 230, 388
armed conflict victims, 358–360
Aroskar, M. A., 317
assault, 210
assessment
  cultural, 474
  as nursing function, 201–202
  of spirituality, 481–482
assisted suicide, 319, 320
attitudes
  empowerment and, 517
  influence of, 495–496
  technology and, 286–287
Augustine (Saint), 14
authoritarian medical model, 298
authority, 143
authority method of fixing belief, 112
autonomy
  advocacy and, 67–68
  confidentiality and, 79–81
  elements of, 60
  explanation of, 59–60, 296
  factors that threaten, 60–61
  of health care workers, 321
  informed consent and, 64–65
  limits of, 298–299
  noncompliance and, 68–69
  of nurses, 136–139, 222
  paternalism and, 65–66, 296–298
  privacy as expression of, 77–78
  recognizing violations of patient,
    62–64
  social issues and, 440–441
axiology, 93
Aydelotte, M., 144

B

Beauchamp, T. L., 49, 50
beliefs
  authority method of fixing, 112
  influence of, 495–496
  methods of fixing, 3–4, 112–113
  values and, 111–113, 471, 474
Belmont Report, 333
beneficence
  as ethical principle, 70–71, 74
  explanation of, 69–70
  implementation and, 202–203
  research and, 334–336
  social issues and, 440
  technology and, 261
Bentham, Jeremy, 40–41
Berthiaume v. Pratt, 210
Bixler, Genevieve, 128–129, 143
Bixler, Roy, 128–129, 143
Blue Cross plans, 373, 374
Bok, S., 75
breach of duty, 199
Buber, Martin, 34, 73
bullying, 242
burns, 206

C

Califano, J. A., Jr., 420
Callahan, S., 161, 162
Canada, national health insurance in,
  376–377
Canadian Nurses Association (CNA),
  70–71, 394. *See also Code of Ethics
  for Registered Nurses* (Canadian
  Nurses Association)
cardiopulmonary resuscitation (CPR), 266,
  270, 271, 283
care management events, 207
caring
  ethic of, 115–116, 120
  gender and, 120, 454–456
  in nursing profession, 134–135, 161
  politics of, 120–121
  technology and, 288
Cartesian philosophy, 22
case presentations
  abuse, 434
  advance directives, 309, 311
  aging, poverty, and illness, 437
  beneficence and nonmaleficence, 72
  cultural diversity, 474
  death/dying, 275, 276
  decision making, 168, 245, 265, 297

distributive justice, 83–84
duty to patients, 236
economic issues, 234
end-of-life decisions, 268–269, 309, 311
ethical decision making, 168, 179
ethical principles, 63, 72
ethics, 30–31, 39, 42, 47
health care choices, 314
health care economics, 415
homelessness, 432
informed consent, 302
lack of care, 238–239
loyalty to profession, 241
mistaken resuscitation, 272
nursing standards, 141
religious beliefs, 486, 487
research, 337, 340, 343
respect for persons, 133
socioeconomic influences on
    health, 430
values conflict, 99–100, 102
values development, 119
wrongful-death lawsuit, 216
categorical imperative, 45
Catholic Church. *See* Roman Catholic
    Church
causation, 200
Certification of Need programs, 419
character ethics, 48–51
cheating, 331
Children's Health Insurance Program
    (CHIP), 421, 429
Childress, J., 49, 50
China, 380
Chinn, P. L., 92, 455
Christianity. *See* Early Christian Era
civil law, 196–197
Civil Rights Act of 1964, 248, 250, 456
Civil Rights Act of 1991, 248, 251
Clinton, Bill, 421
cloning, 281–282
Code of Ethics for Nurses (American
    Nurses Association)
    on accountability, 139
    on autonomy, 137
    background of, 132
    on beneficence, 71
    on confidentiality, 76, 79
    on delegation of activities, 246–247
    on health policy participation, 399–400
    Kantian principles and, 46
    on professional role of nurses, 238
    on racial discrimination, 249
    on responsibilities and duties of nurses,
        235, 313, 506
Code of Ethics for Nurses (International
    Council of Nurses)
    on autonomy, 137
    on beneficence, 70
    on confidentiality, 76
    on racial discrimination, 249
    on responsibilities and duties of nurses,
        233, 235, 399
Code of Ethics for Registered Nurses
    (Canadian Nurses Association)
    on autonomy, 137
    on beneficence, 70–71

confidentiality and, 76
on responsibilities and duties
    of nurses, 235
Code of Federal Regulations, 338–339
codes of ethics
    beneficence and, 70–71
    characteristics of nursing, 131–134
    development of, 127, 131, 132
    Kantian principles and, 46
    noncompliance and, 69
    nurse practice acts and, 142
    professional, 35–36
coercion, 34–36
cognitive development stages (Piaget),
    113–114
Cole, N., 462
common law, 194
communication
    confidentiality of electronic, 217–219
    cultural diversity and, 479–480
    empowerment and, 517–518
    gender issues and, 459–461
    legal issues related to patient, 220–221
    with patients, 220–221, 461
    with physicians, 460–461
    technology and, 287–288
communitarian theories, 418
compassion, 50, 161
complementary therapies
    cultural diversity and, 315–316, 477–478
    dealing with, 479
    as health care options, 315–316
    informed consent and, 316, 478
confidentiality. *See also* privacy
    arguments in favor of, 77–79
    of electronic communications, 217–219
    as ethical principle, 76–77, 322–323
    explanation of, 76, 336
    limits of, 79–81
    technological advances and, 284–286
conflict
    prevention of, 361–362
    related to obligations, 233
    values, 96–101
Confucius, 34
Connelly, L. M., 520
consent, 211, 301. *See also* informed
    consent
consequentialism, 40. *See also* utilitarianism
Constitution, U.S., 193
constitutional law, 193
context, 155
contraception, 318
contract law, 197
contracts, 197
Copernicus, 21
Corcoran-Perry, S. A., 134
cosmology, 9, 109
covert values, 99, 100
Covey, S. R., 329
criminal events, 208
criminal law, 194–195
critical social theory, 5
Crusades, 16
Cruzan, Nancy, 157, 276
cultural assessment, 474
cultural awareness, 469

cultural competence, 469
cultural diversity. *See also* transcultural
    issues
    complementary therapies and, 315–316
    health care and, 379–380
    racism and, 437–439
    in values development, 109–110
cultural sensitivity, 469
culture, 469–470. *See also* transcultural
    issues
Curtin, L., 134, 247, 295, 508, 509

D

Dalai Lama, 449
damages, 200
Dark Period of Nursing, 21
data, ethical treatment of, 343
Davis, A. J., 317
death/dying. *See also* end-of-life care
    issues related to, 262–266
    palliative care and, 277–279
decision making. *See also* ethical
    decision making; ethical
    decision-making model
    data gathering for, 165–166
    features of, 163–164
    patient capacity for, 306–308, 518–520
    problem analysis and, 151–158
    problem articulation in, 164–165
    process of, 158–159
    values and, 95
decision-making capacity
    elements of, 307–308
    empowerment and, 518–520
    explanation of, 306
Declaration of Helsinki, 333
defamation, 212–213
delegation, 246–247
deliberation, 52, 161
deontology
    drawbacks of, 46–47
    explanation of, 44–45, 48
    Kant and, 45–46
    positive aspects of, 47–48
Descartes, René, 22, 23
device events, 207
Diagnostic Related Groups (DRGs), 419
dilemmas
    explanation of, 152
    moral and ethical, 152–154
    practical, 154
Dilley, K. B., 247
disabilities, discrimination against persons
    with, 250–251
disaster preparedness, 358
disaster response, 356–358
discernment, 50
discrimination
    based on sexual orientation, 458–459
    HIV/AIDS and, 320, 321
    overview of, 248
    against persons with disabilities, 250–251
    racial, 248–249
    sexual, 251–253, 452–453, 455–456
disease, 471
disparate impact, 248–249
displaced persons, 358–360

distributive justice
  communitarian theories and, 418
  decisions related to, 81–82
  distribution of resources and, 416–417
  egalitarian theories and, 418–419
  entitlement and, 413–415
  explanation of, 44, 412
  fair distribution and, 416
  health care and, 82
  health care economics and, 412–419
  influenza pandemic of 2009–2010
    and, 83–84
  libertarian theories and, 417–418
  utilitarian theories and, 417
  war and violence and, 360
diversity, 469, 506. *See also* cultural
    diversity; racial issues; transcultural
    issues
Dock, Lavinia Lloyd, 23, 399
doing good. *See* beneficence
Dolan, J. A., 13, 15
domestic violence, 433–434
Donchin, A., 53
do no harm. *See* nonmaleficence
do not resuscitate (DNR) order, 266,
    270–273
Doyle, E. I., 104
durable power of attorney, 305–306
duty of care, 199

E

Early Christian Era, 13–14, 366
Earth Charter, 354–355
Earth ethics, 351–355
ease stage of moral reckoning, 174–176
economics, 269–270, 410. *See also* health
    care economics
egalitarian theories, 418–419
elderly population, 436
electronic communications, confidentiality
    of, 217–219
Ellin, Joseph, 74–75
embryonic stem cells (ESC), 282–283
Emodi, Sylva, 454
emotions, ethical decision making
    and, 161–162
empirical knowledge, 15
employers
  obligations to, 233
  relationships with, 237–240
empowerment
  barriers to, 519–520
  decision-making capacity and, 518–520
  diversity and, 506–508
  ethical decision making and, 161
  nature of, 500–501
  nurse practice acts and, 143
  overview of, 4–5, 499–500
  patient, 516–521
  personal, 501–504
  professional, 222, 504–506
  re-visioning and, 508–509
end-of-life care. *See also* death/dying
  advance directives for, 304–312
  decisions related to, 268–269, 312–313
entitlement
  elements of, 413
  right to health care and, 413–415

environmental events, 208
Equal Employment Opportunity
    Commission (EEOC), 248
equitable treatment, 336–337
ethic, 163
ethical decision making
  approaches to, 158, 160
  attributes for, 160–161
  at bedside, 163
  emotions and, 161–162
  moral distress and, 170–173
  moral outrage and, 173–174
  moral reckoning and, 174–180
  nursing process of, 159–160
  overview of, 151, 158–159
  problem analysis and, 151–158
  as socially and culturally mediated
    process, 121
  values and, 95
ethical decision-making model
  application of, 168–169
  data gathering and moral claims
    identification step in, 165–166
  evaluation step in, 166, 168, 170
  explanation of, 163–164, 167
  problem articulation step in, 164–165
  strategy exploration step in, 166
  strategy implementation step in, 166
ethical dilemmas, 153–154
ethical principles
  applied to social issues, 439–441
  autonomy as, 59–69 (*See also* autonomy)
  beneficence as, 69–71
  confidentiality as, 76–81
  explanation of, 59
  fidelity as, 84–85
  justice as, 81–82
  nonmaleficence as, 71–73
  veracity as, 73–76
ethical theory
  background of, 38–39
  case presentations for, 30–31, 39
  deontology and, 44–48
  moral particularism and, 51–53
  moral philosophy and, 35–38
  naturalism and, 37–38
  overview of, 30, 31
  philosophical basis for, 32–35
  rationalism and, 38
  utilitarianism and, 40–44
  virtue ethics and, 48–51
ethic of caring, 115–116, 120
ethics. *See also* codes of ethics;
    nursing ethics
  controversial technologies and, 281–284
  in disaster situations, 357–358
  Earth, 351–355
  effect of, 4
  empowered decision making and, 4
  explanation of, 35–36
  health care and, 135
  health care policy and, 398
  holistic, 121
  informed consent and, 300–301
  of justice, 120, 121
  law vs., 190–191
  of managed care, 377–378, 422–424
  moral philosophy and, 38

nursing profession and, 31–32
  origin of term, 48
  problem solving and, 234
  reproductive policies and, 318–319
  in research, 333–339, 341–343
  rules of action and, 7
  virtue, 48–51
ethnocentrism, 470
eugenics, 280, 318
euthanasia, 266, 319–320
evaluation, as nursing function, 201–202
expertise, 135–136
expert witnesses, 223–224

F

fair distribution, 416
faith, 116–118. *See also* religion;
    spirituality
false imprisonment, 211–212
fee-for-service system, 411
felony, 195
Ferris v. County of Kennebec, 202
FICA Spiritual History Tool, 482
fidelity, 84–85, 236, 330
Flexner, Abraham, 128, 138
Flexner Report, 128, 129
floating, 234–235
focal virtues, 49–50
Foot, Phillipa, 49
foreign objects, neglecting to remove, 204
foreseeability, 79–80, 199–200
forgery, 331
formalism, 44. *See also* deontology
Fowler, J. W., 110, 113, 116–118
fraud, 209
full disclosure, 336
Fulton, Y., 4

G

Gadow, S., 232
Galileo Galilei, 21
gays, 458–459
gender/gender issues. *See also* men;
    women
  caring and, 120, 454–456
  communication and, 459–461
  healing professions and, 8–9
  on moral decision making, 120
  in nursing, 452–453
  nursing practice and, 8–9, 450–451
  race and, 461–463
  sexism and, 457–458
  sexual orientation and, 458–459
  in women's health, 453–454
gender stereotypes, 9, 451, 455–456
genetic engineering, 280–281
genetic research, 280–281
genetic screening, 280
Gilligan, C., 113, 115–116, 118, 120
Gilloran, A., 452
Gingerich, B. S., 101
golden mean, 49
Golden Rule, 6, 41, 316
Goldsmith, J., 67
grassroots lobbying, 402
Grigsby, K., 455
Group, T. M., 24
Gruending, D. L., 129

H

Habermas, J., 5
Hadley, E., 400
Hardwig, J., 299
harm principle, 80
Hartman Value Profile, 101–102
Harvard Pilgrim Health Care Ethics
    Program, 377
healing professions. *See also* nursing/nursing
    practice
    in ancient cultures, 8–13
    in Early Christian Era, 13–14
    gender influences and, 8–9
    in Middle Ages, 14–20
    in Modern Era, 22–24
    in Renaissance and Reformation, 20–21
health care
    access to, 363–364, 377, 397, 421, 422,
        429, 438
    alternative traditions of, 379–380
    confidentiality in, 322–323
    in contemporary United States, 410–412
    cost of, 363–364, 373
    cultural diversity and, 475–477
    distributive justice and, 412–413
    emergency, 356–358
    environmentally responsible, 352–353
    global issues related to, 375–378
    poverty and, 429–430
    right to, 413–415
health care delivery
    in ancient cultures, 365–366
    background of, 364–365
    expanded coverage and, 374–375
    from Middle Ages to Industrial
        Revolution, 366–367
    physicians and hospitals and, 368
    in rural and urban areas, 381
    significant events in, 369–371
    in twentieth- and twenty-first century,
        369, 371–374
    in United States, 367–375
health care economics
    distributive justice and, 412–419
    health care reform and, 420–422
    managed care and, 422–424
    medical futility and, 269–270
    overview of, 410–412
    recent trends and, 419–422
health care options
    complementary therapies as, 315–316
    controversial, 316–333
    overview of, 312–313
    recommended treatment and, 313
health care reform, 420–422
health care resources, 416–417
health insurance
    background of, 373, 420
    expansion of, 374–375
    in industrialized nations, 376–377
Health Insurance Portability and
    Accountability Act (HIPAA) (1996),
    81, 339
health policy
    circumstances of, 396
    ethics and, 398
    explanation of, 393–395
    formulation of, 395–396
    implementation of, 396
    lobbying and, 402–405
    modification of, 397–398
    nursing and, 399–401
    politics and, 289–393
    research data and, 399
health promotion model, 431–432
hedonistic utilitarianism, 40
Henderson, Virginia, 67
Hesse, H., 29
heterosexism, 458
Hill-Burton Act (1946), 373, 374
Hippocrates, 10, 11, 365
Hippocratic Oath, 10–11, 71, 75, 76
HIV/AIDS
    health policy and, 395–396
    patient self-determination and, 320–322
holistic ethics, 121
homelessness, 429, 431–432, 438
honesty, academic, 330–331
hospitals, 372–373
hostile work environment sexual
    harassment, 252
human dignity, 334, 336
humanism, 21
human rights protection, 334, 335, 339,
    341–342
human trafficking, 435–436
Hurricane Katrina, 43–44, 357
Hurricane Rita, 357

I

ICN. *See* International Council of Nurses
    (ICN)
illness, 471
imperative
    categorical, 45, 46
    of duty, 46
    explanation of, 45
    practical, 45–46
incivility, 242–243
individuals with disabilities, 250–251
Industrial Revolution, 366–367
influenza pandemic of 2009–2010, 83–84
informed consent
    complementary therapies and,
        316, 478
    contemporary practice of, 64–65
    ethical and legal elements of, 300–301
    exceptions to, 299
    explanation of, 64, 299–300
    HIV/AIDS and, 320
    nursing role and responsibilities in,
        301–304
    research and, 65, 338–339
injury, 200
integrity
    explanation of, 50, 96
    moral, 50
intentional torts
    components of, 208, 209
    explanation of, 208
    types of, 208–213
International Council of Nurses (ICN).
    See also Code of Ethics for Nurses
    (International Council of Nurses)
    allocative policy and, 394
    code of ethics development by, 132
    on displaced persons, 360
    on responsibilities of nurses, 233
    on war and violence, 362
intervening factors
    explanation of, 154
    types of, 155–158
intimate partner violence (IPV),
    433–434, 438
invasion of privacy, 209–210

J

Jameton, Andrew, 73, 144, 170, 171, 507,
    508
Jones v. Chicago HMO, 214–215
journals, 97, 98
judicial decisions, 394
justice. *See also* distributive justice
    autonomy and, 298–299, 412–419
    distributive, 44, 81–84, 360
    as ethical principle, 81, 412
    ethic of, 120, 121
    research and, 336–337
    social issues and, 439
    theories of, 417–419

K

Kant, Immanuel, 22, 44–46, 73
Kantianism, 44. *See also* deontology
King, Martin Luther, Jr., 188, 191
Kohlberg, L., 113–115, 118, 120

L

Lachman, V. D., 504
language
    cultural diversity and, 476
    of violence, 441–442
Lao Tsu, 108
lateral violence, 242, 243
law. *See also* legal issues; legal trends
    administrative, 194
    common, 194
    confidentiality and, 80–81
    constitutional, 193
    contract, 197
    ethics vs., 190–191
    explanation of, 189, 394
    functions of, 189–190
    nurse practice acts, 140, 142, 143
    private, 196–197
    public, 194–195
    statutory/legislative, 193
    tort, 197–213
legal issues. *See also* law
    autonomy and empowerment as, 222
    conscientious practice maintenance as,
        221–222
    informed consent as, 303–304
    liability insurance as, 223
    nurses as expert witnesses as,
        223–224
    overview of, 192
    patient communications as, 220–221
    related to advance directives, 308
    related to managed care, 422–423
    related to technology, 274–276
    related to transcultural issues,
        479–480
    risk management as, 219

legal trends. *See also* law
  involving claims against nurses, 215–216
  involving criminalization of nurses'
    professional negligence, 216–217
  involving electronic media confidentiality,
    217–219
  involving managed care organizations,
    214–215
  overview of, 213–214
legislative law, 193
Leininger, M., 134, 471, 473n
lesbian, gay, bisexual and transgender
  (LGBT) patients, 459
lesbians, 458–459
letter writing, 403–404
Lewenson, S. B., 462
liability insurance, 222–223
libel, 212–213
libertarian theories, 417–418
licensure, 84, 143
Lipkin, M., 74
Little, M. O., 51–52, 440
living wills, 305, 306
lobbying
  by American Nurses Association, 401
  choice of words when, 405
  explanation of, 396, 402
  grassroots, 402
  methods of, 402–403
  political campaigns and, 404–405
lobbying campaigns, 403–404
loyalty
  explanation of, 232–233
  institutional demands for, 237–238
  in nurse-patient relationship, 85
  of nurses, 240–241, 497
Luther, Martin, 20

M

Mahowald, M. B., 318
malpractice
  areas of, 202–208
  claims against nurses, 215–216
  components of, 198–199
  data on nurse, 200–201
  explanation of, 198
  risk reduction for, 219, 220
  as tort offense, 200
managed care
  ethics of, 377–378, 422–424
  explanation of, 422
managed care organizations (MCOs),
  214–215
material rules, 413
Matthaei, J., 461
Medicaid, 394, 419, 429
medical futility, 266–270
medicalization, 451
medical profession, 17–18
Medicare, 24, 374, 375, 394, 419
medication errors, 203
Megel, M., 455
men
  caring and, 455–457
  in nursing, 452–453
  in nursing school, 460
mental illness, 16
metaphors, 496–497

Middle Ages
  health care delivery in, 366–367
  philosophy in, 14
  religious influences in, 14–16
  social turmoil in, 18–20
  women in, 17–20
Mill, John Stuart, 22, 41, 73
misdemeanors, 195
Mobe v. Williams, 300
Modern Era, 22–24
Montessori, Maria, 247
Moore, Lawrence, 79
moral courage, 503–504
moral development
  gender and, 120
  Kohlberg's theory of, 114–115
  transcultural considerations in,
    109–110
moral dilemmas, 152–154, 235
moral distress, 170–173
moral integrity, 50, 160–161
moral outrage, 173–174
moral particularism, 51–53
moral philosophy, 35, 38–39
moral problems, 151, 152
moral reasoning, 6
moral reckoning
  ease stage of, 174–176
  explanation of, 174
  methods to anticipate, minimize and
    control, 178–180
  reflection stage of, 178
  resolution stage of, 177–178
  situational binds and, 176–177
morals, effect of, 4
moral theories, 34–35
moral thought, 5–6, 93
moral uncertainty, 152
moral values, 93–94
Mosaic health code, 11
multiple stakeholders, 155–156
Munhall, P. L., 338
Munson, R., 66

N

National Council of State Boards of
  Nursing, 142
National Institutes of Health (NIH), 335
National Practitioner Data Bank (NPDB),
  200–201, 215
National Quality Forum (NQF), 206
naturalism, 37–38
necessity, 210–211
negligence
  criminalization of nurses' professional,
    216–217
  explanation of, 197–198
  institutional vs. individual, 195–196
  malpractice as, 198–199
Newman, M. A., 134
Nietzsche, Friedrich, 82
Nightingale, Florence, 9, 11, 22–23, 51,
  131–132, 135, 367, 456
Nightingale Pledge, 51
noncompliance, 61, 68–69, 313
nonmaleficence
  as ethical principle, 71–73
  explanation of, 71

social issues and, 439
technology and, 261
Nuremberg Code, 333
Nuremberg trials, 65, 333
nurse practice acts, 140, 142, 143
nurses' relationships
  with institutions, 237–240
  with other nurses, 240–243
  with patients, 85
  with physicians, 171–172, 243–244, 246
  with subordinates, 246–247
nursing ethics. *See also* ethics
  autonomy and, 136–139
  caring and, 134–135
  expertise and, 135–136
nursing/nursing practice. *See also* healing
    professions
  accountability and, 139–140, 142–143
  advance directives and, 310, 312
  assessment and evaluation as element
    of, 201–202
  authority and, 143
  communication with physicians, 460–462
  definition of, 450
  elements of conscientious, 221–222
  ethics and, 31–32
  as expert witnesses, 223–224
  gender influences and, 8–9, 450–451
  gender stereotyping and, 9, 451, 455–456
  historical background of, 8–24
  influences on, 495–499
  informed consent and, 301–304
  loyalty of, 240–241, 497
  men as, 452–453
  metaphors of, 496–497
  moral decision making in, 120–121
  origins of, 4, 5, 22–24, 127, 450
  patient empowerment and, 516–518
  perception of, 498–499
  policy goals for, 401
  politics and, 391, 400–401
  professional status of, 128–133
  research and, 142–143
  revisioning, 508–509
  sexual harassment and, 251–253, 456–458
  social responsibility and, 7–8
  standards of, 139–140
  technology and, 284–288
  unity and, 144
  virtue ethics in, 51
nursing process model for decision making,
  4, 159–160
*Nursing's Agenda for Health Care
  Reform* (American Nurses
  Association), 396
Nursing's Social Policy Statement (American
  Nurses Association), 7
nutrition, 273–274

O

Obama, Barack, 422
obligations, 232–233
O'Keefe, M. E., 201
Ondeck, D. A., 101
O'Neill, O., 52
organ transplantation, 283–284
Oswald v. LeGrand, 204–205
overt values, 99

P

palliative care, 277
palliative care conferences, 277–279
partisan, 389
paternalism
    advocacy vs., 68
    autonomy and, 66, 296–298
    explanation of, 65–66, 451
patience, 161
patient health information (PHI), 339
Patient Protection and Affordable Health
        Care Act (2010), 375, 422
patient protection events, 207
patients
    autonomy of, 60–64
    clarifying values with, 102–103
    communication with, 220–221, 461
    decision making at bedside of, 163
    decision-making capacity by, 518–520
    empowerment of, 516–521
    health care choices of, 313, 315–322
    lesbian, gay, bisexual and
        transgender, 459
    obligations to, 233, 236
    paternalistic attitude toward, 296–297
    relationships with, 85
    withholding or withdrawing treatment
        from, 262
Patient Self-Determination Act (PSDA)
        (1991), 308
Paul (Saint), 14
Peer Review Organizations (PROs), 419
Peirce, Charles Sanders, 3–4, 112–113
Pender, N. J., 103, 104
Percival, T., 66
personal health information (PHI), 284–286
philosophy
    in ancient societies, 12–13
    in Early Christian Era, 14
    explanation of, 32–34
    influence on society, 9
    of knowledge, 34
    in Middle Ages, 14
    in Modern Era, 22
    moral, 34–35, 38–39
    of practice, 34
    in Renaissance and Reformation, 20, 21
physicians
    communication with, 460–461
    external constraints placed by, 176–177
    nurses' relationships with, 171–172,
        243–244, 246
Piaget, J., 113
plagiarism, 330–331
plaintiffs, 196
Plato, 2, 11, 12, 14, 23, 48, 51, 111, 112
Poddar, Prosenjit, 79
political, 389
political activism, 402
political campaigns, 389, 404–405
political issues
    examples of, 392–393
    explanation of, 389
    nurses and, 391
political parties, 389
*Position Statement on Cultural Diversity in
    Nursing Practice* (American Nurses
    Association), 470

poverty, 429–430, 436, 438
Powelson, Harvey, 79
power, 499, 502. *See also* empowerment
power imbalance, 156–157
practical dilemmas, 154
practical imperative, 45–46
prayer, 485
precautionary principle, 353–354
precedents, 194
privacy. *See also* confidentiality
    explanation of, 76
    as expression of autonomy, 77–78
    technological advances and, 284–286
privacy rights, 209–210
private law, 196–197
problem analysis
    intervening factors and, 154–158
    moral/ethical dilemmas and, 152–154
    moral uncertainty and, 152
    overview of, 151–152
    practical dilemmas and, 154
problems, 151–152
problem solving
    alternative solutions and, 237
    nature of problem and, 234–237
    obligations and, 232–233
    overview of, 231–232
    personal values and, 232
product events, 207
profession
    explanation of, 129–130
    nursing as, 130–133
professional liability insurance, 223
professional practice standard, 301
Professional Standards Review
        Organizations (PSROs), 419
Protestantism, 20
public law, 194–195

Q

quality of life, 260–261
quid pro quo sexual harassment, 251–252
Quinlan, Karen Ann, 157, 275

R

racial discrimination, 248–249
racial issues, 461–463
racism, 437–439, 462
Rand, Ayn, 34, 240
Raphael, D. D., 37
rationalism, 38
Rawls, J., 418
realm of ends, 46
reasonable person standard, 301
reasoning method of fixing belief, 113
reflection stage of moral reckoning, 178
Reformation, 20–21
refugees, 358–360
refugee settlements, 359
regulations, 394
regulatory policies, 138, 394–395
Reich, W. R., 135
relationships. *See* nurses' relationships
religion
    in ancient cultures, 9–11
    dilemmas related to, 485–486
    in Early Christian Era, 13–14
    explanation of, 482

in Middle Ages, 14–16
    moral thought and, 6
    nursing profession and, 8
    spirituality and, 485
    variations in, 481–484
religiosity, 484
Renaissance, 20–21
reproductive rights, 317–319
reproductive technology, 279–280
research
    beneficence and, 334–336
    ethical issues in, 333–339, 341–343
    informed consent and, 64–65, 338–339
    justice and, 336–337
    overview of, 332–333
    protection of human rights and,
        341–342
    respect for human dignity and, 336
    social issues and, 442–443
    theory and practice derived from,
        142–143
    treatment of data and, 343
    vulnerable populations and, 339–341
research data, 399
resolution stage of moral reckoning,
        177–178
respect. *See also* ethical principles
    for autonomy, 59–60 (*See also* autonomy)
    for human dignity, 334
    for persons, 59, 133
    for vulnerable populations, 340–341
responsibility, 161
Reverby, S., 455
right to fair treatment, 336–337
right to privacy, 209–210
risk management
    autonomy and empowerment and, 222
    conscientious practice maintenance and,
        221–222
    explanation of, 219
    liability insurance and, 223
    nurses as expert witnesses and, 223–224
    patient communications as, 220–221
Robb, Isabel Hampton, 128, 132
Roberts, D., 24, 318
Robertson v. Provident House, 211
Roe v. Wade, 390
Rogers, Martha, 134–135
Roman Catholic Church, 14–21
Roman Empire, 366
rules, 394
rule-utilitarianism, 41, 43–44

S

sacred space, 485
Salgo v. Leland Stanford, Jr., 300
Schessler v. Keck, 213
Schiavo, Terri, 157, 309
*Schloendorff v. The Society of New York
        Hospital*, 300
scientific revolution, 21
Scofield, G. R., 272
Selanders, L. C., 5
self-awareness
    enhancement of, 96–97
    explanation of, 95–96, 502
    journaling and, 97, 98
    spirituality and, 486–487

self-determination, 296–298, 312, 316, 317, 477. *See also* autonomy; health care options
sensitivity, 161
Sewell, M., 468
sexism, 433, 457–458
sexual harassment, 251–253, 456–458
sexual orientation, 458–459
Shakespeare, William, 58
Sime, A. M., 134
Singer, P., 409
situational binds, 176–177
Slater, Victoria, 121
Slater v. Baker & Stapleton, 300
Smith v. Juneau, 202
social issues
   ethical principles applied to, 439–441
   homelessness as, 429, 431–432
   human trafficking as, 435–436
   increasing elderly population as, 436
   intimate partner violence as, 433–434
   personal impediments to addressing, 441–442
   poverty as, 429–430
   racism as, 437–439
   scholarship and, 442–443
   websites for information on, 444–446
social need, 5–8
social responsibility, 7–8
Socrates, 12, 34, 38, 45, 111
Socratic method, 12, 33
spirituality
   assessment of, 481–482
   explanation of, 480–481
   healing professions and, 8, 10
   integrated into nursing care, 481–482
   nurturing and, 486–487
   religion and, 482–486
Squires, T., 453
stakeholders, 155–156
standards of nursing practice, 139–140
Standards of Nursing Practice (American Nurses Association), 140
Statement on a Patient's Bill of Rights (American Hospital Association), 74
statutes, 394. *See also* law
statutory/legislative law, 193
stem cell research, 282–283
stereotyping, 9, 451, 455–456, 470
Stevens, P. E., 4
subjective standard, 301
subordinate relationships, 246–247
Sullivan, E. J., 453
Supreme Court, U. S., 390–391
surgical events, 207
sympathy, 37–38

T

Tafoya, T., 350
Tannen, D., 460
Tarasoff, Tatiana, 79
Task Force on the Prevention of Workplace Bullying, 242
technology
   artificial sources of nutrition and hydration and, 273–274
   benefits and challenges of, 259–262
   cloning, 281–282
   controversial, 281–283
   do not resuscitate orders and, 270–273
   genetic diagnosis, engineering, and screening, 280–281
   issues of life, death, dying, and, 262–266
   legal issues related to, 274–276
   medical futility and, 266–270
   nursing practice and, 284–288
   organ and tissue procurement and transplantation, 283–284
   palliative care and, 277–280
   patient treatment decisions and, 262
   reproductive, 279–280
   stem cell, 282–283
telenursing, 218–219
tenacity method of fixing belief, 112
Teresa (Mother), 426
theories
   derived from research, 142–143
   explanation of, 113
   of justice, 417–419
torts
   explanation of, 297
   intentional, 208–213
   unintentional, 197–208
transcultural care principles, 471–473
transcultural issues. *See also* cultural diversity
   complementary therapies and, 315–316, 477–478
   cultural values and beliefs and, 471–474
   health care system and, 475–477
   legal considerations related to, 479–480
   overview of, 469
   understanding culture and, 469–470
Tressman, S., 507
triage, 357
trust, 331
trustworthiness, 50
truth
   discovery of, 3–4
   ethical principles and, 73–76
Tuma, Jolene, 303–304, 498

U

uncertainty, 155
undue hardship, 250
Uniform Health Care Information Act (UHCIA), 218
unintentional torts, 197–208
unity, 144
Universal Declaration of Human Rights (United Nations), 414
urgency, 158
utilitarianism
   act-utilitarianism, 41, 42
   drawbacks of, 44
   explanation of, 40, 48
   rule-utilitarianism, 41, 43–44
   theories of, 40–41, 417
utility, 40, 78

V

values
   beliefs and, 111–113, 471, 474
   covert, 99, 100
   explanation of, 93
   institutional, 99–102
   moral, 93–94
   overt, 99
   problem solving and personal, 232
   in professional situations, 98–102
   self-awareness and, 95–98
   technology and, 286–287
values clarification
   explanation of, 95
   importance of, 95–96
   with patients, 102–104
   self-awareness and, 96–98
values conflict, 98–101
values development
   explanation of, 94–95
   nursing considerations related to, 120–121
   theoretical perspectives of, 113–118
   transcultural considerations in, 109–110
Vankawala, H., 43
veracity, 73–76, 330
victim blaming, 441
violence
   intimate partner, 433–434
   language of, 441–442
   lateral, 242, 243
   war and, 360–363
virtue, 48–49
virtue ethics
   explanation of, 48–49
   focal virtues and, 49–50
   in nursing, 51
vulnerable populations, 441–442

W

Walker, A., 515
war, 360–363, 372–373
Waterman, H., 460
Watson, J., 134
whistle-blowing, 506–507
Wilkinson, J. M., 170, 176
Williams, C., 451–453
Wilson, H. S., 341
Winston, M. E., 78–79
witch hunts, 18–20
women. *See also* gender/gender issues
   in ancient cultures, 10, 11
   in Early Christian Era, 13–14
   intimate partner violence and, 433–434
   in Middle Ages, 17–20
   in nursing, 450–452
   reproductive rights and, 317–319
   witch hunts and, 18–20
Women's Health Initiative (WHI) (NIH), 335–336
World Health Organization (WHO), 133, 379, 436
World Medical Association, 357
World War I, 373
World War II, 373–374

Z

Zschoche, D., 126
Zurlinden, J., 458